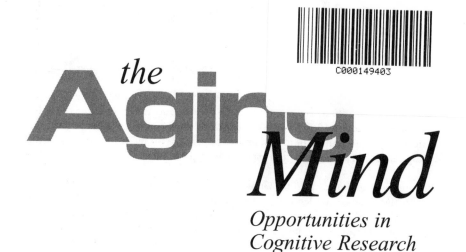

the Aging Mind

Opportunities in Cognitive Research

Committee on Future Directions for Cognitive Research on Aging

Paul C. Stern and Laura L. Carstensen, editors

Board on Behavioral, Cognitive, and Sensory Sciences

Commission on Behavioral and Social Sciences and Education

National Research Council

NATIONAL ACADEMY PRESS
Washington, D.C.

NATIONAL ACADEMY PRESS • 2101 Constitution Avenue, N.W. • Washington, D.C. 20418

NOTICE: The project that is the subject of this report was approved by the Governing Board of the National Research Council, whose members are drawn from the councils of the National Academy of Sciences, the National Academy of Engineering, and the Institute of Medicine. The members of the committee responsible for the report were chosen for their special competences and with regard for appropriate balance.

This work was supported by Task Order 55 under NIH Contract No. N01-OD-4-2139 between the National Academy of Sciences and the National Institutes of Health, U.S. Department of Health and Human Services. Any opinions, findings, conclusions, or recommendations expressed in this publication are those of the author(s) and do not necessarily reflect the view of the organizations or agencies that provided support for this project.

Suggested citation: National Research Council (2000) *The Aging Mind: Opportunities in Cognitive Research*. Committee on Future Directions for Cognitive Research on Aging. Paul C. Stern and Laura L. Carstensen, editors. Commission on Behavioral and Social Sciences and Education. Washington, DC: National Academy Press.

Library of Congress Cataloging-in-Publication Data

The aging mind: opportunities in cognitive research / Committee on Future Directions for Cognitive Research on Aging ; Paul C. Stern and Laura L. Carstensen, editors.
    p. cm.
Includes bibliographical references and index.
    ISBN 0-309-06940-8 (pbk.)
    1. Cognition—Age factors. 2. Ability, Influence of age on. I. Stern, Paul C. II. Carstensen, Laura L. III. National Research Council. Committee on Future Directions for Cognitive Research on Aging. IV. Title.
    BF724.55. C63 A48 2000
    155.67'13—dc21   00-008630

Additional copies of this report are available from National Academy Press, 2101 Constitution Avenue, N.W., Washington, D.C. 20418

Call (800) 624-6242 or (202) 334-3313 (in the Washington metropolitan area)

This report is also available online at **http://www.nap.edu**

THE NATIONAL ACADEMIES

National Academy of Sciences
National Academy of Engineering
Institute of Medicine
National Research Council

The **National Academy of Sciences** is a private, nonprofit, self-perpetuating society of distinguished scholars engaged in scientific and engineering research, dedicated to the furtherance of science and technology and to their use for the general welfare. Upon the authority of the charter granted to it by the Congress in 1863, the Academy has a mandate that requires it to advise the federal government on scientific and technical matters. Dr. Bruce M. Alberts is president of the National Academy of Sciences.

The **National Academy of Engineering** was established in 1964, under the charter of the National Academy of Sciences, as a parallel organization of outstanding engineers. It is autonomous in its administration and in the selection of its members, sharing with the National Academy of Sciences the responsibility for advising the federal government. The National Academy of Engineering also sponsors engineering programs aimed at meeting national needs, encourages education and research, and recognizes the superior achievements of engineers. Dr. William A. Wulf is president of the National Academy of Engineering.

The **Institute of Medicine** was established in 1970 by the National Academy of Sciences to secure the services of eminent members of appropriate professions in the examination of policy matters pertaining to the health of the public. The Institute acts under the responsibility given to the National Academy of Sciences by its congressional charter to be an adviser to the federal government and, upon its own initiative, to identify issues of medical care, research, and education. Dr. Kenneth I. Shine is president of the Institute of Medicine.

The **National Research Council** was organized by the National Academy of Sciences in 1916 to associate the broad community of science and technology with the Academy's purposes of furthering knowledge and advising the federal government. Functioning in accordance with general policies determined by the Academy, the Council has become the principal operating agency of both the National Academy of Sciences and the National Academy of Engineering in providing services to the government, the public, and the scientific and engineering communities. The Council is administered jointly by both Academies and the Institute of Medicine. Dr. Bruce M. Alberts and Dr. William A. Wulf are chairman and vice chairman, respectively, of the National Research Council.

COMMITTEE ON FUTURE DIRECTIONS FOR
COGNITIVE RESEARCH ON AGING

Contents

Preface

Over the past decade, the fields of cognitive science and neuroscience have made major contributions to the study of human cognition. In doing so, these fields have become increasingly interdependent. Arguably, nowhere have these gains been more relevant and substantial than in the areas of cognitive and neuroscience research on aging. Understanding how and why cognitive functioning changes with age offers great promise for improving the lives of older citizens in the United States, who are a growing segment of the population. Recognizing the urgency and the importance of these lines of research to a rapidly aging society, the National Institute on Aging (NIA) called for a "reappraisal of research opportunities that will further our understanding of how cognition develops and changes with age" (statement of Ronald Abeles, NIA, to the National Research Council Board on Behavioral, Cognitive, and Sensory Sciences, August 11, 1998).

In early 1999, the NIA asked the National Research Council (NRC) to evaluate the field of cognitive aging in order to identify areas of opportunity in which additional research would substantially improve basic understanding of cognitive functioning in aging, by drawing on recent developments in behavioral science, cognitive science, and neuroscience that are not yet fully applied to this subject area. The NRC, through the Board on Behavioral, Cognitive, and Sensory Sciences, created the Committee on Future Directions for Cognitive Research on Aging to undertake this task. The committee, which I had the honor of chairing, was asked to identify a small number of significant and promising research opportunities in cognition and aging in neuroscience, cognitive science, and behavioral science, in some cases emphasizing research opportunities that would have the added benefit of linking these three approaches in new ways.

The committee was asked to work very quickly. It held three meetings in June, August, and November 1999, at which it identified a variety of possible research opportunities and considered the promise of each. Without exception, every member of the committee worked diligently toward the requested end. Through informal processes of consultation and deliberation, the committee arrived at its consensus recommendations to the NIA. As the committee considered priorities, it invited the input of a number of outside specialists representing critical areas to make possible a deeper discussion of the more promising areas of opportunity. Some of the guests of the committee discussed these areas at the August meeting and at a committee-sponsored workshop in November 1999. Committee members were, to a person, dedicated scientists concerned about the future of their fields and even more so about the future of the rapidly maturing population.

Richard J. Hodes, director of the NIA, deserves substantial praise for requesting this report. The committee thanks Ronald Abeles, now special assistant to the director of the Office of Behavioral and Social Sciences Research at the National Institutes of Health, for his stewardship as the NIA project officer in support of the study. The committee is also grateful for their efforts and support to Marcelle Morrison-Bogorad, NIA associate director for neuroscience and neuropsychology of aging, and Richard Suzman, NIA associate director for behavioral and social research as well as to Jared Jobe, Andrew Monjan, and Molly Wagster, program officers for the NIA's cognitive research programs.

The committee also received exceptionally wise counsel from Barbara Torrey, executive director of the National Research Council's Commission on Behavioral and Social Sciences and Education, for which we are deeply grateful. Cecilia Rossiter, the project assistant for the committee, was not only efficient and considerate but went far above and beyond the call of duty by offering insights into the report as well. The committee also owes thanks to Christine McShane, who provided thorough, constructive, and efficient editing for the entire volume, and to Carrie Muntean, who readied the manuscript for publication.

However, there is one person and one person alone who made this report possible in the very short time frame allocated. That person is study director Paul Stern. His ability to listen astutely, to integrate committee generated ideas effectively, and to write skillfully and efficiently, allowed us to proceed within the time constraints of our task. Although I owe my deepest thanks to all of the committee members who took up this work, the report you read herein would not exist without Paul Stern.

We also owe special thanks to several experts from outside the committee whose input was valuable. Prominent among these individuals are the authors of the seven background papers for the committee, which appear in Appendixes A-G: John Morrison of Mount Sinai School of Medicine; Carl Cotman of the University of California, Irvine; Ellen Peters, Melissa L. Finucane, Donald MacGregor, and Paul Slovic of Decision Research; Donald Fisher of the University of Massachusetts; Shari Waldstein of the University of Maryland, Baltimore County; Shinobu Kitayama of Kyoto University; and Thomas Albright of the Salk Institute. In addition, we benefited considerably from the comments and presentations by John Breitner of Johns Hopkins University, John Desmond of Stanford University, Roger A. Dixon of the University of Victoria, Ronald McKay of the National Institute of Neurological Disorders and Stroke, John Nesselroade of the University of Virginia, Christian Pike of the University of Southern California, Susan Resnick of the National Institute on Aging, and Esther Thelen of Indiana University, all of whom influenced the committee in important ways.

This report and the background papers in the appendixes have been reviewed by individuals chosen for their diverse perspectives and technical expertise in accordance with procedures approved by the National Research Council's Report Review Committee. The purpose of this independent review was to provide candid and critical comments that would assist the institution in making the published report as accurate and as sound as possible and to ensure that the report meets institutional standards for objectivity, evidence, and responsiveness to the study charge. The review comments and draft manuscripts remain confidential to protect the integrity of the deliberative process.

We wish to thank the following individuals for their participation in the review of this report: Marilyn S. Albert, Departments of Psychiatry and Neurology, Massachusetts General Hospital and Harvard Medical School; Fredda Blanchard-Fields, School of Psychology, Georgia Institute of Technology; Fergus Craik, Department of Psychology, University of Toronto; William Estes, Department of Psychology, University of Indiana; Donald L. Fisher, Department of Mechanical and Industrial Engineering, University of Massachusetts; John Gabrieli, Department of Psychology, Stanford University; Arthur Kramer, Beckman Institute, University of Illinois; Leah L. Light, Department of Psychology, Pitzer College; Richard Shiffrin, Department of Psychology, Indiana University; and Arthur Wingfield, Department of Psychology and Volen National Center for Complex Systems, Brandeis University.

We also wish to thank the following individuals for their participation in the review of the seven papers included as appendices in this volume: Merrill F. Elias, Department of Psychology, University of Maine; John Gabrieli, Department of Psychology, Stanford University; Andrea LeBlanc, Department of Neurology and Neurosurgery, McGill University; George Loewenstein, Department of Social and Decision Sciences, Carnegie Mellon University; Denise Park, Institute for Social Research, Research Center for Group

Dynamics, University of Michigan, Ann Arbor; William Rouse, Enterprise Support Systems; and Wendy Suzuki, Center for Neural Science, New York University.

Although the individuals listed above provided constructive comments and suggestions, it must be emphasized that responsibility for the final content of this report rests entirely with the authoring committee and the institution; responsibility for the papers in the appendices rests entirely with their authors.

The committee has identified some key research directions that will, if vigorously pursued, lead to sharply increased understanding of cognitive change in older adults and new opportunities to improve their functioning and quality of life.

Laura L. Carstensen, *Chair*
Committee on Future Directions for
Cognitive Research on Aging

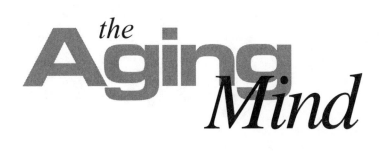

Executive Summary

Now is a time of great promise for learning more about the aging mind and turning that knowledge to the advantage of older people. Neuroscientists are making rapid progress in understanding the neural basis of sensation, memory, language, and other cognitive functions and are poised to understand, at the molecular and cellular levels, neural changes that affect the life course of cognitive capabilities. Behavioral researchers are classifying types of cognitive functioning, measuring them, tracking changes in particular functions over the life cycle, and documenting declines, maintenance, and improvement in these functions over the life span. Researchers in cognitive science are developing detailed models and theories of cognitive processes that can help make sense of observed patterns of change in functioning and link them to observed changes in neural systems. Social scientists are demonstrating the significance of cultural supports and life experiences in shaping cognitive content and processes over the life span. All these scientific developments are making possible new understandings of how normal processes of aging affect cognitive functioning and new interventions to maintain cognitive performance in older people.

In 1999, the National Institute on Aging (NIA) asked the National Research Council to identify areas of opportunity in which additional research support would substantially improve understanding of cognitive functioning in aging. The Committee on Future Directions for Cognitive Research on Aging was formed to identify highly promising opportunities in behavioral science, cognitive science, and neuroscience and at the conjunctions of these fields.

We worked from a conceptual framework that describes the aging mind in terms of three interacting systems that support the performance of cognitive tasks: cognitive structures and processes, neural health, and behavioral context, including task structure and social, cultural, and technological factors. We use the term "the aging mind" to signal a broad conception of cognitive aging that includes not only changes that can be directly observed in the brain or by standard laboratory tests of cognitive function, but also complex and knowledge-based aspects of intelligence, as well as cognitive aspects of the self, personality, and interpersonal functioning. In this conception, people adapt to changes in the body and in the social, cultural, and technological context of behavior in order to perform the tasks of living. Adequate cognitive functioning depends both on the integrity of neural systems and on these contextual factors.

This framework takes seriously recent understandings of plasticity. Neural decline in aging may not be as uniform or as profound as once believed, and various adaptive processes at the neural, behavioral, and social levels may mitigate the behavioral effects of the neural changes that do occur. To understand and assist the aging mind, it is necessary to consider changes in neural health and in behavioral context that occur in later life, as well as to understand inter- and intraindividual differences in cognitive function both cross-sectionally and over time.

We examined recent advances in the relevant science and identified three major areas in which scientific developments are creating significant opportunities for breakthroughs. The committee recommends that the NIA undertake major research initiatives in these three areas.

1. Neural Health. The NIA should undertake a major research initiative to build the scientific basis for promoting neural health in the aging brain.

Recent research shows that, contrary to a conventional belief, neural cell loss may not be the primary cause of cognitive decline in older people who are not suffering from Alzheimer's disease or related dementias. It suggests that aside from neural cell loss, changes in the health of neurons and neural networks play a major role in cognitive function. A new research focus on neural health in aging can improve basic understanding of the aging mind and lead to new health-maintaining interventions. A research initiative on neural health should consist of elements addressed to each of four major goals: developing quantitative functional and performance indicators, including behavioral tests, for neuronal health and neuronal dysfunction; identifying factors that affect neural health during the aging process, especially including imbalances in homeostatic processes, such as apoptosis, inflammation, and oxidative activity; devising interventions for the maintenance of healthy neurons and the rescue and repair of neural networks; and assessing the efficacy of intervention strategies.

2. Cognition in Context. **The NIA should undertake a major research initiative to understand the effects of behavioral, social, cultural, and technological context on the cognitive functioning and life performance of aging individuals and to build the knowledge needed to intervene effectively in these contexts to assist individuals' functioning and performance.**

Current research indicates that aging impairs cognition in some tasks but spares it in others. Until recently, the impairments were thought impossible to prevent or change. However, growing bodies of evidence show that the most impressive feature of the human mind across the life span may be its adaptability. Life experience can bring about lasting changes in the brain that shape the aging mind. In other words, biology and culture codetermine cognitive structure and functioning. Individuals adapt, sometimes with great success, so as to maintain cognitive functioning and task performance in the face of changes in the brain and in their social contexts. Systematically different life experiences yield systematically different cognitive contents and processes. And technology can modify the context of cognition to greatly improve functioning for older people. Much can be learned from increased research attention to the aging mind in its context: to factors such as cultural expectations and differences, changes in living situations and motives in late life, and emerging technologies. A new research initiative on cognition in context would seek to understand such factors and to identify ways to maintain and improve cognitive functioning of older people, taking these factors into account. Research under the initiative would pursue three major goals: understanding adaptive processes that affect cognitive functioning and performance during aging; understanding how differences in sociocultural context bring about systematic variation in cognitive functioning and performance; and developing the knowledge needed to design effective technologies, based on advances in the technology of sensing and information processing, to support adaptivity in older people.

3. Structure of the Aging Mind. **The NIA should undertake a major research initiative to improve understanding of the structure of the aging mind, including the identification of mechanisms at the behavioral and neural levels that contribute to age-related change in cognitive functioning.**

As already noted, research has established that aging affects cognitive functioning and performance of life tasks differently depending on the cognitive operation and the individual. Although the patterns of variation are not yet well understood, some of the differences have been linked to life experience factors, including physical exercise, diet, cognitive training, expertise, and the provision of environmental support; others have been linked to changes in sensory-motor functioning and to chronic diseases. A new research initiative on the structure of the aging mind would aim to specify the patterns of variation in cognitive functioning during the aging process and to identify the mechanisms, at levels of analysis from the molecular to the cultural, that contribute to age-linked stability and change. The research would include stability and change in knowledge and cognitive content that is specific to cognitive aging in humans. Research under the initiative would contribute to the search for effective interventions to assist older people in maintaining cognitive functioning and performance. The initiative should include studies of the full variety of phenomena that have been linked to cognitive aging and should emphasize the use of promising methods of measurement and analysis that are either new or underutilized in cognitive aging research. Research under the initiative should emphasize three method-based research strategies for understanding the aging mind: relating high-resolution measures of neural functioning to measures of cognitive functioning; elaborating theory-based and mathematical models; and conducting and analyzing large-scale, multivariate studies.

Achieving the goals of these research initiatives will require, in addition to financial support for research, special efforts to meet the needs for interdisciplinary research, provide specific infrastructure, and increase collaboration between the NIA and other agencies.

Interdisciplinary research. The study of the aging mind is highly interdisciplinary and becoming more so. Life scientists, behavioral scientists, and social scientists are challenged to seek new levels and forms of collaboration. To achieve the needed collaborations, the NIA should consider new funding mechanisms, including asking scientists from very different fields to work together in selected areas and establishing new research programs, program offices, and special emphasis review panels. In addition:

4. The NIA should support postdoctoral fellowships, conferences, workshops, and summer institutes to encourage individual scientists to broaden their knowledge and technical capability to address interdisciplinary issues that are central to the new research initiatives. It should organize a special competition that would provide multiyear support of a few small multidisciplinary research centers or teams focused on analytical problems that require the simultaneous application of multiple perspectives.

Research infrastructure. Infrastructure is needed in the form of access to aged animals for research; a large longitudinal database on human cognitive aging; and improved capacity for using brain imaging to study the aging mind.

The NIA should support the infrastructure for research on cognitive aging in the following ways:

5a. The NIA should help support the maintenance of colonies of pathogen-free aged animals (including primates, rats, and mice) in regional centers.

5b. The NIA should undertake a major effort to expand or develop large-scale longitudinal studies of cognitive aging. The studies should cover the range of variation in the population and should support research aimed at understanding the relationships among neural, cognitive, behavioral, sensory-motor, health, and life experience variables as they affect cognitive aging. Other institutes of the National Institutes of Health should be invited to cooperate in this effort, as they may benefit from the type of comprehensive longitudinal research being developed.

The NIA and cooperating institutes should engage in structured discussions with the research community, perhaps through a series of workshops, to address the problems involved in using resources effectively to create a broadly useful base of longitudinal data on cognitive function and its neural, behavioral, and experiential correlates.

5c. The NIA should support the capacity for using brain imaging data in the following ways:
—supporting a consensus conference to develop standard procedures for collecting and reporting human brain imaging data, specifically including MRI data, on brain-behavior relationships in aging; and
—working with other institutes at the National Institutes of Health to establish a monkey brain imaging facility with fMRI capability at the National Institutes of Health and to support a few similar centers elsewhere.

Collaboration between the NIA and other agencies. Several of the above recommendations are best advanced through collaborations involving the NIA and other agencies. For example, investments in animal colonies, improved MRI capabilities, and longitudinal research will be widely beneficial, and research on adaptive technology for aging will also help nonaged disabled populations.

6. The NIA should seek additional opportunities to participate with other institutes such as the National Institute of Mental Health, the National Institute of Neurological Disorders and Stroke, and the National Eye Institute to develop initiatives in neuroscience and cognitive aging as a way to increase the power of its research investments.

1

Understanding the Aging Mind

It is well known that the population of the United States is aging. As the proportion of older people in the population grows, it becomes increasingly important to understand age-related changes in cognitive functioning. For the many aging people in good physical condition, cognitive decline is the main threat to their ability to continue enjoying their favorite activities; for those whose physical activities are limited, cognitive decline is a major additional threat to quality of life.

The view that aging is synonymous with universal and rapid cognitive decline is giving way to a recognition that for some aging individuals, mental acuity continues well into advanced age. Moreover, recent scientific findings give growing reason to believe that it may be possible to help older people maintain more of their cognitive function into later years.

Research is showing that the adult brain has much greater capacity for plasticity than previously believed, growing new dendrites and perhaps even new neurons (Kolb and Whishaw, 1998; Buonomano and Merzenich, 1998; Gould et al., 1999b). In addition, adult brains respond positively to a variety of life experiences and to biochemical interventions. In animal studies, administration of nerve growth factor (NGF) has reversed deterioration in adult nerve cells (D.E. Smith et al., 1999). Antioxidants have improved cognitive performance and signal transduction in aged rats (Socci et al., 1995; Joseph et al., 1999). And behavioral interventions with animals, such as training, enrichment of the environment, increased social interaction, and simple physical exercise have increased neurogenesis in adult brains (Gould et al., 1999a; Kempermann et al., 1997, 1998; van Praag et al., 1999). In older people, positive effects on cognitive function have been reported in response to anti-oxidants and to behavioral interventions, such as exercise and training (e.g., Jama et al., 1996; Paleologos et al., 1998; Albert et al., 1995; Kramer et al., 1999). Such findings are suggesting many new possibilities for effective intervention to improve cognitive function in older people.

Much remains unknown, however, about how great the potential is to avoid serious decline in cognitive performance as part of what has been called "usual aging" (Rowe and Kahn, 1998). Little is known about the mechanisms that explain these provocative findings or about how they might be turned into effective interventions to improve human lives.

Now is a time of great promise for learning more about the aging mind and for turning that knowledge to the advantage of aging individuals. Neuroscientists are making rapid progress in understanding the neural basis of sensation, memory, language, and other cognitive functions and are poised to understand, at the molecular and cellular levels, those neural changes that affect the life course of cognitive capabilities. The time is right for developing intervention strategies to maintain the integrity of neuronal function and to rescue and repair malfunctioning neurons. Behavioral researchers are making rapid progress in classifying types of cognitive functioning, measuring them, tracking changes in particular functions over the life cycle, and documenting declines, maintenance, and improvement in these functions over the life span. This research is making it possible to develop behavioral and technological interventions to maintain cognitive performance in older individuals. Researchers in cognitive science are developing detailed models and theories of cognitive processes that can help make sense of observed patterns of change in functioning and link them to observed changes in neural systems. Social scientists are demonstrating the significance of cultural supports and life experiences in shaping cognitive content and processes over the life span.

Much valuable and promising research is already going on in each of these fields of research related to the aging mind. However, the fields do not communicate with each other as much as is probably desirable. Neuroscientists may document a positive or negative neural change but often do not use behavioral tests to determine whether such change makes a difference to the behaving organism. Behavioral researchers may clarify changes in function but often do not investigate the biological basis for the changes. We believe that, given the current state of knowledge, much can be learned from studies with both humans and experimental animals that link recent advances in some of these fields to unresolved problems in other fields. This volume describes a set of highly promising research opportunities—areas in which research over the next several years is likely to yield major advances.

A CONCEPTUAL FRAMEWORK

Much progress is being made by behavioral science, cognitive science, and neuroscience researchers in understanding cognitive changes during the aging process. However, what is being learned from each research perspective has not fully penetrated the work of researchers proceeding from other perspectives. This realization drew the committee to consider the ways that each perspective might illuminate the others—to develop a conceptual framework that would facilitate making these connections.

Such a framework represents the performance of life's cognitive tasks by aging individuals as dependent on three interacting systems: *cognitive structures and processes, neural health,* and *behavioral context,* including task structure and social, cultural, and technological factors. The distinction between performance and cognitive structures and processes is analogous to that between phenotype and genotype: the latter represents a capability for the former that is actualized only under the proper somatic and environmental conditions.

We use the term "the aging mind" to refer to change in cognitive structures, processes, and content. We have adopted this old-fashioned term to enlarge the conception of cognitive aging to include not only changes that can be directly observed in the brain or by standard laboratory tests of cognitive function, but also cognitive aspects of the self, personality, and interactions with other people. This sort of broadening of the concept of cognition is evident in ideas of "situated cognition" and "interactive minds" (e.g., Baltes and Staudinger, 1996) and is consistent with recent work in developmental science showing how minds—in evolution and ontogeny—are adapted and tuned to their particular environments (Gigerenzer et al., 1999). This work also includes a strong focus on the knowledge-based content of the aging mind (Baltes et al., 1999).

Several features of the conceptual framework deserve elaboration.

The framework is intended for understanding the performance of life activities. We presume that research on the aging mind is ultimately directed toward understanding how individuals perform activities of living. Research on the aging mind is motivated not only by curiosity about cognitive functioning, but also by a search for practical ways to maintain and improve the cognitive performance of aging individuals.

We thus conceive of "mind" broadly. It includes the so-called higher-level functions of language, thought, judgment, attention, learning, memory, and decision making, as well as cognitive functions involved in less intellectual activities that depend on neocortex, such as locomotion, perception, and driving a car. It also includes the content and structure of knowledge and other aspects of cognition necessary for functioning in society.

The aging mind is shaped by a conjunction of factors. These include direct changes in the brain, variations in behavioral context (for example, task structure, motives, cultural meanings, social and technological supports), and somatic events (e.g., nonneurological disease, sensory-motor changes). Each of these is driven in part by factors that change over the life course and each may affect cognitive functioning in real-life contexts. Thus, although healthy neurons and the integrity of neural systems are necessary for adequate cognitive functioning, other factors, which affect the brain only indirectly, are important as well. For instance, cultural and social supports are necessary for adequate cognitive functioning in advanced years.

Interactions and mutual causation among neural, behavioral, and somatic phenomena are important topics for study. Discoveries about neural plasticity have put an end to the notion that the brain functions only as an independent variable in brain-behavior relationships. Experience shapes the brain and thus influences cognitive functioning across the entire life span, although these effects may be particularly strong early in life. Certain somatic processes, such as cardiovascular disease and sensory-motor changes, may affect cognitive function indirectly through their direct effects on brain functioning. Systematic differences in life experiences between cultural groups may also affect cognitive aging by altering the brain. Thus, research on the aging mind includes studies to determine the health of aging neurons; the ways in which social, behavioral, and somatic variables affect neural health and cognitive structure, content, and process; and the effects of molecular, cellular, and behavioral interventions on neural health and cognitive functioning.

Adaptive processes are central to understanding the aging mind. A prevalent model has been that of more-or-less inexorable cognitive decline. Normal aging was presumed to inevitably involve loss of neural capabilities, which in turn led automatically to loss of function. The evidence indicates, however, that different cognitive functions have different life courses (Schaie, 1994, 1996; Baltes, 1997; Baltes et al., 1999). Many people retain many cognitive capabilities into very advanced years, indicating that interindividual variation exists in rates of change with aging (Hultsch et al., 1998; Schaie, 1994, 1996; Willis, 1991), although the importance of these variations is still a matter of controversy. Three explanations of the variations can be considered. Neural changes may not be as uniform or as profound as once believed; various adaptive processes at the neural, behavioral, and social levels may mitigate the behavioral effects of the neural changes that do occur; and finally, the cultural and social environments may offer opportunities for adaptation and new growth.

The role of adaptations is particularly important. Older people adapt to changes in their nervous systems and their environments and, at the same time, both types of changes affect their ability to perform cognitive tasks. To separate the various causes of cognitive change, it is necessary to examine inter- and intraindividual differences in cognitive function both cross-sectionally and over time to identify patterns. Such examinations should highlight the roles of dynamic adaptive processes, including changes in neuronal structure and function and in behavioral and social factors (e.g., social opportunity structures, the individual's routines and physical environment, the individual's goals, and the use of social and technological supports) that codetermine an individual's ability to function effectively.

IDENTIFYING RESEARCH OPPORTUNITIES

Our task has been to identify areas of opportunity in which additional research support from the National Institute on Aging (NIA) would substantially improve understanding of cognitive functioning in aging by drawing on recent developments in behavioral science, cognitive science, and neuroscience that are not yet fully applied to this subject area. As already noted, we have adopted a broad definition of cognitive function.

Our focus is on cognitive function in aging people who are not suffering from a dementia-causing disease—that is, on "normal" rather than "pathological" aging. The boundary between normal and pathological aging is hard to define. For one thing, some individuals who are aging "normally" at one point in time may later develop dementia, suggesting that their earlier "normal" functioning was in fact compromised by preclinical signs of that dementia. For another, conditions associated with aging that are not themselves considered as cognitive pathology, such as hypertension, sensory decline, and certain cardiovascular events, may have cognitive effects, as discussed in Chapter 4. People experiencing such conditions who do not suffer from one of the dementias must be considered as aging "normally" for the purposes of research in the near term; however, research may eventually discover that for some of them, a pathological process was directly affecting their cognition. Thus, a population of "normally" aging individuals defined at one time may be determined on the basis of later research or later life events to have included some individuals whose cognition was compromised by a pathological process.

A major difficulty for our task is that there are many promising research directions from which to choose. The aging mind is a topic at the intersection of several active fields of behavioral science, cognitive science, and neuroscience within which research is continually opening new vistas. New research opportunities arise often in these fields, even without special efforts to find them. We have therefore made a special effort to identify opportunities that might not automatically flow from current lines of research. For example, we looked for opportunities that might arise by applying recently developed concepts, methods, or insights in one field to problems in other fields of research on the aging mind in which their implications have not yet been much explored.

We sought particularly to identify research opportunities that would link behavioral science, cognitive science, and neuroscience approaches to cognition and aging in new ways. Thus, in identifying areas of possible research opportunity, we considered the following issues:

(1) Does the research directly address or have clear potential applications to cognitive function in aging?

(2) Can the research improve understanding of cognition and aging by drawing on recent developments in behavioral science, cognitive science, and neuroscience that are not yet fully applied in this area?

(3) Will the research open new possibilities to link these different approaches to cognition and aging?

(4) Will the research lead to fundamentally new and promising directions for investigation, as well as adding to existing knowledge?

(5) Does research progress depend on developing infrastructure, such as new technology or datasets?

Needless to say, the research opportunities we identify in this report are not the only promising ones. Other research directions might also meet the above tests, and there are other possible ways of formulating a research agenda. However, the research opportunities identified in this report appear to us to be particularly compelling. In our view, their vigorous pursuit will lead to significant advances in knowledge.

ABOUT THIS BOOK

Our report consists of the five chapters of this volume. Background papers that provide supportive detail are presented in appendixes. This chapter explains the committee's conceptual framework and the way we went about identifying research opportunities. Chapters 2, 3, and 4 focus on three substantive areas in which we propose major research initiatives, and Chapter 5 addresses implementation issues in pursuing these initiatives. All four of these chapters contain recommendations for action.

Chapter 2 focuses on neural health. It discusses emerging developments in the study of processes in the brain that provide a substrate for age-related change in cognitive functioning. It recommends a major research initiative aimed at understanding processes at the molecular and cellular levels that affect neural health, intervening in these processes to improve cognitive functioning, and relating neural changes to changes in cognitive functioning and behavior.

Chapter 3 focuses on cognition in context. It discusses recent developments in understanding how behavioral, social, cultural, and technological contexts shape the content, structure, and process of cognition throughout the life cycle, including cultural-experiential influences on brain development. It recommends a major research initiative to understand the aging mind in relation to the neurobiological effects of life experience and the effects of cultural difference and cultural and behavioral supports on the aging mind. The initiative would also investigate possibilities for maintaining cognitive functioning by changing life experience or providing supportive technologies.

Chapter 4 is concerned with the structure of the aging mind. It discusses the major interindividual differences in rates and patterns of change in cognitive content, structure, and process during aging and recommends a major research initiative to specify and explain these patterns in relation to age-related changes in the brain, sensory and motor systems, nonneurological diseases, and life experiences that may predispose toward or protect against cognitive decline. The chapter discusses the value of brain-imaging technology for contributing to the needed understanding; the need to develop behavioral indicators that are closely associated with the action of particular neural circuits; and the potential for applying concepts and methods from other areas of cognitive research, particularly cognitive development in early life, to studying the dynamics of cognitive aging.

Chapter 5 discusses implementation of the research initiatives. It addresses the investments needed to build the interdisciplinary literacy and collaborations needed to advance knowledge at the conjunction of established fields and research traditions; to improve the available stock of longitudinal data on cognitive aging; and to develop other kinds of infrastructure that are of broad use to the health sciences as well as essential for understanding the aging mind.

The appendixes include signed papers commissioned by the committee to provide more detailed accounts of the current state of research in fields that we see as leading to exciting advances and to speculate about possible directions in these fields. Although these papers are not the work of the committee, we consider them to be useful aids to thinking about how to move cognitive aging research in several of the directions we recommend.

2

Neural Health

As various jokes about "losing brain cells" illustrate, it has long been supposed that age-related cognitive decline is a result of neurodegeneration: the loss of neurons and synapses. This hypothesis is supported by high-resolution neuroanatomical investigations of the brains of patients with Alzheimer's disease and related dementias, which reveal that the level of cognitive decline and dementia is closely correlated with the extent of neuronal cell loss and synaptic degradation. Moreover, the neurodegeneration occurs selectively in brain regions associated with the functions lost in the dementias (Price et al., 1998).

This view of the neural basis for age-related cognitive decline has led to much productive research on the causes of neural cell death. Recent research developments, however, including provocative reports of neural regeneration in the adult brain (e.g., Gould et al., 1999b), are suggesting the need to expand the science in a new direction, toward understanding the determinants of change in neural health during the aging process. The underlying idea is that the causes of age-related cognitive decline, particularly in individuals who do not suffer from the dementias, may be found in dynamic processes that impair the health and functioning of living neurons. Although these mechanisms may eventually kill neurons, they may have deleterious cognitive effects even without causing neuronal loss, and the processes may begin well before old age. Little is known so far about mechanisms that maintain or impair neural health or that repair or restore unhealthy neurons.

RECENT SCIENTIFIC DEVELOPMENTS

One important line of recent evidence suggests that the mild age-related cognitive decline that occurs in nondemented individuals is different from that occurring in people with Alzheimer's disease and may not be due entirely or even primarily to neuronal loss. The progressive neuronal cell death that is observed in Alzheimer's disease is not characteristic of benign senescent memory loss that occurs frequently with increased aging (Morrison and Hof, 1997; Rapp and Gallagher, 1996; for further discussion and references, see Morrison, Appendix A). In particular, the entorhinal cortex, which displays massive neuronal loss in the brains of patients with advanced Alzheimer's disease, does not undergo any significant neuronal loss with aging in non-demented patients (Morrison, Appendix A). These findings support the hypothesis that the mild memory decline that occurs with age may be due to biochemical shifts in still-intact neural circuitry. Like neuronal loss, these disruptions may involve selective vulnerability in the entorhinal cortex and other brain regions, such as the hippocampus (West, 1993; Peters et al., 1998; Gomez-Isla et al., 1996; Morrison, Appendix A).

If cognitive decline can be attributed even in part to disruptions in the neural network other than cell loss, it is important to identify the responsible mechanisms. Recent research has identified various dynamic processes that occur in the adult brain, indicating that, in general, the brain undergoes more change than previously believed. Among the more dramatic kinds of change that have been observed are increased dendritic growth (Kolb and Whishaw, 1998) and neurogeneration in areas associated with higher cognitive functions (e.g., Gould et al., 1999b). For evidence of lasting changes in the brain as a result of life experiences, see Buonomano and Merzenich (1998), Greenough (1976), Elbert et al. (1995), and Pascual-Leone and Torres (1993). Genetic factors, such as the presence of the APOE-ε4 allele, well known to be associated with Alzheimer's disease, may also influence cognitive outcomes in nondemented older persons. In addition, neural health is likely to be affected by three cellular and molecular processes that contribute to neurodegeneration, in Alzheimer's disease and related dementias: apoptosis (programmed cell death), inflammation (acute phase injury), and the generation of free radicals (oxidative stress). The selective vulnerability of certain brain regions to neuronal loss in dementias is known to match closely with those regions in which these three processes are most active.

Especially intriguing is the fact that although these three processes are implicated in dementia, they are normally beneficial to cognitive functioning: each is involved throughout life in helping to maintain the integrity of healthy neural circuits. Thus, dysfunctions in these processes, even if not leading to cell loss, may provide mechanisms for cognitive decline.

The beneficial functions of apoptosis, inflammation, and free radical release can be briefly summarized as follows. Apoptosis is essential for brain plasticity, synaptic turnover, and selective removal of dysfunctional neurons and glia. A healthy apoptotic response mechanism is critical in the aging brain to allow for efficient adaptive remodeling of neural networks. Inflammation is critical in the acute phase response to provide basic "housekeeping" functions, including the removal of debris from dying cells and their exudates (e.g., amyloid). Reactive glia are the most critical components in maintaining neuronal homeostasis with increasing age. Free radicals released during inflammation by reactive glia are aimed at destroying foreign invaders in the brain and thus comprising a basic immune protection mechanism for brain functioning.

These processes can become detrimental when they go out of balance, for example, shifting from "acute" responses to brain injuries to a "chronic" response pattern. Unbridled apoptosis, inflammation, and free radical release would quickly shift the balance from neural health to neural dysfunction and ultimately to rampant neurodegeneration. Such a shift might either be localized to small subsets of neurons or be widespread, affecting entire neural networks. The extent to which apoptosis, inflammation, and free radical release act as beneficial as opposed to detrimental events in the central nervous system would dictate whether the neural circuit is maintained in a healthy manner or is chronically disrupted, eventually leading to neurodegenerative changes. A hypothesis worthy of investigation is that progressive dysregulation of these processes with age is intimately involved with neural dysfunction and mild cognitive impairment relatively early in life, whereas chronic activity of these events over many years leads eventually to neuronal and synaptic deficits and to dementia.

This hypothesis is described in more detail by Cotman (Appendix B), who discusses the relevant evidence and proposes that although the initiation of acute events of the above-mentioned processes is beneficial for the maintenance of the neural circuitry, problems arise when "initiation" shifts to "propagation." For example, acute apoptosis can facilitate neuronal plasticity in the central nervous system, but chronic apoptosis can promote dysfunctional neurons (e.g., in those undergoing chronic caspase activation and managing to survive with compromised function). Chronic apoptosis would ultimately result in neurodegeneration, leading to major neural network abnormalities. Thus, in the early stages of chronic apoptosis, one would expect the promulgation of dysfunctional neurons and abnormally altered afferent/efferent profiles in the neural network. This would eventually proceed to neurodegenerative events, including neuronal cell loss, requiring robust plastic responses to maintain the integrity of the neural network. Likewise, the nurturing activities of reactive glia can shift from enhancing adaptive mechanisms in the brain to killing neurons (e.g., via free radical release) if acute phase responses become chronic ones.

Such hypotheses illustrate the critical need for investigating the determinants of change in neural health, including the ways in which apoptosis, inflammation, and free radical generation are regulated in the central nervous system over the life course. More specifically, studies are required to address how these processes might reach such an exaggerated level that neural circuits are damaged or neurons are killed rather than maintained. They should also investigate the life histories of the processes, which seem to begin by midlife (see Cotman, Appendix B). A better understanding of the role of homeostatic control of these three cellular processes in maintaining healthy neural functioning with age would also facilitate future attempts to replace lost neurons using differentiated stem cells, possibly including self-repopulation with a patient's own differentiated stem cells.

RESEARCH INITIATIVE ON NEURAL HEALTH

The NIA should undertake a major research initiative to build the scientific basis for promoting neural health in the aging brain.

Recent research opens the possibility that changes in neuronal health play a major role in cognitive function in older persons who are not suffering from Alzheimer's disease or related dementias. Indeed, cell regeneration may occur. Understanding the mechanisms affecting neural health through the life cycle can lead to health-maintaining interventions. Major advances are possible from research aimed at four goals: developing quantitative markers for neuronal health and neuronal dysfunction; identifying factors that affect neural health during the aging process; devising interventions for the maintenance of healthy neurons and the rescue and repair of dysfunctional neurons; and assessing the efficacy of intervention using quantitative biomarkers. This research will identify and evaluate biochemical, behavioral, and other interventions that can help maintain neural health and, by doing that, contribute to maintaining cognitive function in older people. The research initiative should emphasize four elements corresponding to these goals.

1. Developing quantitative functional and performance indicators that are indicative of the functional integrity of neurons with special emphasis on the aging brain.

Studies are needed to identify quantitative markers that can be monitored to assess the overall health of single neurons as well as the function of the neural network. These markers would complement indicators of cell death by providing indicators of degrees of neural health. Developing a catalogue of these markers will require molecular, biochemical, neuroanatomical, imaging, electrophysiological, and behavioral studies; the markers themselves may require all these types of measurements. These markers can be utilized to test the efficacy of interventions aimed at maintaining and recovering neural health.

2. Identifying factors that affect neural health during aging.

Research under this element of the neural health initiative would examine the extent to which changes in brain function are due to neural dysfunction other than neural loss. These studies would examine hypotheses regarding mechanisms that underlie neural dysfunction, especially those affecting brain function and neural health through gene expression and through such homeostatic processes as apoptosis, inflammation, and oxidative activity, which may have either beneficial or detrimental effects.

Research under this element of the initiative would also examine factors in life experience that may affect neural health. These studies would focus on such factors as past cognitive training, occupational experience, mental activity across the life span, and other life history and cultural factors that may affect neural health during the aging process, thus linking the neural health initiative to the initiative on cognition in context (see Chapter 3). This element of the initiative would seek to specify the life course of processes affecting neural health in aging. It would support research to develop and test models of the processes that affect neural health in aging and that link neural health to cognitive perfomance.

3. Devising interventions for the maintenance of healthy neurons and the rescue and repair of neural networks.

Studies are needed to develop strategies for maintaining healthy neurons and recovering dysfunctional neurons. These strategies may involve interventions at the molecular, cellular, and behavioral levels. Studies may involve such diverse interventions as transplantation of differentiated and genetically engineered stem cells; gene delivery by transgenic and viral vector mediated approaches; the administration of drugs and nutritional supplements, especially those predicted to be beneficial from epidemiological studies; and training and other behavioral and cognitive interventions. Government support is particularly necessary for trials aimed at clinically testing the efficacy of nonprescription items, such as over-the-counter drugs and nutritional supplements, that have anti-inflammatory or antioxidant properties. Some of these have been associated with reduced incidence of dementia in epidemiological studies (Breitner, 1996; Morris et al., 1998), but the private sector is unlikely to support clinical trials of inexpensive, freely available therapeutics for which there is no patent protection. The NIA might support some such studies in collaboration with the National Center for Complementary and Alternative Medicine.

4. Assessing the efficacy of intervention strategies using quantitative, functional, and performance indicators.

Research under this element of the neural health initiative would employ a variety of methods to evaluate the success of intervention strategies. These methods will rely heavily on the quantitative markers for neural health identified in the first element of the research initiative. For evaluation purposes, it is imperative to combine molecular, biochemical, imaging, neuroanatomical, electrophysiological, and behavioral assays. Thus, the effects of intervention may be monitored by:

- measuring global and region-specific changes in brain volume and neural activity with such techniques as structural or functional magnetic resonance imaging, positron emission tomography, and magnetoencephalography,
- conducting high-resolution ultra-structural analyses (e.g., with confocal and electron microscopy or magnetic resonance microscopy),
- electrophysiological techniques, including single-unit recording, ensemble recording, and evoked potential studies,
- behavioral assays, including existing and improved cognitive tests designed to be sensitive to the integrity of specific brain regions targeted for repair,
- gene expression profiling using chip technology, and
- biochemical and molecular markers of apoptosis, inflammation, and oxidative stress.

IMPLEMENTATION ISSUES

The neural health initiative will require much more intensive involvement of behavioral scientists than has been typical in past neuroscience research. Behavioral scientists will be needed to develop some of the quantitative markers used to measure neural health and assess the effectiveness of interventions. They will also be needed to develop and test hypotheses about the ways life experience may affect neural health. Some useful behavioral research under this initiative can go on in disciplinary fashion, but some will require true integration of behavioral science and neuroscience. For example, the most fruitful hypotheses about how certain life experiences might protect against cognitive decline are likely to postulate causal mechanisms that involve experiential influences on biochemical processes in the brain. And in order to evaluate some molecular-level and cellular-level interventions, it will be necessary to identify or create behavioral measures of the functions the interventions are intended to improve. The issue of measure development is discussed in some detail in Chapter 4.

The research initiative will also depend on the availability of appropriate infrastructure. For instance, easy access to aged transgenic and naïve animals in the scientific research community is critical, as is the development of standardized behavioral testing paradigms for mice and rats. Emphasis in this latter area has traditionally been placed on attempting to develop behavioral protocols for mice and rats that can be related to human cognition. It is also worth considering ways to murinize behavioral testing paradigms for humans, that is, to use types of cognitive tests with aging humans that can tap specific functions that have also been studied in rodent models (for a recent example, see Kahana et al., 1999). These issues of interdisciplinary collaboration and infrastructure are discussed in more detail in Chapter 5.

3

Cognition in Context

Research on cognition in aging has traditionally sought to develop generalizations about changes associated with age that hold regardless of the context within which a cognitive process operates. However, the most impressive generic feature of the human mind may be its remarkable flexibility in adapting to diverse environments. As the cognitive sciences expand their scope, it becomes increasing clear that minds are adapted and often quite finely tuned to particular environments. To understand cognitive functioning, it is necessary to pay attention to the context of cognition (Super and Harkness, 1986; Goodnow, 1990; Shweder, 1991; Baltes and Staudinger, 1996; D'Andrade, 1981, 1995; Fiske et al., 1998). This context includes not only evolutionary and biological constraints and affordances but the cultures in which minds reside, including culturally shared ideas, expectations, habits of mind, communication patterns, and technologies. Contextual factors that enable some older people to function particularly well may be employed to improve functioning for others.

Recognition of cultural influences on cognition is particularly significant for research on the aging mind because it often seems natural to regard age-related changes in cognition as reflecting biological (e.g., neural, cellular, hormonal) change or activity, and equally natural to seek the sources of this variation in biological systems alone. Yet, if cognitive functioning in fact importantly reflects the contexts and environments within which people engage, some of the most important sources of variation in cognition will be found in the meanings, artifacts, practices, and institutions that structure these contexts and environments (Fiske et al., 1998). Note in this context that "old age" is relatively new as a cultural phenomenon and that as longevity and quality of life for older adults increase, the cultural and social aspects of old age are likely to continue changing.

RECENT SCIENTIFIC DEVELOPMENTS

Recent scientific developments in understanding the aging mind suggest the need to expand research to pay more careful attention to various aspects of the contexts of aging minds. Most important are four growing bodies of evidence: (1) that life experience can change the brain; (2) that individuals adapt in various ways to maintain cognitive functioning and task performance in the face of changes in the brain and in their social contexts; (3) that systematically different life experiences yield systematically different cognitive contents and processes; (4) and that advanced technology can modify the context of cognition to greatly improve functioning for older people.

Neurobiology of Life Experience

The coevolution of brain and culture has long been recognized in the study of human evolution (e.g., Durham, 1991), in which there has been some joining of developmental neuroscience and the behavioral-social developmental sciences. More recently, evidence of neural plasticity has revealed the importance of experiences within an individual's life span as a cause of change in the brain. The concept of "experience" was initially identified as a determining or modulating factor of brain development (e.g., Squire and Kandel, 1999). For example, in developmental work on perception, many studies demonstrated that certain aspects of brain development (such as the size of function-specific locations and the complexity and density of synaptic and dendritic architectures) are conditioned by the nature of early "sensory-input" experiences, such as the richness of an animal's environment (Merzenich and Sameshima, 1993; Kolb and Whishaw, 1998). In addition, experimental studies have shown that training in specific tasks also affects brain structure (see Kolb and Whishaw, 1998, for a review). A good recent example, though nonexperimental, is the finding that players of stringed instruments of the violin family have a larger cortical representation of the fingers of the left hand than of the right hand and that this is particularly true of string players who began musical practice before age 13 (Elbert et al., 1995). The presumed reason is that in playing these instruments, the fingers of the left hand are manipulated individually while those of the right hand, which holds the bow, move together. The evidence suggests that architecture in this area of the brain may be more plastic before age 13. These findings demonstrate links among enriching experiences, improved performance, and change in neural representation. Further research is needed to clarify the relationships between particular kinds and durations of life experience and particular changes in the brain and thus to clarify which aspects of "experience" might be protective against cognitive decline.

The intellectual creations of human culture also leave imprints on the brain. For example, letters and digits are culturally created symbols that can be used to represent the same concepts (e.g., "four" and "4"). Yet letter and digit recognition depend on different neural regions in literate subjects (Polk and Farah, 1998). Handwriting can be selectively impaired by brain damage that does not affect other sensory-motor functions of the hand (Alexander et al., 1992). And bilinguals show regional segregation of their different languages (Ojemann and Whitaker, 1978), illustrating that the products of specific cultures can sometimes be recognized in the brain.

There is evidence that the aging brain continues to change. For example, dendritic growth increases, possibly in compensation for cell loss (Kolb and Whishaw, 1998). New research presents evidence of neurogenesis in adulthood: new neurons continually appear in areas of the adult primate brain associated with higher cognitive functions (Gould et al., 1999b). The role of life experiences in such processes has hardly begun to be investigated.

These lines of evidence that experience changes the brain in lasting ways support the idea that many outcomes of brain development from infancy through old age are the expression of experiential-cultural factors and suggest that simple reductionistic and deterministic models in which cognitive capabilities flow exclusively from brain development are inappropriate. They suggest a program of research to examine in detail the proposition that although evolution-based brain development lays the basic foundation of brain architecture, subsequent differentiation and development of the brain is importantly influenced by how societies are organized and by how individuals live their lives. This research program would aim to clarify the relationships between particular kinds and durations of life experience and particular changes in the brain.

Adaptivity of Cognitive Functioning

Older people often continue to perform well the cognitive tasks of living despite declines in some of the underlying cognitive capabilities. For cognitive tasks that require new learning or that depend on speed of responding, performance diminishes with age (Burke and MacKay, 1997); such performance is also related to the ability to enact certain tasks of everyday life, such as such as paying bills or filling out tax forms (Diehl, 1998; Willis and Marsiske, 1991). However, performance on laboratory tasks that measure cognitive processes does not map perfectly onto performance in many important life domains, such as performance in the workplace and the exercise of "practical intelligence" (e.g., solving social problems, planning meals) (Sternberg, 1986).

The research suggests that the more an everyday problem is complex, ambiguous, and dependent on a variety of skills, the weaker the relationship between traditional measures of intelligence and performance. For instance, older adults do well in performing tasks of wisdom (Baltes and Staudinger, 2000). Wisdom involves the coordinated use in making life choices of factual and procedural knowledge about life; knowledge about life conflicts, contexts, and priorities; and knowledge about recognizing and managing uncertainty. It is measured in this research by the number of criteria people consider when they think aloud about problems of life planning, such as how to advise a 15-year-old girl who wants to get married right away, or what to say to a close friend who is thinking about suicide. Performance on such complex and ambiguous tasks shows only a weak relationship to measures of intelligence; rather, it is primarily associated with indicators of life experience, personality, and cognitive style. Thus, age-related declines in measured cognitive processes may not imply equivalent declines in the ability to perform cognitive tasks of living. Some research actually shows positive age trends, with older people outperforming younger people despite lower performance on some measures of cognitive processing (Marsiske and Willis, 1995).

One reason practical functioning may decline more slowly than some kinds of cognitive capability may be that experience-based procedural and declarative knowledge is relatively well maintained in later life (Baltes et al., 1999; Blanchard-Fields and Hess, 1996). To the extent that people come to old age with greater stores of knowledge, adaptivity in later life benefits from those reserves. Adaptivity may also be promoted because older people consider and rely more on other people in solving problems in everyday life (Sansone and Berg, 1993; Blanchard-Fields, 1997). Memory is known to benefit from social support (Dixon and Gould, 1998), and older people's memories are significantly enhanced when they recall them in the presence of another. Margrett (1999) found that older people's performance on a range of tasks, including understanding medication labels, social dilemmas, and map reading, benefited from collaboration; moreover, those who perceived themselves as needing assistance benefited more. In other words, the people with the poorest independent performance were able to compensate by collaboration.

Researchers in the field of what is now called "everyday competence" have come to adopt a framework of "person-environment fit" (Lawton, 1982), which suggests that functioning in real-world situations is determined by the fit between the individual and the environmental and social context. Although this model is applicable to people of all ages, research suggests that "fit" is more important for people whose cognitive abilities are compromised. For example, among people with serious visual impairment, environmental fit is far more relevant to everyday competence than among people with mild or no visual impairment (Wahl et al., 1999). The strong relationship of sensory functioning to cognitive performance among aging individuals (Lindenberger and Baltes, 1994) is just as relevant to everyday activity competence (Marsiske et al., 1997). It appears that older people can sometimes improve their "fit" and their everyday competence by drawing on other people in their environments.

Another aspect of adaptivity is that people's motivations change as they approach the end of life (Carstensen et al., 1999). One change is that emotional goals are more salient to older as opposed to younger people. Older people's adaptation to their life situation seems to give them a relative advantage in certain kinds of cognitive tasks. For instance, older adults perform better than younger adults when solving social dilemmas involving problems high in emotional salience. They are more likely to generate good solutions and to consider other peoples' feelings in their recommendations (Blanchard-Fields, 1997).

In short, aging people are often successful in using other minds and environmental supports to buffer the effects of cognitive decline. However, the adaptive transactions that occur between persons and environments remain poorly understood. Very little research to date has focused on the ways in which older people actually use environmental resources, including social or cultural resources, to maintain functioning. Relatedly, there is growing recognition of the need to consider the broader sociocultural contexts in which people age (Baltes and Carstensen, 1999). In order to understand everyday functioning, it may be necessary to shift from a conception of cognition as something that occurs entirely within the individual to one that takes into consideration distributed, interactive processes that shape and are shaped by the social world and the technological environment.

Cognitive Effects of Life Experiences

If the brain is shaped by experience, then it should not be surprising that individuals who differ systematically in the kinds of experience that shape the brain differ in their cognitive functioning (for a thorough review of social influences on cognition, see Levine et al., 1993). A reasonable hypothesis is that if experiential differences occur at formative periods or persist throughout the life span, then the cognitive effects will be persistent. Another reasonable hypothesis is that so-called crystallized or pragmatic aspects of cognition are likely to be more strongly influenced by life experience than so-called fluid or mechanical aspects.

Considerable evidence is accumulating of cognitive differences between aging members of social groups that differ systematically in experience through the life cycle: groups defined by occupation, socioeconomic status, ethnicity, race, and culture (e.g., Avolio and Waldman, 1994; Burton and Bengston, 1982; Jackson, 1985). For instance, better cognitive performance in aging individuals is generally associated with higher levels of education (e.g., Birren and Morrison, 1961; Blum and Jarvik, 1974; Denny, 1979; Denny and Palmer, 1981; Green, 1969; Kesler et al., 1976; Ripple and Jaquish, 1981; Schaie and Strother, 1968; Selzer and Denny, 1980), higher-status emploment and higher income levels (e.g., Arbuckle et al., 1986; Schaie, 1983; Gribbon et al., 1980; Owens, 1966), and being white rather than black in the United States (e.g., Fillenbaum et al., 1988). The most precipitous decline in adaptive functioning, which occurs during the eighth decade of life, is far less pronounced in people with greater as opposed to lesser education (Schaie, 1996). The association of education with cognitive functioning in old age varies, however, by country. In Germany, for instance, this association is much weaker than in the United States (Baltes and Mayer, 1999). In addition, there is a growing body of evidence that adult members of sharply different cultures differ systematically in the ways they habitually attend, process, and interpret information as well as in the approaches they take toward the aging process (for a review, see Kitayama, Appendix F).

The true meaning of such associations is not yet understood. However, several interesting hypotheses are available to account for them and to suggest causal mechanisms leading from particular life experiences to their presumed cognitive effects. One set of hypotheses centers on cognitive practice or training. The central idea is that formal education, occupational experience, and the like provide cognitive practice that shapes cognitive abilities and maintains particular ones—perhaps a broad range of abilities for general education and a narrower range for certain occupational experiences. Similarly, cultural differences may provide members of certain cultures with training in ways of thinking that are not practiced in other cultures, resulting in lifelong differences in cognitive skills (Gauvain, 1995). An example from a recent study is the finding that adult native speakers of Italian and English show distinct patterns of brain activation in the temporal regions involved in reading and naming tasks during language processing (Paulesu et al., 2000). This finding is thought to be due to the sharp difference between English and Italian in how closely phonemes (sounds) and graphemes (letter combinations) map onto one another. Importantly, this difference is observed for both words and nonsense words, suggesting that the acquisition of a particular language leads to persistent differences in the processing of new languge input.

Another example is the report that formally schooled children are more likely to use the learning strategy called clustering, in which they group like items together explicitly, making recall much easier (Brislin, 1993). This sort of training may help explain differences in memory associated with educational attainment later in the life span. Formal education and experience in wage-labor occupations have been found to be associated with increased concern for time, punctuality, and planning activities in advance (Inkeles and Smith, 1974). The complexity of work roles has also been associated with general characteristics of cognitive functioning in adults (Kohn et al., 1978, 1982). Technology also shapes cognition through training. Abacus users have been found to make different kinds of errors in solving mathematical problems from people who use Arabic numerals (Stigler, 1984; Stigler et al., 1986). It has been argued that in medieval times, when few people could use writing as a memory aid, memory was much more detailed and rote than it is in advanced societies today (see Yates, 1966; Carruthers, 1990; Olson, 1994). And it has been suggested that television shapes a mind adept in rapid processing of images and comfortable with attending for repeated short periods rather than extended ones (Greenfield, 1984).

Following on reported differences in information processing styles between people from East Asian and European cultural groups (Hsu, 1983; Liu, 1974; Lloyd and Moodley, 1990; Nagashima, 1973), Park and colleagues (1999) found that cues in a memory task had different effects on people from the two groups. Compared with people from European cultures, supportive cues helped the East Asians more, and distracting cues harmed their performance more. The explanation offered was in terms of the previously published claim that memory among East Asians is more sensitive to contextual cues, whereas Europeans focus more narrowly on the object at hand. The same authors offered a contextual-support explanation for their finding that Americans perform better than Chinese on a free recall task involving six words from five natural categories.

A second set of causal hypotheses involves health as an intervening variable between social context and cognitive aging. A central idea is that the shared life experiences of certain social groups may lead them to suffer more from diseases like hypertension, cardiovascular disease, and diabetes that directly affect cognitive functioning (see Waldstein, Appendix E, for a discussion of these health effects). For example, people from lower-status social groups, including low-status ethnic minority groups, have poorer health histories, including a higher incidence of chronic diseases that have cognitive effects (Williams, 2000). Similarly, people lacking in social support—resources available through social ties to other individuals and groups—may suffer more from the effects of stress (Caplan, 1974; Cassel, 1976; Cobbs, 1976; Payne and Jones, 1987; Seeman et al., 1996) and experience negative effects on blood pressure and immune function (Uchino et al., 1996). Differences in social support may help account for poorer health outcomes among black Americans, although there are compensatory effects of cultural factors, such as religion (Jackson et al., 1995; Ortega et al., 1983), and the effects may be moderated by demographic variables such as socioeconomic status, marital status, age, and gender.

Another health-related explanation of group differences in cognitive functioning concerns personal control of life outcomes. Lack of personal control in the form of unemployment and working in high-demand, low-control jobs creates stress that sets predisease mechanisms in motion (Karasek and Theorell, 1990; Rushing et al., 1992; Schnall et al., 1994). In addition, beliefs about personal control, which are associated with educational level (Lachman and Weaver, 1998; Marmot et al., 1998; Markus et al., in press), are also associated with a variety of health-promoting behaviors (see Taylor, 1999, for a review).

Stressful experiences may also help explain individual and group differences in cognitive functioning by way of health effects (for reviews summarizing mechanisms linking stressful experience to impairments of health, see Manuck et al., 1990; Seeman and Robbins, 1994; Seeman et al., 1997; McEwen, 1998). For example, several authors have proposed that the experience of racial discrimination leads to chronic stress-induced sympathetic activation that leads in turn to hypertension (see Clark et al., 1999, for a review). Clark and colleagues (1999) have proposed a biopsychosocial model to account for such effects of the experience of discrimination.

Health-related and practice-related variables may also combine to produce intergroup differences in cognitive outcomes. For example, in a recent study of "successful aging," being white predicted greater maintenance of cognitive performance over time (Albert et al., 1995). Education and strenuous activity were intervening factors, suggesting that both of these factors affect cognitive outcomes regardless of race, and that race-related differences in these mediators may help explain between-group differences in cognitive outcomes. The situation is probably even more complex than this. As already noted, the association of educational level with cognitive functioning in old age varies by country. Moreover, even within a country, educational attainment is not the same variable for all groups because they experience systematic differences in the quality of education (e.g., Anyon, 1980; Giroux, 1981; Sieber, 1982; Oakes, 1985; Willis, 1982).

Yet a third set of hypotheses about intergroup differences in cognitive aging is that they are shaped by different cultural meanings of aging. It has often been claimed, for instance, that the dominant American cultural image of aging is one of people who are losing their faculties and are less than fully competent. In contrast, some other societies are said to value aging individuals as having special qualities that entitle them to be treated with added respect compared with their juniors (see, for example, Kitayama, Appendix F). Such social attitudes may affect aging individuals by leading them to think and function in the ways their cultures expect. This social expectation hypothesis is sufficiently plausible to warrant further study.

The above examples indicate that there are numerous plausible hypotheses about how life experiences might yield the observed intergroup differences in cognitive aging; few of these hypotheses, however, have received detailed examination, and most of the research has focused on children or young adults rather than older people. Yet there is reason to believe that these contextual factors may become even more important with age, affecting ideas and expectations of how to age, norms of when to seek support or help, and decisions about whether to comply with advice, as well as the interpersonal and institutional supports guiding such decisions. Understanding the cognitive effects of life experience may have great practical importance because life experiences can be modified. Improved understanding may therefore lead to promising interventions to improve cognitive outcomes.

Technological Support for the Performance of Cognitive Tasks

Technology has long been used to change the context of behavior to help people adapt to declines in their capability to perform daily life tasks. Eyeglasses, hearing aids, and wheelchairs are among the most obvious examples. Recent developments in information and sensing technology promise to yield revolutionary new technological supports that can help aging individuals adapt to declining capabilities.

As computers become smaller, more powerful, and more easily embedded in other objects and processes (e.g., Norman, 1998), they provide the opportunity to devise new technologies to augment the adaptivity and functionality of the human user. An example is computerized eyeglasses that can enhance the peripheral field of vision (Jebara et al., 1998; see Fisher, Appendix D, for a discussion of additional possibilities). New technologies exist for sensing environmental variables, integrating environmental information (see also Abidi and Gonzalez, 1992), and planning possible actions or facilitating possible decisions in order to make a person's behavior more broadly context sensitive and thereby more adaptive. These technologies hold promise for maintaining the ability of older people to manage such tasks as driving motor vehicles (e.g., Hancock and Parasuraman, 1992) and operating automated teller machines (ATMs) and other technologies in spite of declines in sensory-motor and cognitive capabilities.

New technologies are also becoming available to assist with the information processing aspects of judgment and choice. For example, with the explosion of available information over the Internet, technologies to aid decision-making by reducing information overload are sure to proliferate. Some of these will address important life decisions facing older people, such as choosing health care providers and estate planning. However, these information-reducing technologies must be designed to fit well with users' capabilities and needs.

To make such technologies useful in practice, it is necessary to build understanding of the sensory-motor and cognitive processes the technologies are intended to assist and to address issues of information overload, distribution of control between the device and the user, and user acceptance. It is also important to take seriously the idea that technology, as part of social context, shapes society and cognition (e.g., Mead, 1953; McLuhan, 1964; Sclove, 1995). The technologies must also be compatible with the users' values and motives. For example, if the values of older adults shift from emphasizing task efficacy to emphasizing emotional connectedness (e.g., Carstensen et al., 1999), that shift may affect their willingness to adopt some of the new technologies intended to increase their adaptivity. It is important to consider such reactions, both to predict which technological innovations may be successfully introduced to the population of older adults and to assess the possible sociocultural consequences of adopting them. It is also important to evaluate the possibility that particular technological supports might undermine cognitive functioning by supplanting the use of mental abilities.

RESEARCH INITIATIVE ON COGNITION IN CONTEXT

The NIA should undertake a major research initiative to understand the effects of behavioral, social, cultural, and technological context on the cognitive functioning and life performance of aging individuals and to build the knowledge needed to intervene effectively in these contexts to assist individuals' functioning and performance.

An appropriate fit between person and context is necessary for effective cognitive functioning and performance at any age. If anything, the need for adaptation is greater in old age than in middle adulthood because of major changes in context that tend to accumulate in late life, such as losses of family and friends, chronic illness and physical decline, migration to new living conditions, and the contemplation of death. The recommended research initiative would promote adaptivity by pursuing three major goals: understanding adaptive processes that affect cognitive functioning during aging; understanding how differences in sociocultural context bring about systematic variation in cognitive functioning and performance; and developing the knowledge needed to design effective technologies to support adaptivity in older adults.

1. Understanding adaptive processes that affect cognitive functioning and performance during aging.

Studies are now needed to clarify the ways aging individuals deploy their cognitive faculties to maintain a high level of performance of life tasks despite decline in some abilities and to improve performance on the basis of accumulated knowledge and wisdom. These studies should focus particularly on: the ways older people rely on other people, technological aids, emotion-regulation skills, and task-structuring strategies; the interdependencies among adaptive strategies, cultural contexts, and biological (including health) conditions; and the possibilities for organizing environments to facilitate aging individuals' use of adaptive strategies. Such research would include the development of highly specified models of cognitive tasks in order to identify the component(s) of a task that are affected by particular contextual factors. Knowledge of contextual factors that contribute to good functioning can provide the basis for remedial measures.

One area in particular need of serious investigation concerns the ways in which older people make decisions in everyday life, an area in which scientific research is presently scanty. A few empirical findings about general cognition have been established. Older adults are less flexible in learning and revising judgment and decision strategies than middle-aged adults, they prefer less cognitively demanding strategies, and they are slower and perhaps more cautious than younger adults (see Sanfey and Hastie, 2000, and Appendix C for more thorough review). In addition, recent research on social cognition and aging has revealed considerable evidence that older people solve problems differently than younger people (Hess, 1994). To the extent that older people appraise, process, and recall information about social matters differently than younger people, such differences involve socially embedded and culture-bound knowledge (Blanchard-Fields and Hess, 1999). Interestingly, the relative old age "profile" includes superior performance in some areas, such as the ability to solve emotionally charged social problems (Blanchard-Fields, 1997; Blanchard-Fields et al., 1997, 1995), and poorer performance in other areas, such as memory about the source of information (Hashtroudi et al., 1990, 1994). Relative to younger people, older people are less likely to revise existing knowledge structures or schemas when presented with new contradictory information (Hess and Pullen, 1994; Hess and Tate, 1991), rendering them more influenced by accumulated knowledge than younger people. There is also growing consensus that some age differences in cognitive performance reflect age differences in goals (Hasher and Zachs, 1988; Hess and Pullen, 1994; Isaacowitz et al., 2000). Older people appear to be particularly sensitive to emotional aspects of situations, including interpersonal ramifications of problems (Carstensen and Turk-Charles, 1994; Kramer, 1990). Thus, processing goals may direct older people to different aspects of problems.

Thus, performance on everyday decisions that rely heavily on past experience or emotional sensitivity may be relatively well maintained in older people, but performance on decisions that require the interpretation of new information may present problems. Important life decisions, such as about health care, estate planning, and personal abilities (whether or not to continue driving, for example) require the integration of rapidly changing information, sometimes in bewildering quantity—a task that tends to be increasingly difficult as people age and as information proliferates about the decisions. Any serious age-related decrement in the ability to make any of these kinds of decisions wisely will affect not only the decision makers but also their families and perhaps, at least in the case of financial decisions, the larger economy. Despite great interdisciplinary progress in understanding human judgment and decision making, there has been little application to the study of aging (see Peters et al., Appendix C). Studies are needed to illuminate age-related changes in decision-making processes, strategies, and skills and to clarify how these changes are related to cultural expectations, values, and beliefs, as well as to neural health and basic cognitive capabilites. Such studies can help identify the need for decision aids and inform their development. These studies should compare representative samples of populations of different ages to avoid the selection biases that have been present in some studies.

   2. Understanding how differences in sociocultural context bring about systematic variation in cognitive functioning and performance.

   Empirical research to date shows clear associations between cognitive functioning in old age and social class, education, occupation, language, expertise, and ethnicity. Several kinds of studies are needed to clarify these relationships and address the underlying processes responsible for such differences among individuals and groups.

   • *Unpacking the associations between group membership and cognition.* One focus of this research should be on looking more closely at the relationships between rough sociocultural classifications and specific cognitive outcome variables as a way to develop hypotheses about causal mechanisms that may explain the associations (e.g., effects of training and practice, mediation by health effects, stress-related responses). For example, researchers interested in gender differences in cognitive aging, noting the evidence that higher levels of estrogen are related to superior cognitive functioning in aging (C.A. Smith et al., 1999), have considered the potential impact of estrogen and hormone replacement therapy on memory and other cognitive functioning. Although the specific connections between estrogen and cognitive processes and/or other brain functions are still unclear, there is evidence suggesting links of estrogen to neuronal plasticity and to the modulation of neurotransmitter pathways (Costa et al., 1997; Sherwin, 1994). These results suggest that hormone replacement therapy might yield considerable benefit to cognitive functioning in postmenopausal women, but the limited research so far has generated conflicting conclusions (Erkkola, 1996).
   As another example, educational attainment, measured as years of schooling, is likely to be a poor proxy for what actually happens in school to shape the mind and brain. Closer examination of the kinds of thinking that are practiced in school may help illuminate intergroup differences in cognition

that persist through the life cycle. For example, children from lower-status social groups tend to be tracked into less demanding academic classes and to be taught to follow directions unquestioningly rather than to exercise critical thinking faculties (e.g., Anyon, 1980; Giroux, 1981; Sieber, 1982; Oakes, 1985). If children actually learn these lessons, there may be specific long-term effects on their ways of thinking. Similarly, there is evidence to suggest that race differences in biological markers are mediated by life experiences that cause lasting physiological stress responses (Clark et al., 1999). Such differences need to be traced in time from the younger ages, where they have usually been studied, into older age.

It is important to avoid the temptation to interpret group differences in cognitive functioning, particularly between social groups of unequal status, as reflecting underlying biological capabilities rather than responses to unequal opportunity or different life conditions (see Cauce et al., 1998). Considerable analysis is usually necessary to arrive at an appropriate explanation. One problem is that some of the usual statistical assumptions underlying between-group comparisons are not met for certain intergroup comparisons (e.g., there is more variance in the cognitive scores of blacks than whites; House et al., 1990, 1994). Another is that particular cognitive measures may not be equally reliable or valid in different cultural/ethnic groups: if an item is not equally familiar across groups, responding may require different amounts of mental effort (e.g., Cauce et al., 1998). Intergroup differences in measures of crystallized abilities may not reflect underlying biological differences because these abilities may be strongly influenced by culture (Cattell, 1963). And, as already noted, intervening variables such as education may not be the same for all groups being compared. Thus, some investigators have argued that an accurate understanding of the meaning of intergroup differences cannot be attained without careful analysis of within-group variation, especially among minority groups (e.g, Markides et al., 1990; Whitfield and Baker-Thomas, 1999). Group labels (race, ethnicity, etc.) are no more than proxies for underlying psychological variables—a useful place to begin research, but not very meaningful until the mechanisms are traced that link observed cognitive differences to causative factors that connect them to group membership.

   • *Understanding the cognitive effects of culturally shared values, beliefs, and practices.* This research should describe the relevant values and beliefs (e.g., those concerning age, self, health, relationships, spirituality, technology) and the relevant cultural practices (e.g., communication, health, and everyday activities). It should identify the ways in which these values, beliefs, and practices affect cognitive functioning (including attention, reasoning, memory, and language) and the ways in which cognitive functioning shapes these contexts.

• *Understanding the neurobiology of life experience.* Research should examine and specify the ways that life experiences, operating intensively or over long segments of the life cycle, produce lasting changes in the nervous system. An illustration of this research approach is the recent development of a model for research on the biological effects of the experience of racism (Clark et al., 1999). The model offers plausible links from experienced racism to psychological stress to biological manifestations in the endocrine and cardiovascular systems that may in turn be associated with cognitive functioning. Developments more broadly in psychoneuroimmunology (Ader and Cohen, 1993; Maier et al., 1994) and related fields that link life experiences to health outcomes (e.g., Karasek and Theorell, 1990; Rushing et al., 1992; Schnall et al., 1994; Seeman, 1996; Wang and Mason, 1999) are improving the capability to conduct research on the ways in which behavioral variables affect the complex biological systems that support cognition. Research on the neural effects of training and practice may also suggest causal mechanisms that link life experiences to specific neural changes. Such progress in linking experiential to physiological variables is bringing the field of neurobiology of life experience to the edge of development.

Research in this emerging field should focus on identifying specific kinds and durations of experience that alter the brain in ways that affect the course of cognitive aging and on identifying the mechanisms by which these effects occur. Research under this initiative could include studies of the neural consequences of professional expertise; cognitive training and practice; emotional and motivational activity; education and sociocultural involvement; retirement; changes in family structure; social interactions and social support; experiences associated with social class, race, and ethnic group membership; spirituality; and other experiential factors that may affect cognitive functioning through effects on neural processes. It could also include studies that examine the neural effects of adaptations to the above kinds of experience. Additional studies could test experiential interventions (e.g., types of training) that might affect the brain in ways that help protect against cognitive decline. The studies would include both attempts to establish causal relationships and to develop process models that further clarify chains of causation. They would also aim to specify life experiences that alter the brain, particularly those that protect against cognitive decline and that could be used to prolong the ability of older people to perform cognitive tasks.

It is worth emphasizing that research on the neurobiology of experience turns on its head the usual understanding of how biology relates to behavior. Rather than reducing social categories to neural phenomena, it would attempt to understand how individual and social experiences shape the brain. Progress in this research direction requires new collaborations between social scientists and neuroscientists that focus on a neglected aspect of biology-culture interactions. We believe social scientists will be attracted to studying these questions in cognitive science because the research will allow them to test and refine hypotheses about the ways sociocultural factors shape human behavior and development.

3. Developing the knowledge needed to design effective technologies to support adaptivity in older adults.

As already noted, new sensing and information technology holds promise for revolutionary advances in adapting environments to suit the cognitive needs of aging individuals. To achieve this promise, it is necessary to develop a sufficient understanding of sensory-motor and higher-level cognitive functioning in aging individuals to make it possible to design devices and decision aids to work well with individuals whose level of functioning without assistance has declined. It is also important to assess the society- and culture-shaping potential of new adaptive technologies from the perspective of older adults to guard against undesirable secondary effects of the new technology.

To illustrate the need for basic research, consider a computer-controlled device that can provide information to assist an older person in driving a car. To function well, such a device should be capable of identifying what the person is trying to do—for instance, it should be able to discriminate between a pattern of collision avoidance and one of loss of attention or consciousness. Many new control technologies are being developed that can monitor speech, gaze, head movement, gesture, biopotentials, and the like as inputs (NATO Research and Technology Organization, 1998). These technologies would need to be supplemented with analytic techniques, such as hidden Markov models that yield inferences about the person's strategies and goals (see Fisher, Appendix D). Thus, the new devices would need to combine monitoring and control technology, behavioral understanding of the relevant sensory-motor and cognitive processes, and the appropriate quantitative techniques of data processing to provide the right information to the control mechanism. It would also be necessary to address issues of information display, information overload, distribution of control between the device and the user, and user acceptance.

Designing technologies that interact appropriately with the behavioral needs and capabilities of older adults thus presents a significant research challenge. The challenge includes learning how to design technologies to foster and not supplant mental abilities. Meeting this challenge would bring obvious practical benefits and would also advance science by contributing to basic understanding of how older people search, plan, locomote, navigate, and solve problems in technology-aided contexts. More detail on the nature of the research challenges and opportunities can be found in the discussion of adaptive interfaces in Appendix D.

This research also presents a special challenge of implementation because it requires integrating behavioral science and engineering in a context of product design and development. It will be important to establish good communication between the relevant engineering and behavioral science communities so that technological applications can be designed in tandem with improved understanding of cognitive processes. It will also be important to make prototypes of proposed devices available to researchers espousing various theoretical outlooks to provide good tests both of the devices and of the behavioral theories they apply. Moreover, a successful research program will require viable working relationships between the private-sector organizations that may produce the new technologies and cognitive and behavioral researchers, many of them in universities.

We believe that innovative funding mechanisms will be necessary to encourage basic research in support of technology to extend the adaptivity of older adults. Existing programs have not yet integrated all the necessary elements. For instance, the NIA's Roybal center grants have not thoroughly integrated engineering or focused on building theory for broad application. The National Science Foundation's initiative on Knowledge and Distributed Intelligence has these capabilities but does not focus on aging. We recommend that the NIA consider joint funding of research on adaptive technology with other agencies, such as the NSF, that regularly draw on expertise in technology and engineering.

We also recommend that the NIA explore possibilities to support research by matching industrial support in an appropriate proportion with governmental funding. With this mechanism, industry could benefit from behavioral research that it would not usually conduct, and older adults might see useful adaptive technologies sooner. Also, university researchers would be able to perform basic research in the context of more realistic technological environments than they can usually afford. We recommend that the NIA hold an open meeting with appropriate members of the research and business communities to arrive at a joint plan to fund the needed research on technology for adaptivity and to address related issues of patenting, licensing, protection of proprietary information, and access to scientific results.

4

Structure of the Aging Mind

In contrast to the popular notion that mental decline with age is inevitable, progressive, and general, research presents a more complex picture. Aging individuals vary greatly in the rates at which their cognitive functioning changes over the life span; the trajectory of cognitive aging is different for different cognitive functions (e.g., Baltes et al., 1999; Hultsch et al., 1998; Schaie, 1994, 1996; Willis, 1991); and as already noted, experience, including practice, physical exercise, and the status of sensory-motor systems and health, is associated with systematic differences in cognitive performance among older adults.

Much progress has been made over the past quarter-century in identifying which tasks prove particularly difficult for older adults and which do not, and in modeling age-related change in particular cognitive processes. Still lacking, however, are theories that can explain the overall pattern—why some functions are spared while others are impaired, and why patterns of age-related change differ across individuals. It is now possible to make significant progress in this direction. Improvements in measurement of cognitive and neural functioning, new methods of analyzing the data, and an expansion of longitudinal research now make possible substantial improvement in understanding the nature of cognitive aging, including the identification of mechanisms at the behavioral and neural levels that contribute to age-related changes and to differences between individuals and groups.

RECENT SCIENTIFIC ADVANCES

Variations in the Life Histories of Cognitive Functions

Accumulating data on cognitive functioning in later life are yielding a clearer understanding of the complex patterns of change. The Seattle Longitudinal Study (e.g., Schaie 1983, 1994, 1996) provides typical findings. Cross-sectional data from 5,000 adults from age 25 to 88 show consistent negative age effects on such latent abilities as inductive reasoning, spatial orientation, perceptual speed, and verbal memory (new learning). In contrast, numeric ability (simple arithmetic calculations) and verbal ability (synonyms and recognition tests of meaning) show improvement until midlife and then a plateau until the oldest tested age of 81. People at age 81 performed at a higher level on vocabulary tests than people at age 25. These data are for both speeded and unspeeded vocabulary tests combined. If only speeded vocabulary tests are considered, performance declines start in the 60s, although the rate of decline is still lower than for other cognitive functions. Longitudinal data in the Seattle study show an inverted U-shaped age function for most verbal and numerical abilities, with the highest scores achieved at ages from the 30s to the 60s, depending on the ability. World knowledge is usually found to be stable into old age, for example, as measured by the WAIS information subtest (Salthouse, 1982) or general information questions (Camp, 1989; Nyberg et al., 1996; Small et al., 1995; but see Hultsch et al., 1998).

Schaie's data are from psychometric tests that were not designed to identify mental processes and mechanisms underlying the cognitive functions being measured. Using laboratory techniques from cognitive psychology to investigate semantic memory processes, studies consistently report age invariance in semantic organization and processes, and in a variety of other language processes (see Kemper, 1992; Light, 1991; Burke, 1997). This extends even to discourse-level processes, because consistently higher ratings are given to older compared with younger adults' narratives (e.g., James et al., 1998; Kemper et al., 1990). Recent findings, however, demonstrate that some processes involved in language production decline in old age: older adults suffer more failures in retrieval of phonology (word finding failures) and orthography (spelling errors) than young adults, despite their superior vocabularies (Burke et al., 1991; MacKay and Abrams, 1998). This pattern of dissociation in age effects on language functions is at odds with descriptions of age invariance in crystallized or pragmatic functions. Together with dissociations in age effects in other cognitive domains (e.g., explicit versus implicit memory), these data pose a challenge to models of cognitive aging.

Cognitive functions are not only a matter of the speed and accuracy of information processing. The aging mind also involves cognitive contents, such as ideas of self and the meaning of life, and skills that go beyond speed and accuracy of information processing, some of which are described by the concept of wisdom. Capability in such areas often increases through adulthood at least until the 70s, even when cognitive efficacy in the narrow sense is reduced (e.g., Baltes, 1997).

Recent research shows a less differentiated pattern of cognitive performance in advanced old age, that is, beyond age 85. In this age range, all mental abilities seem to decline for most people. Moreover, this research on the oldest old has also identified a pattern of age-related increases in the correlations among measures of cognitive functions, sensory-motor functions, and general health between ages 70 and 100. This phenomenon, often described as a dedifferentiation of cognitive functions (Baltes and Lindenberger, 1997), may be explainable in part in terms of change in sensory-motor and health status, as discussed in the next section.

Modulation of Cognitive Aging by Experience

The trajectories of cognitive aging are not the same for all individuals, even for highly specific cognitive functions. Life experiences matter.

Behavioral and Cultural Factors

As noted in Chapter 3, there are systematic differences in cognitive status among aging members of social groups defined by such factors as socioeconomic status, education, occupation, culture, race, and ethnicity. A mechanism that may explain some of these differences is expertise, resulting from training and practice. Studies comparing experts in chess, aviation, typing, and piano playing report that cognitive functions based on expert knowledge are preserved in old age. Effects of expertise, however, are highly specific. Tasks that imitate areas of practice show preservation of function; tasks that measure general cognitive functioning do not. For example, Krampe and Ericsson (1996) reported standard age differences in general processing speed for expert and amateur pianists, but no age differences for experts in speed of finger movements while playing. Practice among experts was essential for the maintenance of skills. Thus, lifelong habits or practice may produce structural or process changes in the brain that are protective against decline of the practiced functions. Indeed, there is a growing body of evidence in neuroscience demonstrating that experience can produce changes in brain organization, for example, by expanding or reorganizing the functional region associated with a highly practiced behavior (e.g., Squire and Kandel, 1999; Gilbert and Wiesel, 1992; Buonomano and Merzenich, 1998; Greenough, 1976; Elbert et al., 1995; Pascual-Leone and Torres, 1993).

Cognitive performance among older adults is also associated with a variety of noncognitive experiential factors, including tobacco use, alcohol consumption, diet, intake of antioxidants, and levels of physical activity (see Waldstein, Appendix E). Further investigation of the effect of the mechanisms that link experiential factors on cognitive aging promises to increase our understanding of the mechanisms involved in age-related cognitive changes.

Connections Between Cognitive and Sensory-Motor Changes

Considerable evidence exists that peripheral sensory and motor systems decline with age. The sensory input to an older nervous system is attenuated, spatially blurred, and temporally smeared compared with that of a healthy young sensory system. The motor output of the aged individual is also often slower, less agile, and more variable than that of a younger person. Evidence is mounting that there is a correlation between sensory-motor decline and cognitive decline—that much of the interindividual variation in cognitive decline is associated with sensory-motor decline.

Much of the decline in sensory function with age is due to "wear and tear" on these systems (see Kline and Scialfa, 1997; Schneider and Pichora-Fuller, in press, for reviews). For instance, the hair cells of the inner ear, which transduce sound vibrations into neural impulses, tend to wear out over repeated use, leading to loss of hearing sensitivity and poor ability to resolve frequency differences, which are the major hearing problems associated with aging (presbycusis). Once mammalian hair cells are damaged or lost, they cannot be replaced (see Tsue et al., 1994). Hair cells similar to those in the auditory system are sensory transducers for the vestibular system that controls balance and helps in locomotion. These also deteriorate over time. In vision, structural changes in the tissues of the cornea, iris, lens, and their fluids occur over time, one result being that less light reaches the retina for neural transduction. Similar forms of structural decline have been documented for taste, smell, the sense of balance, and proprioception. For these reasons, the information most older people receive through their senses is degraded relative to that received by younger people. Even when corrections are made (e.g., hearing aids, eyeglasses) for some forms of sensory loss, older people still tend to perform poorer on perceptual and attentional tasks than do younger people, especially in terms of temporal processing.

Strong correlations have been reported among declines in sensory, motor, and cognitive function. Mayer and Baltes (1996, see also Baltes, 1997; Baltes and Lindenberger, 1997) developed a measure of general intelligence as a part of the Berlin Aging Study. This measure of intelligence correlates strongly with age (from 70 to 105 years) with more than 32 percent of the variance accounted for. When simple measures of hearing, vision, and motor balance are treated as covariates, the correlation drops so that almost none (less than 0.4 percent) of the variance in intelligence can be accounted for on the basis of age. Salthouse et al. (1998) also found strong correlations of cognitive and noncognitive measures with age, but also found some differences between the changes in cognitive and noncognitive measures.

Four explanations have been suggested for the correlated trajectories of cognitive and sensory-motor changes with age: (1) sensory-motor decline causes cognitive decline, perhaps by increasing central control of sensory-motor function; (2) cognitive decline adversely affects sensory performance; (3) secondary variables that covary with sensory-motor and cognitive decline are the basis for the correlation; and (4) sensory, motor, and cognitive systems are interrelated parts of a single system, so that as one part declines so must all other parts. It is important to discover which is correct. For instance, if sensory-motor decline causes cognitive decline, then aids to sensory-motor performance might protect against, or even reverse, cognitive decline.

Hypotheses about common causes of sensory-motor and cognitive decline in old age call into question the common practice of treating sensory, motor, and cognitive systems as discrete systems underlying behavior (see Schneider and Pichora-Fuller, in press). They suggest that, contrary to the classic view in which sensory systems feed information to cognitive systems, which then dictate action to motor systems, the neurobiological substrate of behavior in old age is a single system with many interacting and highly overlapping subsystems. In this view, sensory transducers, hippocampal cells, and motor neurons are different points within a single system, and any change to one part of the system is highly likely to affect other parts.

In pursuing common cause hypotheses for correlations between sensory-motor and cognitive decline, genetics may provide some of the possible common causes. The studies of the role of *APOE* genotype in Alzheimer's disease show the potential of investigating such genetic variables. In addition, heritability studies of cognition in older adults offer a window into the phenomenon (e.g., McClearn et al., 1997; Johansson et al., 1999; Baltes et al., 1999). Other possible common causes may include patterns of life experience and somatic disease processes, as noted in the preceding and following sections.

Few studies have directly assessed the causal connections among sensory, perceptual, motor, and cognitive changes at any age. Moreover, existing knowledge is based mainly on laboratory tests of sensory, perceptual, and attentional abilities; much less is known about change in the activities of living as related sensory systems decline. There are important exceptions, however, such as the association found between useful field of view and car accidents in older adults (e.g., Owsley et al., 1998). A growing body of diverse literature models motor control as a function of environmental signals and internal models of task dynamics and temporal patterning (e.g., Ivry, 1996; Jordan, 1996; Levison, 1981). Also, recent research on the relations between motor and cognitive development in early life (e.g., Thelen and Smith, 1994;

L.B. Smith et al., 1999) suggests that motor control, because it involves problem solving, integration of multiple information sources, and the organization of dynamic internal representations, may be a productive model for understanding many aspects of cognitive development. Much is yet to be learned about how different neural systems (sensory, motor, cognitive) interact with one another and how those interactions change with age. This research may have fundamental implications for understanding the neurobiological basis of behavior in addition to improving understanding of cognitive aging.

The study of the relationship among cognitive, sensory, and motor decline requires a multidisciplinary approach. Investigators in the cognitive, sensory, and motor sciences have not typically collaborated, however. Such collaboration is needed to better understand the correlations among age-related changes in cognitive, sensory, and motor measures and their implications. A good example of the possibilities from research concerns age-related declines in hearing, which can have a significant impact on the lives of older people (Kline and Scialfa, 1997). Significant advances have been made recently in hearing-aid technology and in knowledge about attention, language comprehension, and cognitive processing, all of which seem to change in aging in correlation with auditory changes. If investigators studying audition work with those studying cognitive variables, such as language, the results might include better understanding of how these variables interact with age and innovations that might significantly improve older people's ability to communicate and function in their daily lives.

Cognitive Effects of Changes in Health Status

It has been proposed by some that age-related cognitive decline in many individuals is attributable to disease processes that affect the nervous system only indirectly, including cardiovascular diseases and diabetes, among others (Salthouse et al., 1990; Waldstein, Appendix E). Health problems negatively affect cognitive functioning and are more prevalent in the elderly (e.g., Perlmutter et al., 1988). In addition, the effects of neural changes on cognitive functioning may be moderated by health status or specific disease conditions.

High blood pressure is perhaps the most studied of the relevant health conditions. High blood pressure levels are adversely related to many neuropsychological measures of cognitive functioning (e.g., Elias and Robbins, 1991; Elias et al., 1990; Elias et al., 1993; for reviews see Waldstein, 1995; Appendix E). This relationship is quite apparent when normotensive subjects are compared with hypertensive ones, although there are moderating factors—for example, education has been reported to have a protective effect (Elias et al., 1987; see Waldstein, Appendix E). By some measures, blood pressure accounts for half the variance in cognitive performance of older adults (Madden and Blumenthal, 1998; Elias et al., 1998). Cardiovascular disease, for which hypertension is an important risk factor, has also been shown to have a negative impact on cognitive functioning (e.g., Hertzog et al., 1978; Schaie, 1996). Various mechanisms have been proposed, including direct effects of elevated blood pressure, indirect effects through stress-induced cardiovascular and neuroendocrine responses, and third-variable explanations in which common genetic or environmental factors may predispose an individual both to hypertension and to cognitive decline (see Waldstein, Appendix E). Different explanations may apply for different subgroups of hypertensive individuals or at different points in the life span.

Diabetes is among the other disease conditions that appear to be related to cognitive functioning. Most research suggests that diabetes is related to such measures of cognitive functioning as verbal memory, sensory-motor speed, cognitive flexibility, and concept formation (Dey et al., 1997; Elias et al. 1997; Mochizuki et al., 1998; Naor et al., 1997; van Boxtel et al., 1998), although there is also evidence to the contrary (Muqit and Ferdous, 1998; Worrall et al., 1996).

Numerous possible causal mechanisms may explain correlations between disease conditions and particular types of cognitive functioning, and research is just beginning in this area. In addition to having some potential to illuminate some of the causes of cognitive decline, this line of research brings an added benefit: it can strengthen research on other aspects of cognitive aging by promoting controls for health conditions and interpretations that take such conditions into account.

In addition, there is a considerable body of research on the relationship between self-rated health and cognition (e.g., Field et al., 1988; Hultsch et al., 1993; Perlmutter et al., 1988; Perlmutter and Nyquist, 1990; Salthouse et al., 1990). For example, Perlmutter and Nyquist (1990) found that self-reported health accounted for a significant proportion of the variance in cognitive performance (e.g., digit span and fluid intelligence), even after age-related differences in health were statistically controlled. These associations may reflect cognitive effects of subclinical health conditions, although other explanations are also possible. Some researchers, however, have failed to find a link between self-assessed health and cognition (e.g., Salthouse et al., 1990).

Changes in mental health status, such as depression, may also influence cognitive functioning in older people. In addition to the association of depression with poor physical health (Wells et al., 1989) and elevated rates of mortality (Murphy et al., 1987), depressed individuals are also characterized by impaired cognitive functioning (Wright and Salmon, 1990). The assumption made by most researchers in this area is that the poor cognitive performance is related to other symptoms of depression, rather than representing a direct influence of depression on brain functioning. For example, the symptoms of fatigue, diminished energy and motivation, reduced cognitive effort, and increased rumination and self-focus all combine to impair learning and memory performance in depressed individuals (Gotlib and Hammen, 1992). Although there is some recent evidence indicating that depressed individuals actually demonstrate better memory for negative than for positive information (Gotlib et al., in press), it is clear nevertheless that depression interferes globally with cognitive functioning.

Improved explanations of the relationships of somatic disease to cognitive decline may reveal opportunities to use health interventions to improve cognitive functioning. Although only limited evidence exists of cognitive improvement resulting from specific health interventions (see Waldstein, Appendix E), the research is still in its infancy. Opportunities for intervention may be of particular importance for low-income and minority groups that have below-average use of health care services and high rates of chronic illnesses (black Americans, for example, have higher rates of hypertension, diabetes mellitus, and coronary heart disease) (Ferraro and Farmer, 1996; Harper and Alexander, 1990; Marquis and Long, 1996; Miles and Bernard, 1992).

As the above discussion indicates, various noncognitive indicators, including blood pressure, sensory-motor performance, and peak expiratory flow (Albert et al., 1995), account statistically for large proportions of the variance in rates of cognitive decline in normal aging. These proportions are so large as to indicate overdetermination, a condition in which several different factors appear to explain the same variations in cognitive performance. The strongly correlated trajectories of so many variables constitute an important puzzle for research on the structure of the aging mind: Which variables are causally prior to which? Which correlations reflect the operation of underlying common causes? Which correlations present opportunities for noncognitive interventions that can help preserve cognitive function?

Developments in Measurement and Theory

Growing sophistication in theoretical understanding of cognitive functions, advances in measurement of neural phenomena and cognitive functions, and the availability of analytic techniques from related fields are making possible new advances in explaining the patterns of cognitive aging and linking changes in cognitive function to changes in the brain.

Improved Measurement of Neural and Cognitive Phenomena

Advanced neuroimaging and electrophysiological techniques for measuring on-line brain function, such as functional magnetic resonance imagery (fMRI), position emission tomography (PET), magnetoencephalography

(MEG), transcranial magnetic stimulation (TMS), electroencephalography (EEG), event-related brain potentials (ERP), and event-related optical signal (EROS), several of which so far are underutilized for the study of age-related cognitive changes, make breakthroughs possible in understanding brain-behavior links. Techniques such as fMRI and single-unit recording of neural activity are providing unprecedented levels of spatial and temporal resolution in observations of the brain, and other new and emerging techniques may hasten progress. Functional MRI, for example, can provide measurements in the brain with a time resolution of less than 1 second and spatial resolution of about 2 mm; technological advances promise further improvements in resolution (Le Bihan and Karni, 1995; Albright, Appendix G). Such techniques allow for much closer observation of neural phenomena than ever before, making possible much closer analysis of the relationships between neural and cognitive processes (e.g., Gabrieli, 1998).

Behavioral research has developed a rich array of laboratory techniques that isolate and measure specific mental operations that are fundamental to cognition. These techniques offer greater sensitivity and analytic power than traditional neuropsychological tests, which are designed to detect impairments but not to identify underlying processes and mechanisms. For example, experimental techniques have been used to demonstrate the distinct neural bases of implicit versus explicit memory in cognitive neuroscience research with patients (e.g., Gabrieli et al., 1995; Shimamura and Squire, 1984) and using imaging techniques (e.g., Uecker et al., 1997). The research demonstrates that implicit and explicit memory are differently affected by aging (Fleischman and Gabrieli, 1998; LaVoie and Light, 1994). Similarly, techniques for on-line evaluation of language comprehension processes have isolated semantic and syntactic processes required for comprehension (e.g., Marslen-Wilson and Tyler, 1980). These techniques have been central to evaluating the neural basis of comprehension in research with patients (e.g., Kempler et al., 1998) and using imaging techniques (Caplan et al., 1998, 1999). On-line measures of comprehension have provided evidence consistent with the maintenance of semantic comprehension processes in old age (e.g., Madden, 1988; Stine and Wingfield, 1994; see Burke, 1997; Light, 1991), although there is less agreement about syntactic processes (Caplan and Waters, 1999; Kemper and Kemptes, 1999; Stine-Morrow et al., 1996).

In animal research, tasks have been developed that are selectively sensitive to the effects of damage to the hippocampus, the amygdala, the caudate nucleus, the cerebellum, and the frontal cortex in rats. These tasks have since been adapted for the mouse and their research applications are being disseminated to researchers. For example, the Cold Spring Harbor Laboratories established an annual course in mouse behavior in 1998.

Because of the variety of behavioral tasks that are available, it is increasingly possible to use behavioral observations to identify specific brain regions in which age-related changes that affect cognition are occurring. This information will be important to future efforts to intervene at the molecular and cellular level, because it will tell where in the brain to look for the substrate of observed behavioral effects.

As neuroscience research attains higher levels of resolution, it will become possible to identify particular neural circuits believed to be associated with particular cognitive functions. To achieve understanding of brain-behavior links at this level, it is important to build theory and to identify or construct behavioral measures that fit the structure of cognition and can be localized with comparable resolution to neural observations. This implies a search for fine-grained measures of specific cognitive processes and of the operation of particular neural systems. It also implies a continuing co-evolution of behavioral measures and brain measures and a continuing effort to refine both kinds of measures in order to further clarify brain-behavior links.

An important point to recognize with regard to the above issues of measurement is the central role of experimental animals in research on aging. Neural observations are more feasible in animal models, and many findings are likely to generalize across species. Biological research during the past decade has shown the extraordinary extent to which cellular and molecular mechanisms are conserved through evolution. Indeed, even at the level of brain systems and brain-behavior relationships, one finds considerable parallel across species. Recent advances in molecular biology have caused the mouse to become important for behavioral studies. At the present time, one can expect useful work on brain and behavior, in the context of aging research, to be carried out in the mouse, rat, and monkey, and perhaps in other animal species as well.

Advances in Theory Development

Cognitive behavioral science is making progress on the theoretical side. An example is Baddeley's influential theory of working memory, which postulates interrelated components for speech and visual information with separate storage and rehearsal mechanisms. This theory has motivated investigations of working memory in patients (Vallar and Baddeley, 1984) and using imaging techniques (e.g., Smith and Jonides, 1997) that have supported distinctions in the theory and have identified the neural basis for hypothesized working memory mechanisms. A number of studies following the theory have investigated age differences in components of working memory (e.g., Wingfield et al., 1995).

Research based on theoretically justified measures of specific cognitive functions will make it possible to examine more closely the links between functioning of particular neural circuits and performance on the behavioral indicators, as well as between the behavioral indicators and performance of life tasks. This line of research can go far to clarifying the mechanisms linking age-related changes in neural circuitry to change in cognitive functioning and performance. It is likely also to identify opportunities to intervene either at the neural or behavioral levels so as to maintain performance of life activities in the face of neural decline.

Underutilized Analytical Techniques

A number of mathematical techniques that can be used to characterize the structure and evolution of behavior over time are maturing to a point at which they may be of great benefit in the study of cognitive aging. Four of these are dynamical systems theory, hidden Markov models, connectionist models, and dynamic factor analysis.

Dynamical systems theory characterizes the properties of different patterns of stable behavior, as well as transitions among such patterns. In this approach, behavior is typically represented as a continuous trajectory in a state space, i.e., a space whose dimensions are the important variables needed to describe and predict behavior. Stable behavior is not modeled as simply a constant, but is viewed as resulting from the interaction of various abstract forces and perturbations to a behavioral system. These forces may push a system toward a point in the state space, toward a particular oscillation or limit cycle, or toward some more elaborate pattern of stable behavior. Some perturbations can be compensated for by the system; others result in a loss of stability, and perhaps achievement of a new stable state. This abstract, holistic style of description has been applied to various types of behavior ranging from physiological subsystems (e.g., heartbeat; breathing; see Glass and Mackey, 1988) to coordinated limb movements (e.g., Kelso, 1995). In the developmental domain, this approach has been used to describe changes in perceptual-motor performance in children. It has shown how particular changes in underlying behavioral dynamics combine with each other and with characteristics of the environment to produce stable behavioral patterns (Thelen and Smith, 1994).

A number of intriguing possibilities exist for applying this mathematical approach to older adults. For example, it might be applied to developmental declines in the ways it has been applied to developmental advances. It could clarify the implications for overall performance of declines in particular behavioral dynamics and identify specific types of remediation or environmental modification that could maintain performance despite such declines. Also, because dynamical systems theory characterizes the stability of behavior in terms of a process rather than simply approximating it as a constant, it allows the examination of varieties of stability that differ both qualitatively and quantitatively. Some patterns may be too stable (i.e., rigid) and inhibit adaptive changes in behavior; other patterns may be insufficiently stable and result in loss of control. In other words, there may exist optimum levels and types of stability for specific functions (e.g., Beek, 1989; Thelen, 1999). Also, because dynamical systems theory is applicable across many realms of measurement, it may facilitate comparisons of adaptivity at the neural and behavioral levels.

Hidden Markov models typically represent behavioral patterns as a network of discrete states with various probabilities of transition to subsequent states. Such models may be particularly helpful in designing technological interventions for processes that exhibit discrete transitions. For example, a person's interactions with a computer-controlled device might be characterized by the values of a limited set of discrete state variables corresponding to the physical state of the device and the cognitive state of the person (see Fisher, Appendix D). Interactions that can be characterized by finite sets of possible external inputs and available actions can be thoroughly analyzed in terms of transitions from the current state into some new state. The pattern of state transitions will differ across individuals and may provide useful information in diagnosing problems that a particular individual is having in controlling a device (e.g., Miller, 1985; Fisher, Appendix D). The Markov network may indicate what subgoals a person is trying to achieve and what strategies are being used. This information may provide the basis for designing appropriate changes in the device structure and/or computer prompts to adaptively improve the action patterns of older adults. Similar techniques may also be applicable to more continuous control tasks, such as driving a motor vehicle, to describe the transitions between different discrete subgoals in continuous movement patterns and/or co-occurring discrete subtasks that accompany continuous control of vehicular movement (e.g., Baron and Corker, 1989; Levison, 1993). Other modeling techniques involving Bayesian inference and/or neural networks (e.g., Jacobs and Jordan, 1993; see below) may also be useful for modeling how complex tasks are partitioned into subtasks and/or the effects of multiple competing goals on action. All of these techniques address the temporal microstructure of action.

Connectionist models have shown a dramatic resurgence of interest during the 1980s and 1990s. These models include various approaches known as neural networks, neural models, parallel distributed processing systems, localist models, and spreading activation models, and have in common a network of nodes connected by weighted pathways. Connectionist models are sensitive to biological constraints, as nodes can be loosely associated with neurons and their connections with synapses. Connectionist models have been used to simulate brain processes, for example, topographic map formation in the brain (Reggia et al., 1992), the development of receptive fields (Linsker, 1986), and the physiological basis of EEG (Lagerlund and Sharbrough, 1988). At the psychological level, connectionist models have been used to simulate cognitive operations, such as associative memory (Anderson, 1983) and sentence production (Dell, 1986). These models, developed to account for normal brain and cognitive functions, have been widely used as the basis for modeling brain disorders (for example, focal cortical lesions and disconnection syndromes), as well as cognitive disorders (for example, dyslexia, amnesia, and aphasia) (Reggia et al., 1994). In models of cognitive disorders, patterns of symptoms or deficits emerge from damage to the normal system, and these symptoms are compared with the performance of patients on cognitive tasks.

The connectionist approach has been extremely useful in cognitive research, producing better theoretical understanding of brain function and cognitive processes and generating hypotheses about mechanisms underlying important cognitive behaviors. It has led to the identification of fundamental principles of cognitive processing, such as the necessity of parallel processing to achieve the computational power required for cognition, and it has provided a means for both generating and evaluating hypotheses about the functional deficits that underlie cognitive disorders. However, the connectionist approach has had little impact so far on cognitive aging research. Behavioral research on cognitive aging has produced an accumulation of rich datasets, but theory is insufficient to organize and explain them. Connectionist models have been developed for a wide range of cognitive behaviors and impairments and offer a promising approach for identifying mechanisms that can explain existing data on the pattern of cognitive functioning in old age and generate hypotheses for future research.

Dynamic factor analysis provides an expansion of cross-sectional factor analysis, which is normally used to identify a small set of distinct behavioral variables that clarifies the pattern underlying a larger number of measures. With dynamic factor analysis, these variables can be analyzed over time in ways that explore temporally lagged relationships among them. Because of the demands of repeated behavioral measurement, dynamic factor analysis is typically used to analyze changes occurring on time scales of days to months. Dynamic factor analysis has been productive for studying temporal variability within individuals in such personality characteristics as perceived control of one's environment (e.g., Eizenman et al., 1997) and emotional positivity and negativity (e.g., Shifren et al., 1997). The finding that intraindividual variability in perceived control correlates with mortality in older adults over a five-year period (Eizenman et al., 1997) suggests that the method is useful for studying relationships involving life experience variables. Dynamic factor analysis may be useful for analyzing cognitive and behavioral adaptations in aging individuals that occur over appropriate time scales, such as in response to dementia, stroke, or stressful life events (e.g., loss of a spouse, confinement in a hospital or nursing home).

Modeling techniques such as these are important not only for their potential ability to represent particular cognitive phenomena. They may also offer first steps toward the development of process models that would improve understanding of the chains of causation—probably quite complex—that link life experiences, physical and mental health, social and technological context, sensory-motor phenomena, and neural changes to the life course of cognitive capability and performance. It is also important to emphasize that progress in the modeling of cognitive processes depends on continued improvement in understanding of those processes that comes from improved psychometric measures and from experimental research on perception and cognition.

RESEARCH INITIATIVE ON THE STRUCTURE OF THE AGING MIND

The NIA should undertake a major research initiative to improve understanding of the structure of the aging mind, including the identification of mechanisms at the behavioral and neural levels that contribute to age-related change in cognitive functioning.

Research has established that the effect of aging on cognitive functioning and performance of associated life tasks varies for different cognitive operations and for different individuals. It has also revealed that in advanced old age, the correlations increase among measures of different cognitive functions. Furthermore, research has linked a variety of experiences to cognitive performance in older adults, including physical exercise, diet, cognitive training, expertise, and the provision of environmental support; it has also documented relationships of cognitive functions to body systems, including sensory-motor functioning and chronic diseases. The mechanisms underlying these relationships are not yet known; hypotheses are still at an early stage of development.

The recommended research initiative would aim to specify the patterns of variation in cognitive functioning during the aging process and to identify the mechanisms, at levels of analysis from the molecular to the cultural, that contribute to age-linked stability and change. By identifying these mechanisms, the initiative would contribute to the search for effective interventions to assist older adults in maintaining cognitive functioning and performance. For instance, it might document benefits from diet, exercise, cognitive activity, and other interventions and determine whether certain of these have more general or more lasting effects than others.

The research initiative should include studies of the full variety of phenomena identified in this chapter as well as related ones. It should build on a base of psychometric and experimental research on cognitive processes, which should continue to receive NIA support. We believe, however, that the most rapid advances are likely to result from encouraging researchers to expand their portfolio of research approaches by applying and integrating promising methodologies that are either new or underutilized in cognitive aging research, along with continuing research with well-established methods. We therefore recommend that the initiative emphasize three method-based research strategies and their integration.

1. Relating high-resolution measures of neural functioning to measures of cognitive functioning in the aging mind.

The research initiative should support investigator-initiated research that will measure and analyze the reciprocal relations between brain and cognition. This research should utilize the new high-resolution techniques for measuring neural functioning and should link these observations to measures of cognitive functioning that are capable of isolating specific mental operations. The research will investigate age differences in the cortical components and behavioral indicators of cognitive processes as well as the effects of interventions and experience on cortical organization and behavior.

For this research approach to achieve its potential, the research initiative should support studies that address key methodological issues associated with brain imaging techniques. One such issue that requires immediate research is the decoding of the vascular signal of fMRI in ways that allow meaningful comparisons across the life span. As is well known, fMRI signals measure neural function indirectly by measuring blood flow; because blood flows differentially to active regions of the brain, the fMRI is presumed also to reflect neural activity (Le Bihan and Karni, 1995). However, the precise correlation between neural activity and the vascular signal is not known, and it may vary with age because of atrophy and other neuronal changes related to aging, as well as changes in vascularization (D'Esposito et al., 1999; Taoka et al., 1998). Eventually, longitudinal studies with humans may aid interpretation. For the next decade or more, however, the best source of insight may be information from animals, particularly the awake, behaving monkey, in which the relationship between single unit activity and the fMRI signal can be directly explored in the same tasks (Albright, Appendix G). Recently, the feasibility of this approach was demonstrated in the monkey (Stefanacci et al., 1998), and an improved technique for doing such work was demonstrated in monkeys using a custom-designed, vertical bore magnet that allows the monkey to sit in a conventional primate chair within the magnet (Logothetis et al., 1999).

Another methodological problem deserving immediate attention concerns ways to improve the correspondence between behavioral measures and neural observations, such as those that new measurement techniques can provide. Recent advances in the behavioral measurement of specific cognitive functions have already been noted. The research initiative should support studies to identify or develop focused behavioral indicators that connect closely to high-resolution neural observations. It is to be expected that simple behaviors will yield more easily to this approach than complex ones, which are more likely to involve distributed neural activity.

This line of research requires two kinds of knowledge that rarely exist in the same investigator: knowledge of cognitive techniques for isolating mental operations and of neuroimaging or electrophysiological techniques for measuring on-line brain function. We therefore recommend that the NIA support workshops to provide basic training to investigators. The goal of the workshops would be to provide training on techniques for measuring and decomposing phenomena at both the cognitive-behavioral and the neurological levels in order to encourage investigators to develop relevant research applications. We also recommend that the NIA support research to develop or modify behavioral and neural measures so as to improve the correspondence between these types of measurement.

2. Elaborating theory-based and mathematical models of the aging mind.

The research initiative should support theory-driven research that develops models of cognitive aging effects that will increase our understanding of patterns of stability and change among mental processes in the aging mind, as well as complex interactions among cognitive and other systems. Existing findings from cognitive aging research provide a wealth of data that demonstrate both impaired and preserved cognitive functions in old age. Theories to explain this pattern, however, have been slow to develop.

This research strategy should take advantage of theoretical and mathematical tools that have proved useful in related fields. To illustrate, connectionist models of language and knowledge representation and production system models of executive functions and memory have been very influential in improving understanding of basic cognitive processes; they can be productively extended to account for age-related changes in these processes. Also, research should be encouraged that applies various types of statistical and mathematical models (e.g., structural equation models, dynamic factor analysis, Markov models, dynamical systems models, adaptive control theory) to understanding short-term variability, long-term stability and change, and multisystem causal linkages involving or affecting cognitive functioning in older adults (e.g., sensory-motor functioning and cognition).

3. Conducting and analyzing large-scale, multivariate studies of the aging mind.

To achieve the objectives of this research initiative, it will be necessary to expand the use of large-scale, multivariate, longitudinal studies. It is necessary to expand and improve on previous longitudinal research by including variables reflecting high-resolution cognitive and neural measures; indicators of health status and sensory-motor functioning; and measures of relevant life experience. Analysis of multiple measures can help explain patterns of correlations, such as that in which several different physiological variables appear to explain the same variations in cognition. It is also important to examine a broad representative sample of the population, sometimes oversampling in subgroups whose health status or responses to life experiences are expected to illuminate important theoretical questions, and to encompass a wide age range. Moreover, by following individuals into very old age, promising new findings suggesting the existence of unexpected linkages between cognitive functioning and survival could be investigated. The requirements for long-term longitudinal studies are discussed in more detail in Chapter 5.

The conjunction of improved measurement, advances in modeling, and the comprehensive collection of longitudinal data on cognitive functioning and associated factors can have a synergistic effect in advancing knowledge. Longitudinal studies can make a quantum improvement by employing new fine-grained neural and behavioral measures; renewed attention to modeling can make better sense of the patterns that underlie associations between these neural and behavioral measures and that can be drawn from the longitudinal data.

5

Implementation

The preceding chapters identify three major research initiatives that can yield breakthroughs in understanding the aging mind and practical applications for improving the functioning of older adults. In some instances, we have identified issues of implementation specific to particular research initiatives (for example, the need to develop innovative funding mechanisms for basic cognitive research needed to develop new technology to improve the adaptivity of older adults). This chapter addresses a set of implementation issues that cut across the research initiatives and offers some specific recommendations. They concern the organization of research support under the initiatives and the needs to promote interdisciplinary research, support infrastructure, and collaborate across agencies.

ORGANIZATION OF RESEARCH SUPPORT

In our judgment, the best way to support research under the three initiatives will vary. In some research areas (for example, the application of new mathematical techniques to cognitive aging), it may be sufficient at first to request proposals from individual investigators. In other areas, it may be advisable to organize competitions that require applicants to work together across disciplines. For example, the NIA might ask cognitive psychologists and engineers to work together on proposals for research on technological supports for cognitive performance in older adults, or neuroscientists and behavioral scientists to work together to propose research linking neural and behavioral phenomena at high resolution. This strategy may also prove useful for encouraging the early stages of research on other topics that are likely to require unusual interdisciplinary collaborations (e.g., the neurobiology of training and practice). Appendix D offers a detailed discussion of the need for interdisciplinary collaboration on research on technological support, the benefits that may be gained, and some of the challenges.

In certain areas it may be worthwhile to hold competitions for small research teams or centers that would bring together cognitive scientists, behavioral scientists, and neuroscientists around a common problem. It is especially worth considering this support option for the initiative on cognition in context. An emerging interdisciplinary field such as the neurobiology of life experience might develop most rapidly as the result of the work of such interdisciplinary research groups.

To pursue the research initiatives successfully, it may be advisable for the NIA to establish some new research programs or program offices, or at least to establish special emphasis panels to review the proposals. The initiative on cognition in context may be an example, as it encompasses an unusually wide range of disciplines. We encourage the NIA to consider these organizational issues carefully and to consult with the research community as it develops the research initiatives and to seek forms of organization that will encourage the needed interdisciplinary integration (see next section).

PROMOTING INTERDISCIPLINARY RESEARCH

As this report makes clear, the study of cognitive aging is highly interdisciplinary and becoming more so. Each of the recommended research initiatives requires collaborations among neuroscientists, cognitive scientists, and behavioral scientists. Progress on each initiative depends on the development of research from multiple points of view (multidisciplinary research) and on efforts to integrate these points of view into comprehensive understandings of cognitive aging (interdisciplinary research). These needs extend even beyond the already interdisciplinary field of cognitive science, which has developed by linking such diverse specialties as linguistics, artificial intelligence, and neuroscience with behavioral science.

A great diversity of approaches is appropriate given the research problems, but it presents challenges of training and coordination because of the required breadth of knowledge. The field of cognitive neuroscience in particular requires the rethinking of traditional disciplinary training programs. The investigation of the relationship between cognition and brain processes demands knowledge of behavioral techniques for identifying cognitive processes and architecture, as well as techniques for measuring structural and functional aspects of brain. This interdisciplinary approach is especially germane to cognitive aging research for which age-related changes highlight the dynamic relationship between brain and cognitive processes.

Recent advances in imaging technology have generated enormous interest in brain-behavior relationships, increasing the importance of training for neuroscientists in experimental techniques for investigating cognitive processes. Graduate training in neuroscience, however, often emphasizes techniques for investigating brain structure and process with little emphasis on behavioral techniques that are fundamental to the investigation of memory, language, attention, and other cognitive functions and less on linking neural phenomena and fundamental cognitive processes to adaptive behavior in real-life situations.

The NIA should support postdoctoral fellowships, conferences, workshops, and summer institutes to encourage individual scientists to broaden their knowledge and technical capability in order to address interdisciplinary issues that are central to the new research initiatives.

For example, these mechanisms should be used to encourage neuroscientists and neuropsychologists to increase their training in cognitive experimental techniques and cognitive models. They should be used to encourage applicants with graduate degrees in cognitive psychology, linguistics, artificial intelligence, and the study of socioeconomic, educational, and cultural differences to strengthen their knowledge of brain structure and their ability to use techniques for investigating brain function.

The NIA, perhaps in conjunction with other institutes, should organize a special competition that would provide multiyear support of a few small multidisciplinary research centers or teams focused on analytical problems posed by the research initiatives that require the simultaneous application of multiple perspectives (e.g., neurobiology of training or cultural difference, development of adaptive technology).

The mechanism of interactive research program grants may also be useful for encouraging collaboration on common problems by researchers approaching them from different disciplinary perspectives.

RESEARCH INFRASTRUCTURE

Progress on the three major research initiatives depends on supportive research infrastructure, as already noted. For example, we have noted the need for access to aged animals for research. To ensure adequate access to such animals requires support beyond that provided for individual research projects. Such support is a public good for research.

The NIA should help support the maintenance of colonies of patho-

gen-free aged animals (including primates, rats, and mice) in regional centers.

This support should probably be in collaboration with other research funding agencies. It will involve a long-term commitment, especially for primates, and the support of highly skilled researchers and animal care staff. The research community should be consulted for advice on which animal strains are most important to keep available for research purposes.

The rest of this section discusses two major types of infrastructure that require support for the benefit of research on all the recommended initiatives: general-use databases, and brain imaging research capability.

Building General-Use Databases

Strategic investments in general-use data can support research on all three recommended initiatives. In our judgment, the greatest opportunity for such support lies in developing and expanding long-term, longitudinal studies.

There is little dispute that longitudinal research is essential to investigate processes of age-related change directly, rather than indirectly in the form of cross-sectional differences that may reflect a mixture of the products of change and of preexisting differences. Nevertheless, largely because of the greater time and expense, there are currently far more reports of cross-sectional comparisons of cognitive variables than longitudinal comparisons.

For many years the dominant interpretation has been that cross-sectional and longitudinal comparisons in cognition yield substantially different results, with much smaller, and later-occurring, age-related declines in longitudinal contrasts than in cross-sectional contrasts. However, some recent data call this view into question (e.g., Hultsch et al., 1998; Zelinski and Burnight, 1997; Sliwinski and Buschke, 1999). It is clear that the relation between cross-sectional and longitudinal age trends is still not fully understood, and thus it is important to have more linkages between the two major methods of investigating age differences. Longitudinal studies are certainly not the only type of research that can yield valuable information about aging, but they provide unique information that is not available from other research designs.

Several high-quality longitudinal studies focusing on cognition are currently under way in the United States (e.g., Baltimore, Seattle, Los Angeles) and elsewhere (e.g., Victoria, British Columbia; Manchester, England; Berlin, Germany). However, there are a number of features not represented in most existing studies that would be very desirable to include in future longitudinal studies.

First, at least in the initial assessment, the sample of participants should reflect major demographic variations in the population, and not just healthy middle-class whites as is the case in most current U.S. studies. Obtaining a truly representative sample may require that the same protocol be implemented in several different sites, but the benefits of a broader base of generalization are likely to justify the additional costs and effort. In addition, it will be valuable for some purposes to oversample groups of particular interest, such as members of ethnic and racial minority groups, people with particular life experiences (e.g., certain occupations) or health conditions believed to predispose to cognitive changes, people with known risk factors for dementia, and the oldest old. Knowledge about cognitive change in the oldest old is limited because most past longitudinal research started in middle age, with the result that by ages 85 and beyond, samples were too small to allow good generalizations. It might therefore be valuable to expand some longitudinal studies by adding respondents at older ages.

Second, to examine precursors to changes and to allow more complete investigation of trajectories over time, the research participants should span a broad age range, ideally beginning in the 20s instead of the 50s or later, and extending to the end of life so as to investigate reported associations of cognitive status with mortality. Beginning the longitudinal assessments at early ages seems warranted because cross-sectional analyses have revealed substantial age-related differences in some cognitive abilities before age 50 (e.g., see the meta-analysis in Verhaeghen and Salthouse, 1997). Furthermore, at least one recent report found that cognitive variables in early adulthood predicted cognitive status more than 50 years later (Snowden et al., 1996). In addition, as noted in Chapter 2, there is reason to believe that neural changes occurring in early or mid-adulthood may be the first signs of cognitive changes that are not clinically observable until much later.

Third, a wider variety of variables should be obtained from the research participants than has been typical in past research. Within the cognitive domain, several different types of cognitive abilities should be assessed, not just memory or intellectual abilities, as in some current projects. It is also desirable to include variables reflecting specific theoretical processes in attention, memory, and language instead of only psychometric variables that probably reflect an unknown mixture of processes. It is essential, of course, that these theoretically more precise variables be established to have high levels of reliability in order to be included in longitudinal research protocols.

In order to relate changes in cognitive tasks to changes in daily functioning, it would be valuable to include some measures of everyday, or ecologically valid, activities. These should include a mixture of activities for which a neural substrate has been identified and others known to require cognitive activity, but for which the neural substrate remains unknown. Data should also be collected on life experience factors that may affect cognitive aging. These include basic sociodemographic information (ethnicity, education, socioeconomic status, etc.), but also more specific experiential factors that may underlie group differences in cognitive aging (see Chapter 3).

Other types of variables should also be included in future longitudinal studies. Several existing longitudinal studies include assessments of physical health, personality, lifestyle, hormone levels, and genetic markers, and new studies should continue and expand on those efforts to understand the mind through the life course, including influences from the prenatal environment and correlated physical conditions (e.g., blood pressure, respiratory flow, use of medications). This effort would support the research initiative on cognition in context. Including measures of brain structure and function along with the cognitive and physical assessments would support the research initiatives on the structure of the aging mind and on neural health. Among the possibilities that might be considered are volume estimates from structural MRIs (e.g., Raz et al., 1998) and variables obtained from event-related potentials (ERPs) or functional MRIs.

As noted in Chapter 4, moderate to strong correlations have been reported between cognitive variables and sensory-motor variables in cross-sectional studies (e.g., Anstey et al., 1993, 1997; Baltes and Lindenberger, 1997; Lindenberger and Baltes, 1994; Salthouse et al., 1996, 1998). To pursue the research opportunity afforded by examining these correlations, it would be helpful for new longitudinal studies to include assessments of sensory and motor capabilities.

A body of longitudinal studies that includes this variety of variables would provide the fundamental database for a successful research initiative on the structure of the aging mind, as well as significant support to the other two research initiatives. Analyses of the data could focus not only on changes in mean levels of performance in individual variables, but also on changes in the interrelations among variables. Researchers could examine change in various cognitive measures to determine which antecedent conditions predict cognitive change. They could also examine changes in associations among variables, particularly after temporal lags. For example, they could consider whether a change in the relation between two variables from one measurement occasion to the next is predictive of later change in a third variable. This sort of analysis would be particularly interesting when the early and late variables are from different domains, such as neural and cognitive.

Research on rich longitudinal datasets could clarify where in the structure of variables age-related changes are most pronounced. Some research has suggested that longitudinal change operates on a general factor (e.g., Hertzog and Schaie, 1988; Hultsch et al., 1998). However, relatively little research has been conducted attempting to investigate the structure of change across different types of variables. Information of this type is potentially very important because it can clarify how specific or broad an explanation will be needed to account for age-related cognitive changes. Finally, powerful new analytical models, such as latent growth modeling and latent change analysis, could be applied that might yield insights not possible with cross-sectional data.

The NIA should undertake a major effort to expand or develop large-scale longitudinal studies of cognitive aging. The studies should cover the range of variation in the population and should support research aimed at understanding the relationships among neural, cognitive, behavioral, sensory-motor, health, and life experience variables as they affect cognitive aging. Other institutes of the National Institutes of Health should be invited to cooperate in this effort, as they may benefit from the type of comprehensive longitudinal research being developed.

This recommendation is for an expansion of research activity and is not intended to detract from existing laboratory-based research on cognitive aging. In fact, longitudinal research may require an expansion of laboratory research in order to develop, validate, and continually improve measures of cognitive processes that are essential for use in longitudinal and other research on cognitive aging.

Considerable attention needs to be devoted from the outset to how best to implement this recommendation. We are recommending the study of a very large number of variables in a very broad population, and practical limitations will severely restrict the number of variables that can be measured for each individual participant in a study. There are trade-offs to be made between the needs for in-depth analysis of particular cognitive functions and for understanding these functions in context (e.g., the roles of sensory-motor, health, and cultural variables). In addition, it is necessary for any measure to pass screens of reliability and validity to be included in a major longitudinal study.

The NIA and cooperating institutes should engage in structured discussions with the research community, perhaps through a series of workshops, to address the problems involved in using resources effectively to create a broadly useful base of longitudinal data on cognitive function and its neural, behavioral, physical, and experiential correlates.

These discussions should address the following issues, among others:

—effective ways to combine large-scale and more focused research so as to continually strengthen the base and the value of general-use data;
—selection of which neural, behavioral, physical, experiential, and other variables to include in large-scale longitudinal studies and which to use in smaller, focused studies;
—assessment of the adequacy of particular measures or indicators for the variables selected for inclusion in longitudinal studies;

—priorities for developing and validating measures and indicators that might be included in future longitudinal studies;

—the value of adopting standard procedures for screening or categorizing research participants with regard to status on key health and cognitive variables so as to increase comparability across studies;

—appropriate evaluation methods, including the possibility of special review, for research proposals within the effort to expand longitudinal research, particularly in light of possible tensions between the needs of long-term longitudinal research and the evaluation criteria traditionally employed by study sections.

Building Research Capability for Using Data from Brain Imaging

The potential of brain imaging technology for research on cognitive aging will not be realized without focused investments in infrastructure. Three key elements of infrastructure are missing.

A Common Database for Human Brain Imaging Data Linked to Behavioral Characteristics

The research community could greatly benefit from an effort to standardize measures made from human brain imaging data, particularly MRI data, that can be used for brain-behavior research so that data collected for different purposes can be combined into a growing general database. To achieve this benefit, standard procedures would have to be developed for collecting and reporting such data, which would probably begin with records that contain structural brain imaging data, particularly MRI data, and behavioral characteristics of the same individuals.

The NIA should support a consensus conference that would discuss limitations and concerns specific to functional imaging and aging and develop standard procedures for collecting and reporting human brain imaging data, specifically including MRI data, usable for studying brain-behavior relationships during the aging process.

The conference would aim to identify and reach consensus about specific problems, including age effects on the coupling of neural and hemodynamic responses, time of day for MRI observations (e.g., the inappropriateness of testing older adults at night), the need for a stereotaxic atlas for the brains of older adults, and the implications of structural images for interpreting functional images. The conference would publish a report recommending certain procedures as standard, thus making a common database possible. The approach could be similar to one used to develop standards for electrophysiological measurement of event-related potentials (Donchin et al., 1977; Picton et al., in press).

Centers for Monkey Brain Imaging Research

At the present time, the most pressing need is for centers that include capability for fMRI research on monkeys. Because such research is best carried out in a custom-designed, vertical bore magnet, progress in all research fields that can benefit from real-time imaging of the aging brain depends on the availability of this expensive equipment. The cost of the equipment provides the rationale for establishing research centers, possibly in collaboration with other institutes at the National Institutes of Health (NIH). Centers would presumably be established in places where there is existing expertise in cognitive neuroscience and in the techniques needed for research with awake, behaving monkeys. Optimally, the monkey facilities would be sited in close approximation to human fMRI facilities, so as to permit the sharing of core personnel and computer software.

The NIA, working with other institutes at NIH, should establish a monkey brain imaging facility with fMRI capability at NIH and support a few similar centers elsewhere.

Adequate Access to MRI Physicists

The rapidly increasing amount of MRI research underlines the shortage of qualified MRI physicists to work on research teams studying cognition in aging. Although this problem is broader in scope than the research concerns of the NIA, it is likely to slow research progress unless appropriate action is taken. The NIA should work with other federal agencies on ways to address the problem.

COLLABORATION ACROSS INSTITUTES

We have specifically recommended that the NIA collaborate with other institutes to establish research centers, including one at NIH, where monkey brain imaging procedures, specifically including fMRI, can be carried out in a custom-designed, vertical bore magnet. We believe that this is a single example of a more general point.

The NIA should seek additional opportunities to participate with other institutes such as the National Institute of Mental Health, the National Institute of Neurological Diseases and Stroke, and the National Eye

Institute to develop initiatives in neuroscience and cognitive aging as a way to increase the power of its research investments.

Several examples illustrate the kinds of collaborations that are likely to be beneficial. The NIA might share in the support of animal colonies and benefit by improved access to aging animals for research purposes. Research to clarify the interpretation of fMRI signals and to develop protocols for recording data and statistical techniques for analyzing them would be beneficial not only to the NIA but also to other institutes that support research that relies on these signals. Collaborations with other NIH institutes that deal with disabled populations (e.g., the National Institute of Neurological Diseases and Stroke, the National Institute of Arthritis and Musculoskeletal and Skin Diseases, the National Institute of Deafness and Other Communication Disorders) would probably help advance research on adaptive technology. And interinstitute collaborations can also help in carrying out the large-scale longitudinal studies recommended in this chapter. These studies, sometimes with the inclusion of a few additional variables in the research protocol, can provide valuable information on a range of issues relating to health and well-being. Collaboration with other institutes and agencies may make possible studies that could not be fielded with NIA support alone.

References

Abidi, M.A., and R.C. Gonzalez, eds.
  1992   *Data Fusion in Robotics and Machine Intelligence.* Boston: Academic Press.
Ader, R., and N. Cohen
  1993   Psychoneuroimmunology: Conditioning and stress. *Annual Review of Psychology* 44:53-85.
Albert, M.S., K. Jones, C.R. Savage, L. Berkman, T. Seeman, D. Blazer, and J.W. Rowe
  1995   Predictors of cognitive change in older persons: MacArthur Studies of Successful Aging. *Psychology and Aging* 10(4):578-589.
Alexander, M.P., R.S. Fischer, and R. Friedman
  1992   Lesion localization in apractic agraphia. *Archives of Neurology* 49(3):246-251.
Anderson, J.
  1983   Cognitive and psychological computation with neural models. *IEEE Transactions on Systems, Man, Cybernetics* 13:799-815.
Anstey, K.J., S.R. Lord, and P. Williams
  1997   Strength in lower limbs, visual contrast sensitivity, and simple reaction time predict cognition in older women. *Psychology and Aging* 12:137-144.
Anstey, K.J., L. Stankov, and S.R. Lord
  1993   Primary aging, secondary aging, and intelligence. *Psychology and Aging* 8:562-570.
Anyon, J.
  1980   Social class and the hidden curriculum of work. *Journal of Education* 162:67-92.
Arbuckle, T.Y., D. Gold, and D. Andres
  1986   Cognitive functioning of older people in relation to social and personality variables. *Psychology and Aging* 1:55-62.
Avolio, B.J., and D.A. Waldman
  1994   Variations in cognitive, perceptual, and psychomotor abilities across the working life span: Examining the effects of race, sex, experience, education, and occupational type. *Psychology and Aging* 9(3):430-442.

64

Baltes, M.M., and L.L. Carstensen
  1999   Social psychological theories and their applications to aging: From individual to collective. Pp. 209-226 in *Handbook of Theories of Aging*, V. Bengtson and K.W. Schaie, eds. New York: Springer.
Baltes, P.B.
  1997   On the incomplete architecture of human ontogeny: Selection, optimization, and compensation as foundation of developmental theory. *American Psychologist* 52(4):366-380.
Baltes, P.B., and U. Lindenberger
  1997   Emergence of a powerful connection between sensory and cognitive functioning across the adult life span: A new window to the study of cognitive aging? *Psychology and Aging* 12:12-21.
Baltes, P.B., and K.U. Mayer, eds.
  1999   *The Berlin Aging Study: Aging from 70 to 100.* New York: Cambridge University Press.
Baltes, P.B., and U.M. Staudinger, eds.
  1996   *Interactive Minds.* New York: Cambridge University Press.
Baltes, P.B., and U.M. Staudinger
  2000   Wisdom: A metaheuristic to orchestrate mind and virtue toward excellence. *American Psychologist* 55:122-136.
Baltes, P.B., U.M. Staudinger, and U. Lindenberger
  1999   Lifespan psychology: Theory and application to intellectual functioning. *Annual Review of Psychology* 50:471-507.
Baron, S., and K. Corker
  1989   Engineering-based approaches to human performance modeling. Pp. 203-217 in *Applications of Human Performance Models to System Design*, G.R. McMillan, D. Beevis, E. Salas, M.H. Strub, R. Sutton, and L. van Breda, eds. New York: Plenum.
Beek, P.J.
  1989   Timing and phase locking in cascade juggling. *Ecological Psychology* 1:55-96.
Birren, J.E., and D.F. Morrison
  1961   Analysis of the WAIS subtests in relation to age and education. *Journal of Gerontology* 16:363-369.
Blanchard-Fields, F.
  1997   The role of emotion in social cognition across the adult life span. *Annual Review of Geriatrics and Gerontology* 17:238-266.
Blanchard-Fields, F., Y. Chen, and L. Norris
  1997   Everyday problem solving across the adult life span: Influence of domain specificity and cognitive appraisal. *Psychology and Aging* 12:684-693.
Blanchard-Fields, F., and T.M. Hess, eds.
  1996   *Perspectives on Cognitive Change in Adulthood and Aging*, 4th ed. San Diego: Academic.
  1999   *Social Cognition and Aging.* New York: Academic Press.
Blanchard-Fields, F., H.C. Jahnke, and C. Camp
  1995   Age differences in problem-solving style: The role of emotional salience. *Psychology and Aging* 10:173-180.
Blum, J.E., and L.F. Jarvik
  1974   Intellectual performance of octogenarians as a function of education and initial ability. *Human Development* 17:364-375.

Breitner, J.C.S.
  1996   Inflammatory processes and anti-inflammatory drugs in Alzheimer's disease: A cur-
          rent appraisal. *Neurobiology of Aging* 17:789-794.
Brislin, R.
  1993   *Understanding Culture's Influence on Behavior.* Fort Worth, TX: Harcourt Brace
          Jovanovich.
Buonomano, D.V., and M.M. Merzenich
  1998   Cortical plasticity: From synapses to maps. *Annual Review of Neuroscience* 21: 149-
          186.
Burke, D.M.
  1997   Language, aging and inhibitory deficits: Evaluation of a theory. *Journal of Gerontol-
          ogy: Psychological Sciences* 52B:254-264.
Burke, D.M., and D.G. MacKay
  1997   Memory, language, and ageing. *Philosophical Transactions. Royal Society of London.
          Series B. Biological Sciences* 352:1845-1856.
Burke, D.M., D.G. MacKay, J.S. Worthley, and E. Wade
  1991   On the tip of the tongue: What causes word finding failures in young and older
          adults. *Journal of Memory and Language* 30:542-579.
Burton, L.M., and V.L. Bengston
  1982   Research in elderly minority communities: Problems and potentials. Pp. 215-222 in
          Minority Aging: Sociological and Social Psychological Issues, R.C. Manuel, ed.
          Westport, CT: Greenwood.
Camp, C.J.
  1989   World-knowledge systems. Pp. 457-482 in *Everyday Cognition in Adulthood and Late
          Life*, L.W. Poon, D.C. Rubin, and B.A. Wilson, eds. Cambridge, England: Cam-
          bridge University Press.
Caplan, C.
  1974   *Support Systems and Community Mental Health.* New York: Behavioral Publications.
Caplan, D., N. Alpert, and G. Waters
  1998   Effects of syntactic structure and propositional number on patterns of regional cere-
          bral blood flow. *Journal of Cognitive Neuroscience* 10(4):541-552.
  1999   PET studies of syntactic processing with auditory sentence presentation. *Neuroimage*
          9(3):343-351.
Caplan, D., and G.S. Waters
  1999   Verbal working memory and sentence comprehension. *Behavioral and Brain Sci-
          ences* 22:77-126.
Carruthers, M.J.
  1990   *The Book of Memory: A Study of Memory in Medieval Culture.* Cambridge, England:
          Cambridge University Press.
Carstensen, L.L., D.M. Isaacowitz, and S.Turk-Charles
  1999   Taking time seriously: A theory of socioemotional selectivity. *American Psychologist*
          54(3):165-181.
Carstensen, L.L., and S. Turk-Charles
  1994   The salience of emotion across adult life span. *Psychology and Aging* 9:259-264.
Cassel, J.
  1976   Psychosocial processes and stress: Theoretical formulation. *International Journal of
          Health Services* 4:471-482.
Cattell, R.B.
  1963   Theory of fluid and crystallized intelligence: A critical experiment. *Journal of Educa-
          tional Psychology* 54:1-22.

Cauce, A.M., N. Coronado, and J. Watson
   1998   Conceptual, methodological, and statistical issues in culturally competent research.
          Pp. 305-331 in *Promoting Cultural Competence in Children's Mental Health Services*,
          M. Hernandez and M.R. Isaacs, eds. Baltimore, MD: Paul H. Brookes Publishing
          Co.
Clark, R., N.B. Anderson, V.R. Clark, and D.R. Williams
   1999   Racism as a stressor for African Americans: A biopsychosocial model. *American
          Psychologist* 54(10):805-816.
Cobbs, S.
   1976   Social support as a moderator of life stress. *Psychosomatic Medicine* 35(5):300-314.
Costa, A., R.E. Nappi, E. Sinforiani, G. Bono, A. Poma, and G. Nappi
   1997   Cognitive function at menopause: Neuroendocrine implications for the study of the
          aging brain. *Functional Neurology: New Trends in Adaptive and Behavioral Disorders*
          12(3-4):175-180.
D'Andrade, R.G.
   1981   The cultural part of cognition. *Cognitive Science* 5:179-195.
   1995   *The Development of Cognitive Anthropology*. Cambridge, England: Cambridge Uni-
          versity Press.
Dell, G.
   1986   A spreading-activation theory of retrieval and sentence production. *Psychological
          Review* 93:283-321.
Denny, N.W.
   1979   Problem solving in later adulthood: Intervention research. Pp. 37-66 in *Lifespan
          Developmental Behavior*, 2d vol., P.B. Baltes and O.G. Brim, Jr., eds. New York:
          Academic Press.
Denny, N.W., and A.M. Palmer
   1981   Adult age differences on traditional and practical problem-solving measures. *Jour-
          nal of Gerontology* 36:323-328.
D'Esposito, M., E. Zarahn, G.K. Aguirre, and B. Rypma
   1999   The effect of normal aging on the coupling of neural activity to the bold hemody-
          namic response. *Neuroimage* 10:6-14.
Dey, J., A. Misra, N.G. Desai, A.K. Mahapatra, and M.V. Padma
   1997   Cognitive function in younger type II diabetes. *Diabetes Care* 20(1):32-35.
Diehl, M.
   1998   Everyday competence in later life: Current status and future directions. *Gerontologist*
          38:422-433.
Dixon, R., and O. Gould
   1998   Younger and older adults collaborating on retelling everyday stories. *Applied Devel-
          opmental Science* 2:160-171.
Donchin, E., E. Callaway, R. Cooper, J.E. Desmedt, W.R. Goff, S.A. Hillyard, and S. Sutton
   1977   Publication criteria for studies of evoked potentials (EP) in man: Methodology and
          publication criteria. Pp. 1-11 in *Progress in Clinical Neurophysiology: Vol. 1. Atten-
          tion, Voluntary Contraction and Event-Related Cerebral Potentials*, J.E. Desmedt, ed.
          Basel: Karger.
Durham, W.H.
   1991   *Coevolution: Genes, Culture and Human Diversity*. Stanford, CA: Stanford University
          Press.
Eizenman, D.R., J.R. Nesselroade, D.L. Featherman, and J.W. Rowe
   1997   Intraindividual variability in perceived control in an older sample: The MacArthur
          Successful Aging Studies. *Psychology and Aging* 12:489-502.

Elbert, T., C. Pantev, C. Wienbruch, B. Rockstroh, and E. Taub
1995 Increased cortical representation of the fingers of the left hand in string players. *Science* 270(5234):305-307.
Elias, M.F., and M.A. Robbins
1991 Cardiovascular disease, hypertension, and cognitive function. Pp. 249-285 in *Behavioral Aspects of Cardiovascular Disease*, A.P. Shapiro and A. Baum, eds. Hillsdale, NJ: Erlbaum.
Elias, M.F., M.A. Robbins, P.K. Elias, and D.H.P. Streeten
1998 A longitudinal study of blood pressure in relation to performance on the Wechsler Adult Intelligence Scale. *Health Psychology* 17:486-493.
Elias, M.F., M.A. Robbins, N.R. Schultz, and T.W. Pierce
1990 Is blood pressure an important variable in research on aging and neuropsychological test performance? *Journal of Gerontology: Psychological Sciences* 45:128-135.
Elias, M.F., M.A. Robbins, N.R. Schultz, D.H.P. Streeten, and P.K. Elias
1987 Clinical significance of cognitive performance by hypertensive patients. *Hypertension* 9:192-197.
Elias, M.F., P.A. Wolf, R.B. D'Agostino, J. Cobb, and L.R. White
1993 Untreated blood pressure level is inversely related to cognitive functioning: The Framingham Study. *American Journal of Epidemiology* 138:353-364.
Elias, P.K., M.F. Elias, R.B. D'Agostino, L.A. Cupples, P.W. Wilson, H. Silbershatz, and P.A. Wolf
1997 NIDDM and blood pressure as risk factors for poor cognitive performance. *Diabetes Care* 20:1388-1395.
Erkkola, R.
1996 Female menopause, hormone replacement therapy, and cognitive processes. *Maturitas* 23(Suppl):S27-S30.
Ferraro, K.F., and M.M. Farmer
1996 Double jeopardy to health hypothesis for African-Americans: Analysis and critique. *Journal of Health and Social Behavior* 37:27-43.
Field, D., K.W. Schaie, and E.V. Leino
1988 Continuity in intellectual functioning: The role of self-reported health. *Psychology and Aging* 3(4):385-392.
Fillenbaum, G., D.C. Hughes, A. Heyman, L.K. George, and D.G. Blazer
1988 Relationship of health and demographic characteristics to Mini Mental State Examination score among community residents. *Psychological Medicine* 18:718-726.
Finch, C.E., and R.E. Tanzi
1997 Genetics of aging. *Science* 278:407-411.
Fiske, A.P., S. Kitiyama, H.R. Markus, and R.E. Nisbett
1998 The cultural matrix of social psychology. Pp. 915-981 in *The Handbook of Social Psychology*, 4th ed., D.T. Gilbert, S.T. Fiske, and G. Lindzey, eds. Boston: McGraw-Hill.
Fleischman, D.A., and J.D. Gabrieli
1998 Repetition priming in normal aging and Alzheimer's disease: A review of findings and theories. *Psychology and Aging* 13(1):88-119.
Gabrieli, J.D.E.
1998 Cognitive neuroscience of human memory. *Annual Review of Psychology* 49:87-115.
Gabrieli, J., D.A. Fleischman, M.M. Keane, S.L. Reminger, and F. Morrell
1995 Double dissociation between memory systems underlying explicit and implicit memory in the human brain. *Psychological Science* 6:76-82.

Gauvain, M.
1995   Thinking in niches: Sociocultural influences on cognitive development. *Human Development* 38(1):152-180.
Gigerenzer, G., P. Todd, and the ABC Research Group
1999   *Simple Heuristics that Make Us Smart.* New York: Oxford University Press.
Gilbert, C.D., and T.N. Wiesel
1992   Receptive field dynamics in adult primary visual cortex. *Nature* 356:150-152.
Giroux, H.A.
1981   Schooling and the myth of objectivity: Stalking the politics of the hidden curriculum. *McGill Journal of Education* 16:282-303.
Glass, L., and M.C. Mackey
1988   *From Clocks to Chaos: The Rhythms of Life.* Princeton, NJ: Princeton University Press.
Gomez-Isla, T., J.L. Price, D.W. McKeel, Jr., J.C. Morris, J.H. Growdon, and B.T. Hyman
1996   Profound loss of layer II entorhinal cortex neurons occurs in very mild Alzheimer's disease. *Journal of Neuroscience* 16:4491-4500.
Goodnow. J.J.
1990   Using sociology to extend psychological accounts of cognitive development. *Human Development* 33:81-107.
Gotlib, I.H., E. Gilboa, and B.K. Sommerfeld
In   Cognitive functioning in depression: Nature and origins. In R.J. Davidson, ed. *Wis-*
press   *consin Symposium on Emotion,* 1st vol. New York: Oxford University Press.
Gotlib, I.H., and C.L. Hammen
1992   *Psychological Aspects of Depression: Toward a Cognitive-Interpersonal Integration.* Chichester, U.K.: Wiley.
Gould, E., A. Beylin, P. Tanapat, A. Reeves, and T.J. Shors
1999a   Learning enhances adult neurogenesis in the hippocampal formation. *Nature Neuroscience* 2:260-265.
Gould, E., A.J. Reeves, M.S.A. Graziano, and C.G. Gross
1999b   Neurogenesis in the neocortex of adult primates. *Science* 286:548-552.
Green, R.F.
1969   Age-intelligence relationship between ages sixteen and sixty-four: A rising trend. *Developmental Psychology* 34:404-414.
Greenfield, P.M.
1984   *Mind and Media: The Effects of Television, Video Games, and Computers.* Cambridge, MA: Harvard University Press.
Greenough, W.T.
1976   Enduring brain effects of differential experience and training. Pp. 255-278 in *Neural Mechanisms of Learning and Memory,* M.R. Rosenzweig and E.L. Bennett, eds. Cambridge, MA: MIT Press.
Gribbon, K., K.W. Schaie, and I. Parham
1980   Complexity of life style and maintenance of intellectual abilities. *Journal of Social Issues* 36:47-67.
Hancock, P.A., and R. Parasuraman
1992   Human factors and safety in the design of intelligent vehicle-highway systems (IVHS). *Journal of Safety Research* 23:181-198.
Harper, M.S., and C.D. Alexander
1990   Profile of the black elderly. Pp. 193-222 in *Minority Aging: Essential Curricula Content for Selected Health and Allied Health Professions,* M.S. Harper, ed. Rockville, MD: U.S. Department of Health and Human Services, Public Health Service, Health Resources and Services Administration.

Hasher, L., and R.T. Zacks
  1988   Working memory, comprehension, and aging: A review and a new view. Pp. 193-
          225 in *The Psychology of Learning and Motivation: Advances in Research and Theory*,
          22nd vol., G.H. Bower, ed. San Diego, CA: Academic Press.
Hashtroudi, S., M.K. Johnson, and L.D. Chrosniak
  1990   Aging and qualitative characteristics of memories for perceived and imagined com-
          plex events. *Psychology and Aging* 5:119-126.
Hashtroudi, S., M.K. Johnson, N. Vnek, and S.A. Ferguson
  1994   Aging and the effects of affective and factual focus on source monitoring and recall.
          Psychology and Aging 9:160-170.
Hertzog, C., and K.W. Schaie
  1988   Stability and change in adult intelligence: 2. Simultaneous analysis of longitudinal
          means and covariance structures. *Psychology and Aging* 3:122-130.
Hertzog, C., K.W. Schaie, and K. Gribbin
  1978   Cardiovascular disease and changes in intellectual functioning from middle to old
          age. *Journal of Gerontology* 33(6):872-883.
Hess, T.M.
  1994   Social cognition in adulthood: Aging-related changes in knowledge and processing
          mechanisms. *Developmental Review* 14:373-412.
Hess, T.M., and S.M. Pullen
  1994   Adult age differences in impression change processes. *Psychology and Aging* 9:237-
          250.
Hess, T.M., and C.S. Tate
  1991   Adult age differences in explanations and memory for behavioral information. *Psy-
          chology and Aging* 6:86-92.
House, J.S., R.C. Kessler, A.R. Herzog, R.P. Mero, A.M. Kinney, and M. Breslow
  1990   Age, socioeconomic status, and health. *The Milbank Quarterly* 68:383-411.
House, J.S., J.M. Lepkowski, A.M. Kinney, R.P. Mero, R.C. Kessler, and A.R. Herzog
  1994   The social stratification of aging and health. *Journal of Health and Social Behavior*
          35:213-234.
Hsu, F.L.K.
  1983   *Rugged Individualism Reconsidered*. Knoxville, TN: University of Tennessee Press.
Hultsch, D.F., M. Hammer, and B.J. Small
  1993   Age differences in cognitive performance in later life: Relationships to self-reported
          health and activity life style. *Journal of Gerontology* 48(1):1-11.
Hultsch, D.F., C. Hertzog, R.A. Dixon, and B.J. Small
  1998   *Memory Change in the Aged*. New York: Cambridge University Press.
Inkeles, A., and D. Smith
  1974   *Becoming Modern*. Cambridge, MA: Harvard University Press.
Isaacowitz, D., S.T. Charles, and L.L. Carstensen
  2000   Emotion and cognition. Pp. 593-631 in *Handbook of Aging and Cognition*, 2nd ed.,
          F.I.M. Craik and T. Salthouse, eds. Mahwah, NJ: Lawrence Erlbaum Publishers.
Ivry, R.B.
  1996   The representation of temporal information in perception and motor control. *Cur-
          rent Opinion in Neurobiology* 6(6):851-857.
Jackson, J.J.
  1985   Race, national origin, ethnicity, and aging. Pp. 264-303 in *Handbook of Aging and
          Social Sciences*, R.H. Binstock and E. Shanas, eds. New York: Van Nostrand-
          Reinhold.

Jackson, J.S., T.C. Antonucci, and R.C. Gibson
1995 Ethnic and cultural factors in research on aging and mental health: A life-course perspective. Pp. 22-46 in *Handbook on Ethnicity, Aging, and Mental Health*, D.K. Padgett, ed. Westport, CT: Greenwood Press.

Jacobs, R.A., and Jordan, M.I.
1993 Learning piecewise control strategies in a modular neural network architecture. *IEEE Transactions on Systems, Man, and Cybernetics* 23:337-345.

Jagacinski, R.J.
1996 Control theoretic approaches to age-related differences in skilled performance. Pp. 65-81 in *Aging and Skilled Performance: Advances in Theory and Applications*, W.A. Rogers and A.D. Fisk, eds. Mahwah, NJ: Lawrence Erlbaum Associates, Publishers.

Jama, J.W., L.J. Launer, J.C. Witteman, et al.
1996 Dietary antioxidants and cognitive function in a population-based sample of older persons: The Rotterdam Study. *American Journal of Epidemiology* 144:275-280.

James, L.E., D.M. Burke, A. Austin, and E. Hulme
1998 Production and perception of verbosity in young and older adults. *Psychology and Aging* 13:355-367.

Jebara, T., B. Schiele, N. Oliver, and A. Pentland
1998 *DyPERS: Dynamic Personal Enhanced Reality System, Vision and Modeling*. Technical Report #463. Cambridge, MA: Media Lab, MIT.

Johansson, B., K. Whitfield, N.L. Pedersen, S.M. Hofer, F. Ahern, and G.E. McClearn
1999 Origins of individual differences in episodic memory in the oldest-old: A population-based study of identical and same-sex fraternal twins aged 80 and older. *Journal of Gerontology: Psychological Sciences* 54B(3):P173-P179.

Jordan, M.I.
1996 Computational aspects of motor control and motor learning. Pp. 71-120 in *Handbook of Perception and Action*, 2d vol., H. Heuer and S.W. Keele, eds. San Diego: Academic Press.

Joseph, J.A., B. Shukitt-Hale, N.A. Denisova, D. Bielinski, A. Martin, J.J. McEwen, and P.C. Bickford
1999 Reversals of age-related declines in neuronal signal transduction, cognitive, and motor behavioral deficits with blueberry, spinach, or strawberry dietary supplementation. *Journal of Neuroscience* 19:8114-8121.

Kahana, M.J., R. Sekuler, J.B. Caplan, M. Kirschen, and J.R. Madsen
1999 Human theta oscillations exhibit task dependence during virtual maze navigation. *Nature* 399:781-784.

Karasek, R., and T. Theorell
1990 *Healthy Work: Stress, Productivity, and the Reconstruction of Working Life*. New York: Basic Books.

Kelso, J.A.S.
1995 *Dynamic patterns: The Self-Organization of Brain and Behavior*. Cambridge, MA: MIT Press.

Kemper, S.
1992 Language and aging. Pp. 213-270 in *The Handbook of Aging and Cognition*, F.I.M. Craik and T.A. Salthouse, eds. Hillsdale, NJ: Lawrence Erlbaum Associates.

Kemper, S., and K.A. Kemptes
1999 Limitations on syntactic processing. Pp. 79-106 in *Constraints on Language: Aging, Grammar and Memory*, S. Kemper and R. Kliegl, eds. Boston: Kluwer Academic Publishers.

Kemper, S., S. Rash, D. Kynette, and S. Norman
  1990   Telling stories: The structure of adults' narratives. *European Journal of Cognitive Psychology* 2:205-228.
Kempermann, G., H.G. Kuhn, and F.H. Gage
  1997   More hippocampal neurons in adult mice living in an enriched environment. *Nature* 386:493-495.
  1998   Experience-induced neurogenesis in the senescent dentate gyrus. *Journal of Neuroscience* 18:3206-3212.
Kempler, D., A. Almor, L.K. Tyler, E.S. Andersen, and M.C. MacDonald
  1998   Sentence comprehension deficits in Alzheimer's disease: a comparison of off-line vs. on-line sentence processing. *Brain and Language* 64(3):297-316.
Kesler, M.S., N.W. Denny, and S.E. Whitney
  1976   Factors influencing problem solving in middle-aged and elderly adults. *Human Development* 19:310-320.
Kline, D.W., and C.T. Scialfa
  1997   Sensory and perceptual functioning: Basic research and human factors implications. Pp. 27-54 in *Handbook of Human Factors and the Older Adult*, A.D. Fisk and W.A. Rogers, eds. New York: Academic Press.
Kohn, M.L., et al.
  1978   The reciprocal effects of the substantive complexity of work and intellectual flexibility: A longitudinal assessment. *American Journal of Sociology* 84(1):24-52.
  1982   Job conditions and personality: A longitudinal assessment of their reciprocal effects. *American Journal of Sociology* 87(6):1257-1286.
Kolb, B., and I.Q. Whishaw
  1998   Brain plasticity and behavior. *Annual Review of Psychology* 49:43-64.
Kramer, A.F., S. Hahn, N.J. Cohen, M.T. Banich, E. McAuley, C.R. Harrison, J. Chason, E. Vakil, L. Bardell, R.A. Boileau, and A. Colcombe
  1999   Ageing, fitness and neurocognitive function. *Nature* 400(6743):418-419.
Kramer, D.A.
  1990   Conceptualizing wisdom: the primacy of affect-cognition relations. Pp. 279-313 in *Wisdom: Its Nature, Origins, and Development*, R.J. Sternberg, ed. Cambridge: Cambridge University Press.
Krampe, R.T., and K.A. Ericsson
  1996   Maintaining excellence: Deliberate practice and elite performance in young and older pianists. *Journal of Experimental Psychology: General* 125: 331-359.
Lachman, M.E., and S.L. Weaver
  1998   Sociodemographic variations in the sense of control by domain: Findings from the MacArthur studies of midlife. *Psychology and Aging* 13: 553-562.
Lagerlund, T., and F. Sharbrough
  1988   Computer simulation of neural circuit models of rhythmic behavior in the electroencephalogram. *Computers in Biology and Medicine* 18:267-304.
La Voie, D., and L.L. Light
  1994   Adult age differences in repetition priming: A meta-analysis. *Psychology and Aging* 9(4):539-553.
Lawton, M.P.
  1982   Competence, environmental press and the adaptation of older people. Pp. 33-59 in *Aging and the Environment*, M.P. Lawton, P.O. Windley and T.O. Byerts, eds. New York: Springer.
Le Bihan, D., and A. Karni
  1995   Applications of magnetic resonance imaging to the study of human brain function. *Current Opinion in Neurobiology* 5:231-237.

Levine, J.M., L.B. Resnick, and E.T. Higgins
1993   Social foundations of cognition. *Annual Review of Psychology* 44:584-612.
Levison, W.H.
1981   A methodology for quantifying the effects of aging on perceptual-motor capability. *Human Factors* 23(1):87-96.
1993   A simulation model for the driver's use of in-vehicle information systems. *Transportation Research Record* 1403:7-13.
Light, L.L.
1991   Memory and aging: Four hypotheses in search of data. *Annual Review of Psychology* 42:333-376.
Lindenberger, U., and P.B. Baltes
1994   Sensory functioning and intelligence in old age: A strong connection. *Psychology and Aging* 9(3):339-355.
Linsker, R.
1986   From basic network principles to neural architectures. *Proceedings of the National Academy of Sciences* 83: 7508-7512, 8390-8394, 8778-8783.
Liu, S.H.
1974   The use of analogy and symbolism in traditional Chinese philosophy. *Journal of Chinese Philosophy* 1:313-338.
Lloyd, K., and P. Moodley
1990   Psychiatry and ethnic groups. *British Journal of Psychiatry* 156:907.
Logothetis, N.K., H. Guggenberger, S. Peled, and J. Pauls
1999   Functional imaging of the monkey brain. *Nature Neuroscience* 2(6):555-562.
MacKay, D.G., and L. Abrams
1998   Age-linked declines in retrieving orthographic knowledge: Empirical, practical and theoretical implications. *Psychology and Aging* 13:647-662.
Madden, D.J.
1988   Adult age differences in the effects of sentence context and stimulus degradation during visual word recognition. *Psychology and Aging* 3:167-172.
Madden, D.J., and J.A. Blumenthal
1998   Interaction of hypertension and age in visual selective attention performance. *Health Psychology* 17(1):76-83.
Maier, S.F., L.R. Watkins, and M. Fleshner
1994   Psychoneuroimmunology: The interface between brain, behavior, and immunity. *American Psychologist* 49:1004-1017.
Manuck, S.B, A.L. Kasprowicz, and M.F. Muldoon
1990   Behaviorally-evoked cardiovascular reactivity and hypertension: Conceptual issues and potential associations. *Annals of Behavioral Medicine* 12(1):17-29.
Margrett, J.A.
1999   Collaborative Cognition and Aging: A Pilot Study. Unpublished dissertation. Department of Psychology, Wayne State University.
Markides, K.S., J. Liang, and J.S. Jackson
1990   Race, ethnicity, and aging: Conceptual and methodological issues. Pp. 112-129 in *Handbook of Aging and the Social Sciences*, 3rd ed., R.H. Binstock and L.K. George, eds. San Diego: Academic Press.
Markus, H.R., C.D. Ryff, and K.L. Barnett
In   In their own words: Well-being at midlife among high school and college-educated
press   respondents. In *A Portrait of Midlife in the U.S.*, C.D. Ryff and R.C. Kessler, eds. Chicago: The University of Chicago Press.

Marmot, M.G., R. Fuhrer, S.L. Ettner, N.F. Marks, L.L. Bumpass, and C.D. Ryff
  1998   Contribution of psychosocial factors to socioeconomic differences in health. *Milbank Quarterly* 76:403-440.
Marquis, M.S., and S.H. Long
  1996   Reconsidering the effect of Medicaid on health care services use. *Health Services Research* 30:791-808.
Marsiske, M., P. Klumb, and M. Baltes
  1997   Everyday activity patterns and sensory functioning in old age. *Psychology and Aging* 12:444-457.
Marsiske, M., and S.L. Willis
  1995   Dimensionality of everyday problem solving in older adults. *Psychology and Aging* 10:269-283.
Marslen-Wilson, W., and L.K. Tyler
  1980   The temporal structure of spoken language understanding. *Cognition* 8(1):1-71.
Mayer, K.U., and P.B. Baltes, eds.
  1996   *Die Berliner Altersstudie* [The Berlin Aging Study]. Berlin, Germany: Akademie Verlag.
McClearn, G.E., B. Johansson, S. Berg, N.L. Pedersen, F. Ahern, S.A. Petrill, and R. Plomin
  1997   Substantial genetic influence on cognitive abilities in twins 80 or more years old. *Science* 276:1560-1563.
McEwen, B.S.
  1998   Protective and damaging effects of stress mediators. *New England Journal of Medicine* 338:171-179.
McLuhan, M.
  1964   *Understanding Media: The Extensions of Man.* New York: McGraw-Hill.
Mead, M.
  1953   *Cultural Patterns and Technical Change.* Paris: UNESCO.
Merzenich, M.M., and K. Sameshima
  1993   Cortical plasticity and memory. *Current Opinion in Neurobiology* 3(2):187-196.
Miles, T.P., and M.A. Bernard
  1992   Health status of black American elderly. *Journal of the American Geriatrics Society* 40:1047-1054.
Miller, R.A.
  1985   A systems approach to modeling discrete control performance. Pp. 177-248 in *Advances in Man-Machine Systems Research*, W.B. Rouse, ed. Greenwich, CT: JAI Press.
Mochizuki, Y., M. Oishi, Y. Hayakawa, M. Matsuzaki, and T. Takasu
  1998   Improvement of P300 latency by treatment in non-insulin-dependent diabetes mellitus. *Clinical Electroencephalography* 29(4):194-196.
Morris, M., L. Bechett, P. Scherr, et al.
  1998   Vitamin E and Vitamin C supplement use and risk of incident Alzheimer disease. *Alzheimer Disease and Associated Disorders* 12:121-126.
Morrison, J.H., and P.R. Hof
  1997   Life and death of neurons in the aging brain. *Science* 278:412-419.
Muqit, M.M., and H.S. Ferdous
  1998   Cognitive impairment in elderly, non-insulin dependent diabetic men in Bangladesh. *Bangladesh Medical Research Council Bulletin* 24(2):23-26.
Murphy, J.M., R.R. Monson, D.C. Olivier, A.M. Sobol, and A.H. Leighton
  1987   Affective disorders and mortality. *Archives of General Psychiatry* 44:473–480.
Nagashima, N.
  1973   A reversed world: Or is it? Pp. 92-111 in *Modes of Thought*, R. Horton and R. Finnegan, eds. London: Faber and Faber.

Naor, M., H.J. Steingruber, K. Westhoff, Y. Schottenfeld-Naor, and A.F. Gries
1997   Cognitive function in elderly non-insulin-dependent diabetic patients before and after inpatient treatment for metabolic control. *Journal of Diabetes and its Complications* 11(1):40-46.

NATO Research and Technology Organization
1998   Alternative control technologies: Human factors issues. RTO Lecture Series 215, RTO-EN-3, AC/323(HFM)TP/1, Bretigny, France and Wright-Patterson Air Force Base, Ohio.

Norman, D.A.
1998   *The Invisible Computer.* Cambridge, MA: MIT Press.

Nyberg, L., L. Backman, K. Erngrund, U. Olofsson, and L. Nilsson
1996   Age differences in episodic memory, semantic memory, and priming: Relationships to demographic, intellectual, and biological factors. *Journal of Gerontology* 51B:234-240.

Oakes, J.
1985   *Keeping Track.* New Haven, CT: Yale University Press.

Ojemann, G.A., and H.A. Whitaker
1978   The bilingual brain. *Archives of Neurology* 35(7):409-412.

Olson, D.R.
1994   *The World on Paper: The Conceptual and Cognitive Implications of Writing and Reading.* New York: Cambridge University Press.

Ortega, S.T., R.D. Crutchfield, and W.A. Rushing
1983   Race differences in elderly personal well-being: Friendship, family, and church. *Research on Aging* 5:101-118.

Owens, W.A.
1966   Age and mental abilities: A second adult follow-up. *Journal of Educational Psychology* 57:311-325.

Owsley, C., K. Ball, G. McGwin, M.E. Sloane, D.L. Roenker, M.F. White, and E.T. Overley
1998   Visual processing impairment and risk of motor vehicle crash among older adults. *Journal of the American Medical Association* 279:1083-1088.

Paleologos, M., R.G. Cumming, and R. Lazarus
1998   Cohort study of vitamin C intake and cognitive impairment. *American Journal of Epidemiology* 148:45-50.

Park, D.C., R. Nisbett, and T. Hedden
1999   Aging, culture, and cognition. *Journal of Gerontology: Psychological Sciences* 54B(2):75-84.

Pascual-Leone, A., and F. Torres
1993   Plasticity of the sensorimotor cortex representation of the reading finger in Braille readers. *Brain* 116:39-52.

Paulesu, E., et al.
2000   A cultural effect on brain function. *Nature Neuroscience* 3:91-96.

Payne, R.L., and G.J. Jones
1987   Measurements and methodological issues in social support. Pp. 167-205 in *Stress and Health: Issues in Research Methodology*, S.V. Kasl and C.L. Cooper, eds. New York: John Wiley.

Perlmutter, M., C. Adams, J. Berry, M. Kaplan, D. Persons, and F. Verdonik
1988   Memory and aging. Pp. 57-92 in *Annual Review of Gerontology and Geriatrics*, K.W. Schaie, ed. New York: Springer.

Perlmutter, M., and L. Nyquist
1990   Relationships between self-reported physical and mental health and intelligence performance across adulthood. *Journal of Gerontology* 45:145-155.

Peters, A., J.H. Morrison, D.L. Rosene, and B.T. Hyman
1998   Are neurons lost from the primate cerebral cortex during aging? *Cerebral Cortex* 8:295-300.
Picton, T.W., S. Bentin, P. Berg, E. Donchin, S.A. Hillyard, R. Johnson Jr., G.A. Miller, W. Ritter, D.S. Ruchkin, M.D. Rugg, and M.J. Taylor
In   Guidelines for using human event-related potentials to study cognition: Recording
press   standards and publication criteria. *Psychophysiology.*
Polk, T.A., and M.J. Farah
1998   The neural development and organization of letter recognition: Evidence from functional neuroimaging, computational modeling and behavioral studies. *Proceedings of the National Academy of Sciences* 95:847-852.
Price, D.L., et al.
1998   Alzheimer's disease: Genetic studies and transgenic models. *Annual Review of Genetics* 32:461-493.
Rapp, P.R., and M. Gallagher
1996   Preserved neuron number in the hippocampus of aged rats with spatial learning deficits. *Proceedings of the National Academy of Sciences* 93:9926-9930.
Raz, N., F.M. Gunning-Dixon, D. Head, J.H. Dupuis, and J.D. Acker
1998   Neuroanatomical correlates of cognitive aging: Evidence from structural magnetic resonance imaging. *Neuropsychology* 12:1-20.
Reggia, J.A., R.S. Berndt, and C.L. D'Autrechy
1994   Connectionist models in neuropsychology. Pp. 297-333 in *Handbook of Neuropsychology*, 9th vol., F. Boller and J. Grafman, eds. New York: Elsevier.
Reggia, J., C. D'Autrechy, G. Sutton, and M. Weinrich
1992   A competitive distribution theory of neocortical dynamics. *Neural Computation* 4:287-317.
Ripple, R.E., and G.A. Jaquish
1981   Fluency, flexibility, and originality in later adulthood. *Educational Gerontology* 7:1-10.
Rowe, J.W., and R.L. Kahn
1998   *Successful Aging.* New York: Pantheon Books.
Rushing, B., C. Ritter, and R.P.D. Burton
1992   Race differences in the effects of multiple roles on health: Longitudinal evidence from a national sample of older men. *Journal of Health and Social Behavior* 33:126-139.
Salthouse, T.A.
1982   *Adult Cognition.* New York: Springer-Verlag.
Salthouse, T.A., D.Z. Hambrick, and K.E. McGuthry
1998   Shared age-related influences on cognitive and non-cognitive variables. *Psychology and Aging* 13:486-500.
Salthouse, T.A., H.E. Hancock, E.J. Meinz, and D.Z. Hambrick
1996   Interrelations of age, visual acuity, and cognitive functioning. *Journal of Gerontology: Psychological Sciences* 51B:317-330.
Salthouse, T.A., D.H. Kausler, and J.S. Saults
1990   Age, self-assessed health status, and cognition. *Journal of Gerontology* 45(4):156-160.
Sanfey, A.G., and Hastie, R.
2000   Judgment and decision making across the adult life span: A tutorial review of psychological research. In *Aging and Cognition: A Primer*, D. Park and N. Schwarz, eds. Philadelphia: Psychology Press.

Sansone, C., and C. Berg
1993   Adapting to the environment across the life span: Different process of different inputs? *International Journal of Behavioral Development* 16:215-241.
Schaie, K.W.
1983   The Seattle longitudinal study: A twenty-one year exploration of psychometric intelligence in adulthood. Pp. 64-135 in *Longitudinal Studies of Adult Psychological Development*, K.W. Schaie, ed. New York: Guilford Press.
1994   The course of adult intellectual development. *American Psychologist* 49:304-313.
1996   *Intellectual Development in Adulthood: The Seattle Longitudinal Study*. New York: Cambridge University Press.
Schaie, K.W., and C.R. Strother
1968   A cross-sequential study of age changes in cognitive behavior. *Psychological Bulletin* 70:671-680.
Schnall P.L., P.A. Landisbergis, and D. Baker
1994   Job strain and cardiovascular disease. *Annual Review of Public Health* 15:381-411.
Schneider, B., and M. Pichora-Fuller
In   Implications of perceptual deterioration for cognitive aging research. In *The Hand-*
press   *book of Cognitive Aging*, F.I.M. Craik and T.A. Salthouse, eds. Mahwah, NJ: Erlbaum.
Sclove, R.
1995   *Democracy and Technology*. New York: Guilford Press.
Seeman, T.E.
1996   Social ties and health: The benefits of social integration. *Annals of Epidemiology* 6:442-451.
Seeman, T.E., M.L. Bruce, and G.J. McAvay
1996   Social network characteristics and onset of ADL disability: MacArthur Studies of Successful Aging. *Journals of Gerontology Series B—Psychological Sciences and Social Sciences* 51B(4):S191-S200.
Seeman T.E., and R.J. Robbins
1994   Aging and hypothalamic-pituitary-adrenal response to challenge in humans. *Endocrinology Review* 15:233-260.
Seeman, T.E., B. Singer, R. Horwitz, and B.S. McEwen
1997   The price of adaptation—allostatic load and its health consequences: MacArthur Studies of Successful Aging. *Archives of Internal Medicine* 157:2259-2268.
Selzer, S.C., and N.W. Denny
1980   Conservation abilities among middle aged and elderly adults. *International Journal of Aging and Human Development* 11:135-146.
Sherwin, B.B.
1994   Estrogenic effects on memory in women. Pp. 213-231 in *Hormonal Restructuring of the Adult Brain: Basic and Clinical Perspectives. Annals of the New York Academy of Sciences*, 743rd vol., V.N. Luine and C.F. Harding, eds. New York: New York Academy of Sciences.
Shifren, K., K. Hooker, P. Wood, and J.R. Nesselroade
1997   Structure and variation of mood in individuals with Parkinson's disease: A dynamic factor analysis. *Psychology and Aging* 12:328-339.
Shimamura, A.P., and L.R. Squire
1984   Paired-associate learning and priming effects in amnesia: a neuropsychological study. *Journal of Experimental Psychology: General* 113(4):556-570.
Shweder, R.A.
1991   *Thinking Through Cultures: Expeditions in Cultural Psychology*. Cambridge, MA: Harvard University Press.

Sieber, T.
  1982   The politics of middle-class success in an inner-city public school. *Journal of Education* 164:30-47.
Sliwinski, M., and M. Buschke
  1999   Cross-sectional and longitudinal relationships among age, cognition, and processing speed. *Psychology and Aging* 14:18-33.
Small, B.J., D.F. Hultsch, and M.E.J. Masson
  1995   Adult age differences in perceptually based, but not conceptually based implicit tests of memory. *Journal of Gerontology: Psychological Sciences* 50B:162-170.
Smith, C.A., C.A. McCleary, G.A. Murdock, T.W. Wilshire, D.K. Buckwalter, P. Bretsky, L. Marmol, R.L. Gorsuch, and J.G. Buckwalter
  1999   Lifelong estrogen exposure and cognitive performance in elderly women. *Brain and Cognition* 39(3):203-218.
Smith D.E., J. Roberts, F.H. Gage, and M.H. Tuszynski
  1999   Age-associated neuronal atrophy occurs in the primate brain and is reversible by growth factor gene therapy. *Proceedings of the National Academy of Sciences* 96:10893-10898.
Smith E.E., and J. Jonides
  1997   Working memory: A view from neuroimaging. *Cognitive Psychology* 33(1):5-42.
Smith, L.B., E. Thelen, R. Titzer, and D. McLin
  1999   Knowing in the context of acting: The task dynamics of the A-not-B error. *Psychological Review* 106:235-260.
Snowdon, D.A., S.J. Kemper, J.A. Mortimer, L.H. Greiner, D.R. Wekstein, and W.R. Markesbery
  1996   Linguistic ability in early life and cognitive function and Alzheimer's disease in late life. *Journal of the American Medical Association* 275:528-532.
Socci, D.J.C., B.M. Crandall, and G.W. Arendash
  1995   Chronic antioxidant treatment improves the cognitive performance of aged rats. *Brain Research* 693(1-2):88-94.
Squire, L., and E. Kandel
  1999   *Memory: From Mind to Molecules.* New York: Freeman.
Stefanacci, L., P. Reber, J. Costanza, E. Wong, R. Buxton, S. Zola, L. Squire, and T. Albright
  1998   fMRI of monkey visual cortex. *Neuron* 20(6):1051-1057.
Sternberg, R.J.
  1986   A framework for intellectual abilities and theories of them. *Intelligence* 10(3):239-250.
Stigler, J.W.
  1984   Mental abacus: The effect of abacus training and Chinese children's mental calculations. *Cognitive Psychology* 16:145-176.
Stigler, J.W., L. Chalip, and K. Miller
  1986   Consequences of skill: The case of abacus training in Taiwan. *American Journal of Education* 94:477-479.
Stine, E.A.L., and A. Wingfield
  1994   Older adults can inhibit high-probability competitors in speech recognition. *Aging and Cognition* 1:152-157.
Stine-Morrow, E.A.L., M.K. Loveless, and L.M. Soederberg
  1996   Resource allocation in on-line reading by younger and older adults. *Psychology and Aging* 11:475-486.
Super, C., and S. Harkness
  1986   The developmental niche: A conceptualization at the interface of child and culture. *International Journal of Behavioral Development* 9:545-569.

Taoka, T., S. Iwashaki, H. Uchida, A. Fukusmi, H. Nakagawa, K. Kichikawa, K. Takayama, T. Yoshioka, M. Takewa, and H. Ohishi
1998   Age correlation of the time lag in signal change on EPI-fMRI. *Journal of Computer Assisted Tomography* 22(4):514-517.

Taylor, S.E.
1999   *Health Psychology*, 4th ed. New York: McGraw-Hill.

Thelen, E.
1999   Potential Impact of Dynamic Systems Theory of Research in Cognitive Aging. Outline prepared for the Committee on Future Directions for Behavioral and Social Sciences Research at the National Institutes of Health, National Research Council, Washington, D.C.

Thelen, E., and L. Smith
1994   *A Dynamic Systems Approach to the Development of Cognition and Action.* Cambridge, MA: Branford Books/MIT Press.

Tsue, T., E. Oesterle, and E. Rubel
1994   Hair cell regeneration in the inner ear. *Otolaryngology Head and Neck Surgery* 111:281-301.

Uchino, B.N., J.T. Cacioppo, and J.K. Keicolt-Glaser
1996   The relationship between social support and physiological processes: A review with emphasis on underlying mechanisms and implications for health. *Psychological Bulletin* 119(3):488-531.

Uecker, A., E.M. Reiman, D.L. Schacter, M.R. Polster, L.A. Cooper, L.S. Yun, and K. Chen
1997   Neuroanatomical correlates of implicit and explicit memory for structurally possible and impossible visual objects. *Learning and Memory* 4:337-355.

Vallar, G., and A.D. Baddeley
1984   Fractionation of working memory: Neuropsychological evidence for a phonological short-term store. *Journal of Verbal Learning and Verbal Behavior* 23:151-161.

van Boxtel, M.P., F. Buntinx, P.J. Houx, J.F. Metsemakers, A. Knottnerus, and J. Jolles
1998   The relation between morbidity and cognitive performance in a normal population. *Journals of Gerontology. Series A, Biological Sciences and Medical Sciences* 53(2):M147-154.

van Praag, H., G. Kempermann, and F.H. Gage
1999   Running increases cell proliferation and neurogenesis in the adult mouse dentate gyrus. *Nature Neuroscience* 2:266-270.

Verhaeghen, P., and T.A. Salthouse
1997   Meta-analyses of age-cognition relations in adulthood: Estimates of linear and non-linear age effects and structural models. *Psychological Bulletin* 122:231-249.

Wahl, H.W., F. Oswald, and D. Zimprich
1999   Everyday competence in visually impaired older adults: A case for person-environment perspectives. *Gerontologist* 39:140-149.

Waldstein, S.R.
1995   Hypertension and neuropsychological function: A lifespan perspective. *Experimental Aging Research* 21:321-352.

Wang, S., and J. Mason
1999   Elevations of serum T3 levels and their associations with symptoms in World War II veterans with combat-related posttraumatic stress disorder: Replication of findings in Vietnam combat veterans. *Psychosomatic Medicine* 61(2):131-138.

Wells, K.B., A. Stewart, R.D. Hays, M.A. Burnam, W. Rogers, M. Daniels, S. Berry, S. Greenfield, and J. Ware
1989   The functioning and well being of depressed patients: Results from the Medical Outcome Study. *Journal of the American Medical Association* 262:914-919.

West, M.J.
   1993   Regionally specific loss of neurons in the aging human hippocampus. *Neurobiology of Aging* 14:287-293.
Whitfield, K.E., and T.A. Baker-Thomas
   1999   Individual differences in aging among African-Americans. *International Journal of Aging and Human Development* 48(1):73-79.
Williams, D.R.
   2000   Racial variations in adult health status: Patterns, paradoxes and prospects. In *America Becoming: Racial Trends and Their Consequences*, N. Smelser, W.J. Wilson, and F. Mitchell, eds. Washington D.C.: National Academy Press.
Willis, P.
   1982   *Learning to Labor: How Working Class Kids Get Working Class Jobs.* New York: Columbia University Press.
Willis, S.L.
   1991   Cognition and everyday competence. Pp. 80-129 in *Annual Review of Gerontology and Geriatrics,* 11th vol., K.W. Schaie and M.F. Lawton, eds. New York: Springer.
Willis, S.L., and M. Marsiske
   1991   Life span perspective on practical intelligence. Pp. 183-197 in *The Neuropsychology of Everyday Life: Issues in Development and Rehabilitation,* D.E. Tupper and K.D. Cicerone, eds. Boston, MA: Kluwer.
Wingfield, A., P.A. Tun, and M.J. Rosen
   1995   Age differences in veridical and reconstructive recall of syntactically and randomly segmented speech. *Journals of Gerontology. Series B, Psychological Sciences and Social Sciences* 50(5):257-266.
Worrall, G.J., P.C. Chaulk, and N. Moulton
   1996   Cognitive function and glycosylated hemoglobin in older patients with type II diabetes. *Journal of Diabetes and its Complications* 10(6):320-324.
Wright, J.H., and P.G. Salmon
   1990   Learning and memory in depression. Pp. 211-236 in *Depression: New Directions in Theory, Research, and Practice,* C.D. McCann and N.S. Endler, eds. Toronto: Wall and Thompson.
Yates, F.
   1966   *The Art of Memory.* Chicago: University of Chicago Press.
Zacks, R.T., L. Hasher, and K.Z.H. Li
   In   Human memory. In *Handbook of Aging and Cognition,* F.I.M. Craik and T.A.
   press   Salthouse, eds. Mahwah, NJ: Lawrence Erlbaum Publishers.
Zelinski, E.M., and K.P. Burnight
   1997   Sixteen-year longitudinal and time lag changes in memory and cognition in older adults. *Psychology and Aging* 12:503-513.

Appendixes

A
Age-Related Shifts in Neural Circuit Characteristics and Their Impact on Age-Related Cognitive Impairments

John H. Morrison

INTRODUCTION

Increasing chronological age carries with it a heightened risk for diseases such as Alzheimer's disease, as well as functional decline associated with senescence in the absence of any specific neurologic disease, such as age-related memory impairment. Alzheimer's disease leads to a catastrophic decline in cognitive abilities and memory performance in the affected individual. Age-related memory impairment in the context of senescence is far less catastrophic than Alzheimer's disease with respect to the quality of life, but it has a surprisingly high incidence and thus also represents a significant health problem associated with aging. With the increased life expectancy that has already occurred over the last century, let alone the projected further increase, it has become clear that one of the most important goals for neuroscientists over the next several decades will be to develop means of maintaining a high level of cognitive and memory performance in the aged population. The focus of this paper is to outline and to illustrate a circuit-based approach aimed at both revealing the neurobiological basis of age-related memory impairment and identifying targets for intervention.

A MULTITIERED NEUROANATOMIC APPROACH TO AGING

The Link Between Neurochemistry and Neuroanatomy

Traditionally, a given cell class or circuit has been defined and/or categorized on the basis of its physiological and anatomic characteristics, i.e., the information being transmitted and the origin and termination of its connections, respectively. More recently, both neuroanatomical and electrophysiological characterizations of neural circuits have incorporated biochemical and molecular biological information in order to develop a more comprehensive portrayal of the essential qualities of a circuit that relate to its role in brain function. The key biochemical attributes of a given circuit or cell class are largely a reflection of the particular gene expression patterns, dynamics of protein synthesis, degradation and distribution, and selective activation of signaling cascades that are predominant in the neurons that furnish the circuit. The resultant biochemical profile essentially represents the *neurochemical phenotype* of a circuit or cell class. Operationally, one might define neurochemical phenotype as the complement of specific molecules, particularly proteins and their enzymatic products, that are enriched in and utilized by a given class of neurons in a manner that is not shared by other cell classes. The neurochemical phenotype of a neuron includes molecules related to synaptic transmission (e.g., receptors, neurotransmitters, and related enzymes), structural attributes, metabolic processes, or any characteristic that is uniquely well developed in that neuron and critically important to its designated role in brain function.

For example, a cortical neuron that uses GABA, the major inhibitory neurotransmitter, has a neurochemical phenotype that differs in many fundamental ways from a cortical neuron that uses glutamate, the major excitatory neurotransmitter. As implied in the definition of neurochemical phenotype, gene expression and protein distribution patterns are not uniform across the brain or even across a single brain region. In fact, brain circuits are highly heterogeneous with respect to which genes are expressed over time and space, and the intracellular distribution of gene products (i.e., proteins) is highly regulated. Therefore, a comprehensive neuroanatomic analysis of a circuit must address its particular neurochemical profile as well as its anatomic connections, since both will impact that circuit's functional characteristics and role in behavior.

With respect to the task at hand, the goal is to link age-related shifts in neurochemical phenotype and neuroanatomic characteristics in key cortical and hippocampal circuits to functional decrements in memory that occur with aging. Why place the emphasis for studies of aging on cell classes and circuits rather than on brain regions? More specifically, if memory is the issue and the hippocampus is critical to memory, why not address the issue of age-related pathology at the level of the entire hippocampus, rather than isolated cells, circuits, and synapses?

As described below, there are important reasons to identify and consider the brain region of interest as an important step in such analyses. However, the main rationale for bringing the analysis to a higher level of resolution and focusing on distinct cell classes and circuits is that it more accurately reflects neuronal vulnerability to aging and Alzheimer's disease. A given brain region does not generally suffer as a whole; it is more likely that vulnerable circuits in a given region tend to suffer while other circuits are unaffected. Even a region as vulnerable to Alzheimer's disease as the hippocampus has cell classes and circuits that are highly resistant to degeneration as well as those that are vulnerable.

We suspect that normal aging will exhibit an even higher degree of selectivity in affected circuits than does Alzheimer's disease, thus it is even more important to address the question of age-related neuronal vulnerability at the highest possible level of cellular and circuit resolution. In turn, as interventions are developed to prevent age-related decline, they should be targeted to the vulnerable cell classes and circuits, not to a given region. Ideally, the goal should be to sustain the health of vulnerable circuits without impacting those that are resistant to age-related decrements, and in order to do this we must first clarify the neurobiological underpinnings of age-related functional decline at the level of the selectively vulnerable cells, circuits, and synapses.

In addition, it is critical that the cellular and neuroanatomic analyses be quantitative. Qualitative impressions of age-related cell loss, morphologic aberrations, or down-regulation of a particular receptor will not allow for a sufficiently precise or accurate depiction of age-related changes, nor will qualitative judgments possess the requisite statistical power to test many hypotheses. In contrast, quantitative descriptions of structural and biochemical attributes can be readily correlated with quantitative assessments of physiological and behavioral output, allowing for direct links to be established between neurobiological indices and function. This is perhaps most important when testing the effectiveness of an intervention, since one would like to be able to equate any improvement in functional output with a measurable reflection of increased neuronal viability. Throughout this article, the emphasis will be on microscopic approaches to cell and circuit analysis rather than electrophysiological approaches; however, the electrophysiological approach to the hippocampus, aging, and memory is a critical partner to the microscopic data, particularly with respect to delineating complex properties that emerge from the activity of hippocampal neurons.

Targeting Multiple Levels of Resolution: From the Brain Region to the Synapse

The Brain Region

In any such analysis, the first task is to define the brain region(s) and circuits to be analyzed, by virtue of their hypothesized role in the neural function or behavior that is compromised by aging. In addition, the process of neural circuitry analysis becomes more focused as the behavioral measures are improved and refined in their sensitivity and quantitative power. The great advances over the last few decades in the analysis of memory offer an excellent example of the manner in which behavioral data can guide neuro-anatomic analysis toward a given brain region, e.g., the hippocampus, and in turn certain circuits, e.g., the perforant path (discussed below). Defining the brain region(s) of interest is particularly important if one of the experimental goals is to obtain estimates of neuron number, glial cell number, or synapse number, since such estimates are not useful if the region of interest cannot be clearly and precisely defined or its boundaries recognized. In fact, the accurate determination of neuron number in key hippocampal fields such as CA1 and the adjacent entorhinal cortex is what led to the realization that neuron death is unlikely to be at the root of age-related impairment in memory and cognition (Rapp and Gallagher, 1996; Morrison and Hof, 1997; Peters et al., 1998a), challenging the accepted dogma that people inevitably "lose nerve cells" as they age. The use of modern stereological techniques for determining neuron number in a defined brain region has been invaluable for establishing the sustained viability of neurons during aging. One of the many attributes of the stereological techniques that make them particularly valuable for analyses of aging and neurodegenerative disorders is that they generate estimates of neuron or synapse number that are not confounded by tissue or cellular shrinkage, two major potential confounds in studies of aging (West, 1993a, 1993b). The stereologic approach (West, 1993a, 1993b, 1999; Geinisman et al., 1996; Coggeshall and Lekan, 1996) to estimates of neuron number, synapse number, axon length, etc., will continue to be powerful for such studies, particularly as a quantitative database of neuroanatomic information relevant to aging develops.

Cell Classes and Circuits

The next level of resolution beyond that of brain region is the analysis of specific circuits and related cell classes. With respect to the hippocampus and memory, attention is drawn to the neurons in layer II of the entorhinal cortex, which provide the perforant path that connects the entorhinal cortex to the dentate gyrus (Van Hoesen and Pandya, 1975). This circuit is highly vulnerable in aging and Alzheimer's disease (Hyman et al., 1984; Morrison and Hof, 1997; Hof et al., 1999). The entorhinal cortex receives convergent inputs from multiple neocortical association areas and in turn provides the major cortical input to the hippocampus, and thus along with associated parahippocampal and perirhinal areas, it is positioned for a critical role in memory (Squire and Zola-Morgan, 1991; Zola-Morgan and Squire, 1993). The analysis of any key circuit such as the perforant path moves quickly into the issue of cell classes or cell types with respect to the cells of origin of such a projection. While cell type has been traditionally defined exclusively by morphologic criteria (size, shape, extent of neuritic arborization), a more comprehensive definition of cell type might be a designated class of neurons that share key characteristics with regard to morphology, location, connectivity, and neurochemical phenotype. In fact, the concepts of cell type and neurochemical phenotype bear a critical relationship to *selective vulnerability* in aging or neurodegenerative diseases.

Selective vulnerability is most readily appreciated in the context of neurodegenerative disorders such as amyotrophic lateral sclerosis, Parkinson's disease, and Alzheimer's disease. Each disease is characterized by its own, unique pattern of degeneration, with amyotrophic lateral sclerosis involving the loss of upper and lower motor neurons, Parkinson's disease noted for the selective degeneration of dopaminergic neurons in substantia nigra, and Alzheimer's disease characterized primarily by the degeneration of key cortical circuits. In many cases, the vulnerable neurons in a given disorder share particular neurochemical characteristics that can be linked to their selective vulnerability. For example, both the neurons that provide the perforant path from the entorhinal cortex and the neurons that provide the long corticocortical interconnections are highly vulnerable in Alzheimer's disease, and both are marked by a particular cytoskeletal profile that can be linked to their vulnerability (Morrison et al., 1987; Hof et al., 1990: Hof and Morrison, 1990; Hof et al., 1999).

In order to define and understand the determinants of selective vulnerability in neurodegenerative diseases as well as in normal aging, it will be important to determine neuron number according to specific classes of neurons wherein class is based on morphology, connectivity, and neurochemical phenotype. In this way, hypotheses can be tested at a finer level of cell-type resolution, and links can be drawn between a particular element of the neurochemical phenotype and vulnerability. Quantitative analyses using chemically specific approaches (e.g., immunohistochemistry, in situ hybridization) allow for direct investigation of the molecular determinants of selective vulnerability, as reflected, for example, in intracellular biochemical changes in neurons as they change with age or begin to degenerate. This approach is particularly important with respect to links to gene expression, with the goal being a quantitative dataset that links gene expression patterns with circuits, vulnerability, and, potentially, with age-related changes in cognition.

Neuronal Compartments

Beyond the analysis of cell class(es), it is important to determine the degree to which biochemical characteristics of neuronal compartments in individual neurons are affected by age. Given that neuron death is unlikely to be the substrate for age-related memory impairment, it has become increasingly important to investigate more subtle changes in cellular morphology and neurochemical phenotype that would impact function, but not be lethal. This step will require careful quantitative analyses of individual neurons, both in terms of morphometric measures as well as in terms of subcellular analyses of protein distribution patterns. For example, age-related changes in dendritic spine number have been described that could impact neuronal function (Coleman and Flood, 1987), and in fact, in primate neocortex it appears that spine density decreases with age with no change in dendritic length or branching patterns (Duan et al., 1999), and such changes may predominate in the most distal portion of the dendrite (Peters et al., 1998b). In addition, changes in receptor distribution can affect a single portion of the dendritic tree that receives a particular input, leaving the rest of the neuron unaffected (Gazzaley et al., 1996a). Moreover, some age-related changes might preferentially affect the nerve terminal rather than the dendrite, or vice versa. Such subtle changes could profoundly affect circuits and neural transmission with no evidence of generalized cell death.

The Synapse

The highest-resolution morphologic analysis is directed at the synapse and represents a search for potential changes in synapse structure or molecular constituents of the synapse that are related to age and might impact circuit function and behavior. Neocortical synapse loss clearly occurs in Alzheimer's disease and correlates well with degree of cognitive impairment (DeKosky and Scheff, 1990; Terry et al., 1991). High-resolution structural analyses of the synapse suggest that there are synaptic changes in the hippocampus with normal aging in the rat (Geinisman et al., 1995), although such changes may not occur in aged primate (Peters et al., 1996). In addition, the dendritic spine is more plastic than previously thought, and structural changes in the dendritic spine may occur on a time course consistent with induction of changes in synaptic function underlying memory, such as long-term potentiation (Toni et al., 1999). Thus, age-related spine loss or loss of spine plasticity could lead to age-related decline in memory and/or learning.

While purely structural analyses of the aging synapse have been and will continue to be illuminating (Geinisman et al., 1995; Tigges et al., 1996; Peters et al., 1996), perhaps the most exciting applications of electron microscopy to studies of aging will emerge from the use of immunogold postembedding electron microscopy. This immunohistochemical technique has extremely high resolution, in that the molecule of interest is identified by the presence of a discrete gold particle that is 10-25 nanometers in diameter and is highly quantifiable (Chaudhry et al., 1995). In addition, multiple antibodies bound to gold particles of different sizes can be used simultaneously to localize multiple synaptic molecules in a single synapse (He et al., 2000). The number of gold particles can be equated to the number of molecules of the targeted protein in a very small, discrete region, such as a single synapse (see Figure A-1). Such an approach allows for a very high-resolution analysis of the molecular constituents of identified synapses and presumably will be able to reveal shifts in the molecular constituents with experimental manipulations and/or aging at a quantitative level. When such studies are done in behaviorally characterized aged animals, we will be able to draw direct correlations between the distribution of key synaptic molecules and age-related behavioral impairment. No such studies have been completed to date, but they are now under way.

As is apparent from the above discussion, key studies of aging have been and will continue to be directed at questions requiring different levels of resolution in the analysis. The illustrations cited below will focus on the microscopic delineation of vulnerable circuits and cell classes, as well as changes in protein distribution in specific cell classes, circuits, and neuronal compartments. While these examples will hopefully highlight the power of a circuit-based approach, they will also illuminate the present shortcomings of the data, such as a paucity of chemically specific synaptic data and the need for more interdisciplinary analyses. Electrophysiological data will be crucial in the interdisciplinary context, since they are particularly powerful at revealing the emergent properties and information content of hippocampal circuits coding for memory (Barnes et al., 1997a, 1997b; Eichenbaum et al., 1999; Shapiro and Eichenbaum, 1999; Wood et al., 1999). As the data emerge, it will be crucial to develop a set of models and/or databases that link data across studies, such that the synaptic and cellular data will be in a context that is easily linked to the functional role of a known circuit, in a region that is clearly implicated in a function that is compromised in aging, such as memory.

DIFFERENTIATING ALZHEIMER'S DISEASE FROM SENESCENCE: THE CRITICAL ROLE OF THE ENTORHINAL CORTEX AND ITS PROJECTION TO DENTATE GYRUS

At the outset, it is important to draw a distinction between the neurobiological events underlying the dementia of Alzheimer's disease and those that underlie age-related memory impairment (Morrison and Hof, 1997). In Alzheimer's disease and neurodegenerative disorders in general, neuron death occurs that results in circuit disruption and profound impairment of the neural functions dependent on the degenerating circuits (see Hof et al., 1999, for a review). As mentioned above, neuron death is not ubiquitous in neurodegenerative disorders, in that neurons display a particular pattern of selective vulnerability in each disorder. In Alzheimer's disease, the highly vulnerable circuits are: (1) neurons that interconnect functionally linked neocortical areas (Pearson et al., 1985; Rogers and Morrison, 1985; Lewis et al., 1987); (2) the projection from the entorhinal cortex to the hippocampus, referred to

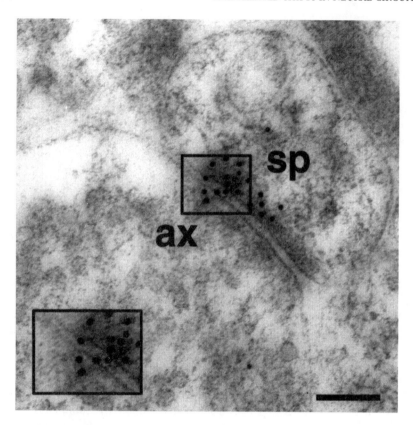

FIGURE A-1 This is a photograph of an electron microscope image that illustrates the postembedding immunogold method. The tissue has been treated with a primary antibody directed against the NMDA receptor subunit NR2A, followed by a secondary antibody that is both conjugated to a gold particle of 10 nanometer diameter, and binds to the primary antibody, thereby forming a bridge and revealing the location of the receptor protein NR2A.

This electron micrograph demonstrates intense NR2A immunogold localization between an axon terminal(ax) and dendritic spine(sp) forming an asymmetric (Type 1) synapse on the dendrites of pyramidal cells in CA1 of monkey hippocampus. The majority of the gold particles, each of which probably represents an individual receptor, are associated with the postsynaptic specialization of the dendritic spine and synaptic cleft, and thus are in a position to mediate NMDA receptor activity at this particular synapse. In addition, two particles are clearly associated with the presynaptic axon terminal, suggesting that NR2A may also participate in autoreceptors that modulate glutamate release presynaptically. Thus, with this approach we can resolve the molecular constituents of the synapse and quantify their relative distribution in specific regions of the synapse. The boxed area is represented at higher magnification in lower left corner (Scale bar = 0.13μm). The author thanks William Janssen and Prabhakar Vissavajjhalla for providing this illustration.

as the perforant path, as well as certain circuits intrinsic to the hippocampus (Hyman et al., 1984); and (3) key diffuse projections to the cerebral cortex, such as the cholinergic projection from nucleus basalis (Whitehouse et al., 1982; for a review, see Kemper, 1999). In contrast to the selective but extensive neuron loss reflective of Alzheimer's disease, neuron death is minimal in the regions classically associated with cognition and memory in the normal course of aging (Peters et al., 1998a). The lack of significant hippocampal and neocortical neuron death in normal aging has now been demonstrated in humans, monkeys, and rats (West et al., 1993b; Gomez-Isla et al., 1996; Rapp and Gallagher, 1996; Gazzaley et al., 1997; Peters et al., 1998a), although some neuron loss appears to occur in humans in the hilus of the dentate and in the subiculum (West, 1993b).

However, a lack of quantifiable neuron loss does not necessarily mean that no degenerative changes are occurring in a given brain region, and it does not rule out more subtle changes that lead to compromised function without cell loss. The entorhinal cortex is a particularly instructive case in this regard. It appears that the neurons within layer II of entorhinal cortex, which serve as a neocortical conduit to the hippocampus through the perforant path, are likely to be the single most vulnerable class of neurons in the brain with respect to both aging and Alzheimer's disease. While these neurons are clearly devastated early in Alzheimer's disease, their status in cognitively normal, aged individuals and those with mild cognitive impairment has been more difficult to pinpoint. Neuron counts in neurologically normal individuals suggest that there is no neuron loss in the entorhinal cortex (Gomez-Isla et al., 1996; West, 1993b). However, analyses of neurofibrillary tangles (NFT), the classic reflection of a degenerating neuron in Alzheimer's disease, suggest that virtually all humans over the age of 55 have some NFT in layer II of entorhinal cortex (Vickers et al., 1992; Bouras et al., 1994).

How does one reconcile these two findings and draw a distinction between age-related degenerative events in the entorhinal cortex that are progressive and those that are not? While the answer to this question continues to be elusive, one approach that appears promising is the use of a comprehensive panel of antibodies in a quantitative experimental design in order to distinguish and quantify transitional events in the neurons within the entorhinal cortex that can be correlated with the clinical dementia rating scale. This approach has led to a focus on patients with a rating of 0.5 that have mild cognitive impairment, yet it is unclear whether their condition represents early Alzheimer's disease or a more stable condition that might be referred to as age-related memory impairment.

The key to reconciling the presence of NFT in this region with the fact that there does not appear to be neuron loss is that the various neuronal profile counts that have been done have not taken into consideration "transitional neurons," i.e., neurons that are still intact and included in an analysis of total neuron counts, yet have transitional intraneuronal pathology resembling an NFT. Such neurons are confusing in that they could be misconstrued as "normal neurons" in a Nissl stain or NFTs in a tau immunohistochemical stain, the two stains that are most commonly used to quantify total "healthy" neurons and NFT, respectively. But these neurons may actually be the key to understanding the difference between early Alzheimer's disease and senescence.

For example, when neurons in layer II of the entorhinal cortex are counted in three categories—ghost tangles, transitional neurons, and healthy neurons—the data are far more revealing with respect to early pathologic events in layer II of entorhinal cortex, and it is quite clear that there might be significant "transitional" pathology in neurologically normal individuals or individuals with a clinical dementia rating of 0.5 in the absence of quantifiable neuron death and in the absence of massive NFT formation (Gimmel et al., 1998; Bussière et al., 1999; see Figure A-2).

These estimates of neuron number in three classes can also be related to each other as ratios in a given case, establishing a case-by-case "index of neurodegeneration" that is not hampered by the individual variability in raw number of neurons that invariably occurs in studies of neuron number. It will be very important to continue to study patients with a clinical dementia rating of 0.5 to try and determine whether this condition is a precursor to Alzheimer's disease or whether it is a condition that can be sustained and stabilized over a long period of time without cascading to Alzheimer's disease. It will be even more enlightening to do these kinds of neuropathologic analyses in patients with prospective neuropsychological assessment. In addition, other molecules linked to degeneration (e.g., neurofilament, presenilin) can be incorporated into the analyses of transitional neurons to obtain even more discrete molecular information on the changes that occur in these neurons in aging and the nature of their selective vulnerability. However, even a more precise delineation of the events surrounding degeneration will not provide a full understanding of the vulnerability of this circuit, since, as described below, the entorhinal-hippocampal connections display age-related changes short of degeneration that could also impact function.

AGE-RELATED NEUROCHEMICAL SHIFTS
IN IDENTIFIED CIRCUITS AND CELL CLASSES

Introduction and Technical Considerations

Modern neuroanatomy is often centered on circuit analysis within the context of biochemical attributes, as described earlier. The most common methods used to link gene expression patterns with cell classes and circuits are immunohistochemistry and in situ hybridization, the localization of proteins

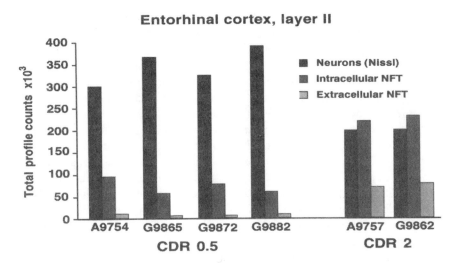

FIGURE A-2   This histogram represents a stereological analysis of the number of neuronal profiles in three different categories in layer II of the human entorhinal cortex, in one hemisphere. These are the neurons that form the perforant path, projecting to the dentate gyrus in the hippocampus proper. The three categories represent three different stages across the spectrum from healthy to degenerated. "Neurons (Nissl)" represent the number of neurons that are intact and appear healthy in a Nissl stain, without a trace of tau-accumulation. "Intracellular NFT" refers to neurons that are still intact as reflected by the Nissl stain, but are also immunoreactive for hyperphosphorylated tau, suggesting that a degenerative process is occurring, leading to tau accumulation and early stages of neurofibrillary tangle (NFT) formation. Extracellular NFTs, often called ghost NFTs, refer to a fully formed NFT with essentially no associated Nissl staining, suggesting that nothing remains of the neuron except the remnants of degeneration. These are end-stage NFTs that can be viewed as a dead neuron.

Six individual cases are shown, four with a clinical dementia rating (CDR) of 0.5, representing very mild cognitive impairment, and two with a CDR of 2, representing early Alzheimer's disease. Note the rather strong correlation between the CDR scores and the increase in transitional, intracellular NFT and extracellular NFT. In the CDR 0.5 cases, at least 75 percent of the layer II entorhinal cortex neurons remain free of pathology, and there are virtually no end-stage extracellular NFTs. However, the 25 percent that are transitional clearly suggest that a degenerative process is well under way in a significant proportion of these neurons. In CDR 2 cases, there is the beginning of an inversion in total numbers of NFT-bearing and NFT-free neurons, with the largest category being transitional intracellular NFTs, and 20 percent having progressed to end-stage NFTs. This may represent a pivotal stage in the development of dementia. How this pattern may be related to other aspects of neurochemical phenotype that may be linked to selective vulnerability will be investigated further in multiple labeling stereologic studies using other antibodies. The author thanks Patrick Hof for providing this illustration.

and mRNA, respectively. This is a crucial level of understanding of brain organization, since it is estimated that over half of the 100,000 genes in the mammalian genome are expressed exclusively or predominantly within the brain, however, many of them are not expressed ubiquitously or in a uniform pattern. In fact, the selective and nonuniform expression of genes is a critical element in each brain region, cell type, or neural circuit's particular neurochemical phenotype, i.e., the set of proteins that are required for that region, cell class, or circuit to perform its unique role in brain function. The regional and cellular delineation of gene expression patterns is thus important as a reflection of function, but it is also increasingly critical as a background for analysis of genetic manipulations, particularly in mouse transgenic models.

While in situ hybridization and several biochemical approaches have been applied in a quantitative fashion on the regional level to reveal relative mRNA levels in one brain region compared with another, the analysis of mRNA or protein levels on a quantitative cellular level has presented special problems with respect to obtaining quantitative data. Just as we need quantitative databases that define neuronal structure, we need quantitative data on gene expression patterns, otherwise we will not be able to measure the effect of a genetic manipulation in the context of neural circuits. This will require precise measurements of protein concentration and/or mRNA levels in specific regions, identified circuits, cell classes, neuronal compartments, and at the level of the synapse. There is little doubt that the emerging gene chip technology will augment efforts to obtain regional data on gene expression patterns, and the single-cell mRNA amplification approaches pioneered by Eberwine and colleagues have already been useful to obtain mRNA expression data on the single-cell level (Eberwine et al., 1992; Kacharmina et al., 1999). In addition, quantitative immunocytochemical analyses of protein levels on a cellular level have been fruitful, although the measurements generally are interpreted as relative protein levels rather than absolute molar measurements (Gazzaley et al., 1996a, 1996b). These quantitative cellular measurements are crucial if we are to obtain data at the desired level of resolution (see earlier discussion) that can be linked to individual cell classes and circuits. The analyses of putative age-related or experimentally induced shifts in glutamate receptors (GluRs) offer an excellent example of this approach, particularly in the hippocampus, where information flow through the trisynaptic circuit is highly ordered anatomically and mediated through glutamate receptors, with the NMDA receptor in particular strongly implicated in memory and age-related changes in memory (Caramanos and Shapiro, 1994; Barnes, 1994; Barnes et al., 1997a, 1997b).

NMDA Receptors, Hippocampal Circuits, and Aging

Both the available data and the missing data on changes in NMDA receptor distribution with aging offer an excellent example of the importance of microscopic analyses at several levels of resolution, as outlined in an earlier section. At the regional level, receptor binding studies have been used to study potential age-related changes in hippocampal GluRs in several species. While several studies have reported decreases in NMDA binding in the hippocampus of mice, rats, and monkeys (Wenk and Walker, 1991; Clark et al., 1992; Magnusson and Cotman, 1993; Le Jeune et al., 1996), other studies suggested that there is no change in NMDA receptors with aging (Nicolle et al., 1996) or perhaps even an increase in humans without Alzheimer's disease (Johnson et al., 1996).

In studying age-related changes in receptors or any of the key synaptic molecules, it is particularly important to be able to take the analysis from the regional level to that of cell classes, circuits, individual neuronal compartments, and synapses, since the changes are very likely to be cell, circuit, and synapse specific and therefore difficult to resolve at the regional level. In the case of multisubunit receptors like the NMDA and AMPA GluRs, it is optimal for the immunohistochemical data to be available at high anatomic resolution and with the highest molecular specificity, since receptor composition at the synapse is a crucial determinant of the functional characteristics of synaptic transmission.

In the same vein, it is best if shifts in GluR expression are detected at the level of GluR families (e.g., AMPA, kainate, NMDA receptors) and subunits within a family (e.g., for the AMPA receptor, GluRs1-4; for NMDA receptors, NR1 and NR2A-D), given that the subunit composition profoundly impacts function (see Hollman and Heinemann, 1994, for a review). Thus, for multisubunit receptor studies in aging, the demands are particularly high in that we want the localization to: (1) have the highest level of molecular specificity, (2) be linked to identified cells and circuits, (3) be available at a quantitative level, and (4) precisely describe the receptor composition at the synaptic level. Furthermore, if the analysis is to be truly comprehensive, then a given circuit needs to be characterized beyond the receptor subunits themselves to the associated proteins that modulate receptor function (e.g., PSD-95).

We have been able to get a start on such a comprehensive analysis, although it is still in its infancy. Motivated by the importance of both the entorhinal cortex projection to the dentate gyrus and the NMDA receptor in age-related changes in memory, we investigated the GluR distribution and immunofluorescence intensity within the dentate gyrus of juvenile, adult, and aged macaque monkeys with the combined use of subunit-specific antibodies and quantitative confocal microscopy (Gazzaley et al., 1996a).

This circuit has great advantages for such an analysis because the projection from the entorhinal cortex to the dentate gyrus is strictly confined to the outer molecular layer, i.e., the distal dendrites of granule cells, whereas other excitatory inputs terminate in a nonoverlapping fashion in the inner molecular layer, the proximal dendrites (Rosene and Van Hoesen, 1987; Witter and

Amaral, 1991). This strict laminar organization allows for putative changes in GluR distribution at the laminar level to be interpreted at the level of intraneuronal compartmentalization (i.e., distal versus proximal dendrites) and with reference to an isolated excitatory circuit (i.e., the perforant path). This quantitative analysis demonstrated that aged monkeys, compared with young adult monkeys, exhibit a decrease in the fluorescence intensity for the subunit NR1 in the outer molecular layer of the dentate gyrus compared with the inner molecular layer. Given the tight laminar organization of these circuits, this suggests that the decreased NR1 levels impact the input from the entorhinal cortex, but not the other excitatory inputs to the dentate gyrus, again, pointing to the entorhinal input to the hippocampus as a key element in age-related changes. Since NR1 is the obligatory subunit for the NMDA receptor, this shift probably represents a general shift in NMDA receptor localization. Parallel qualitative and quantitative studies with antibodies to AMPA and kainate subunits demonstrated that the intradendritic alteration in NR1 occurs without a similar alteration of non-NMDA receptor subunits, even though all three classes of GluRs are colocalized within these dendrites (Siegel et al., 1995). Further analyses, using markers for presynaptic terminals and dendritic markers, demonstrated that these elements were structurally intact in these aged animals.

These findings suggested that, in aged monkeys, a circuit-specific alteration in the intradendritic concentration of NR1 occurs without concomitant gross structural changes in dendritic morphology or a significant change in the total synaptic density across the molecular layer, suggesting that the intradendritic distribution of a neurotransmitter receptor is modifiable in an age-related and circuit-specific manner. Such a shift would lead to compromised NMDA receptor-mediated transmission, which could explain age-related shifts in long-term potentiation and spatial memory (Barnes et al., 1997a, 1997b) in the absence of any purely structural damage.

While these results are compelling, in that they represent a particularly high level of both molecular and anatomic specificity for age-related shifts in circuit attributes, they also are limited in two important ways. First, the animals were not behaviorally characterized, so these neurobiological changes cannot be directly linked to functional change. Second, the aged animals were all females, and their endocrine status was not carefully monitored, although they were presumably all postmenopausal. Given that estrogen is known to affect circuit characteristics in the hippocampus (McEwen and Alves, 1999), perhaps the endocrine status of the aged animals contributed to the receptor changes as much or more than chronological age. Presently, the data are not available from aged primates to clarify this potential confound, but we investigated the cellular mechanisms of estrogen-induced NMDA receptor regulation at the protein and mRNA levels in ovariectomized (OVX) rats with and without estrogen replacement therapy (ERT), using immunocytochemical and in situ hybridization techniques (Gazzaley et al., 1996b). Quantitative confocal microscopy was used to quantify alterations in immunofluorescence intensity levels of NR1 subunit proteins within neuronal cell bodies and dendrites of discrete hippocampal fields. In parallel, in situ hybridization was used to examine NR1 mRNA levels in corresponding hippocampal regions.

The data indicate that ERT in OVX rats significantly increases immunofluorescence intensity levels in comparison to nonsteroid-treated OVX rats within the cell bodies and dendrites of CA1 pyramidal cells and to a lesser extent within the granule cells of the dentate gyrus, without affecting CA3. In contrast, such alterations in immunofluorescence intensity occur without concomitant changes in mRNA hybridization levels. These data demonstrate a substantial degree of GluR plasticity in response to ERT over a fairly short period of time, since the ERT was initiated only one week after OVX, and the animals were sacrificed after only two days of ERT. These data are consistent with the estrogen-induced augmentation of NMDA receptor-mediated transmission by electrophysiological measurements (Woolley, 1999).

As compelling as these data are with respect to E-induced plasticity in the NMDA receptor, they are incomplete, in that we cannot comment on the effects on other related proteins (e.g., other NMDA receptor subunits, other GluRs.). In addition, we do not know how an increase in NR1 at the level of the soma and dendritic shafts translates into a change at the synapse. Moreover, these experiments were performed on young rats. Thus, while the receptor analyses on aged monkeys and estrogen-manipulated young rats suggest that both aging and endocrine status can alter NMDA receptors in a profound and circuit-dependent manner, the appropriate multidisciplinary analyses have yet to be carried out to determine if such alterations directly impact age-related memory decline. Studies of young and aged primates that are closely monitored both behaviorally and endocrinologically will need to be done to properly extend these studies. In addition, these studies will have to be extended to the ultrastructural level, in order to determine whether or not such dendritic shifts in NR1 are manifested at the synapse. Thus, while certain NMDA receptor-mediated hippocampal circuits are excellent targets for gene/circuit/behavioral links to be established in the context of age-related cognitive decline, most of the data needed to solidify such links are still missing.

INTERDISCIPLINARY APPROACHES

While neuroanatomic datasets and behavioral datasets can be compared across experiments, it is most powerful when the neuroanatomic and cellular analyses are done in the same animals that have been behaviorally characterized. This has been particularly powerful in the hands of investigators that behaviorally screen aged animals so that the behaviorally impaired aged animals can be considered as a distinct group from those that are not behaviorally impaired (Rapp and Gallagher, 1996; Gallagher and Rapp, 1997; Peters et al., 1998b). In addition, when the neurobiological data are quantitative and derived from behaviorally characterized animals, direct correlations can be drawn in individual subjects between a given neurobiological index (e.g., synapse number) and behavioral performance (Rapp and Gallagher, 1996; Peters et al., 1998b). Such studies should be encouraged in animal models as well as in human studies; large interdisciplinary teams have begun to develop brain banks from subjects that have had extensive premortem longitudinal assessment.

Recently, an interdisciplinary team carried out a comprehensive analysis of several neurochemical indices in the hippocampus of behaviorally characterized young and aged rats, using quantitative immunohistochemical procedures to examine the hypothesis that changes in the connectional organization of the hippocampus contribute to age-related learning impairment (Smith et al., 1999b). Immunohistochemical markers were used for key pre- and postsynaptic proteins as well as structural proteins that would reveal the degree to which the circuits were affected by shifts in protein distribution as differentiated from frank degeneration. Young and aged rats were tested on a hippocampal-dependent version of the Morris water maze, which revealed substantial variability in spatial learning ability among aged rats (Gallagher and Rapp, 1997). A quantitative confocal method was used to quantify changes in immunofluorescence staining for the presynaptic vesicle glycoprotein, synaptophysin (SYN), which is an established marker for presynaptic terminals and is required for synaptic release. The intensity of specific immunoreactivity was measured in inner (IML), middle (MML) and outer (OML) portions of the dentate gyrus molecular layer, stratum lucidum (SL) and stratum laconosum-moleculare (LM) of CA3, and CA1 stratum radiatum (SR) and LM.

This approach allowed us to link neurochemical changes with specific cell classes and circuits in a very comprehensive fashion involving all three elements of the trisynaptic circuit through the hippocampus, as well as multiple sites of termination of the entorhinal input to the hippocampus. Comparisons based on chronological age alone failed to reveal a reliable difference in SYN staining intensity in any region examined. In contrast, aged subjects with robust spatial learning deficits displayed significant reductions in SYN immunoreactivity in CA3-LM relative to either young controls or age-matched rats with preserved learning. In addition, across all aged rats, individual differences in spatial learning capacity correlated with levels of SYN staining in three of the regions examined: the OML and MML of the dentate gyrus and CA3-LM. These changes in relative SYN levels occurred in the absence of any evidence of structural degeneration of the innervated dendrites, and thus would impact synaptic transmission, perhaps though compromised glutamate release rather than degeneration of pre- or postsynaptic elements.

Most importantly, all three of the regions displaying decreased levels of SYN receive a major projection from layer II of entorhinal cortex, offering further evidence that this circuit is exquisitely sensitive to aging. These findings suggest that circuit-specific alterations in glutamate release in the hippocampus may contribute to the effects of aging on learning and memory, in the absence of frank degeneration. This is a compelling example of the power of using quantitative, chemically specific approaches in behaviorally characterized animals in order to pinpoint the subtle circuit-specific neurobiological substrates of age-related memory impairment.

In these same animals, we investigated the AMPA receptor subunit, GluR2, and the NMDA receptor subunit NR1 to determine whether or not postsynaptic shifts in receptors might also be occurring in the context of aging that would further impact the functional status of the entorhinal inputs to dentate gyrus and CA3 (Adams et al., 1999). Interestingly, there was no statistically significant decrease in NR1 directly associated with age-related memory impairment. However, there was a positive correlation between performance on the Morris water maze and NR1 fluorescence intensity levels regardless of age, and this correlation was present only in CA3. AMPA receptors did not show such a correlation.

Could performance on a memory task be so clearly linked to one particular GluR in a small subset of hippocampal circuits? Clearly, it is too early to draw any causal inference from these data; however, recent transgenic mouse experiments support the notion of a direct relationship between the NMDA receptor proteins and memory performance. First, mice that have the NR1 gene knocked out in a manner that is confined to the hippocampus have impaired learning and memory performance (Tsien et al., 1996). In addition, mice that have a different NMDA receptor subunit, NR2B, overexpressed in the forebrain display enhanced memory and learning in several behavioral paradigms (Tang et al., 1999).

Clearly, these data represent a powerful example of gene/circuit/behavior links that will help to illuminate the role of the NMDA receptor in the hippocampus in age-related memory decline, and they further reinforce the power of multidisciplinary approaches as we move forward in our investigations of the neurobiology of aging. These latter experiments in mice also demonstrate the power of genetically manipulated mice as models for the investigation of memory and, potentially, age-related memory impairment. The required mouse genetics is sufficiently advanced; however, mouse neurophysiology, neuropsychology, and neuroanatomy lag far behind, making detailed interdisciplinary analyses difficult. With respect to mouse neuroanatomy, an important goal for the future will be to develop the quantitative datasets that will link gene products with specific circuits so that genetic manipulations that affect learning and memory can be linked to brain structure in a precise manner. It will also be crucial to avoid the syndrome of "looking for your keys under the street lamp." If one is manipulating gene X to affect behavior Y, one cannot assume that targeted circuits will react in a simple predictable fashion. Analyses of genetically manipulated mice must be comprehensive and quantitative, casting a wide net with respect to affected circuits and behaviors.

The nonhuman primate is also an increasingly important animal model, particularly for studies of cognition (Rapp and Amaral, 1992; Moss et al., 1999) and studies of hormonal effects (Abel et al., 1999). The issues of estrogen, menopause, and the effects of ERT on the hippocampus will be particularly important to analyze in a primate model, given the similarities between nonhuman primate reproductive physiology and that of humans, as well as the advanced cognitive abilities of the nonhuman primate compared with rodent models. In addition, given the extraordinary resource that aged primates represent, these studies should be multidisciplinary whenever possible in order to ensure that interactive datasets are obtained and that the animals are used as fully as possible.

RESTORING CIRCUITS

Given that both normal aging and neurodegenerative disorders disrupt selectively vulnerable circuits, it would appear that the most successful interventions will be those that have a sufficient degree of circuit selectivity. Is there any evidence that damaged or degenerating circuits can be restored in the brain, and if so how successful and selective is the restoration? There is a long history of such attempts and a large resultant literature that is beyond the scope of this review; however, it is informative to the present discussion on aging and neurodegenerative disorders to highlight several of the key approaches that have been attempted, such as tissue transplantation, transplanting engineered cells or viral vectors for gene therapy, the promise of stem cells, and the potential for exploiting the natural neurogenesis that occurs in the adult brain.

Transplantation Strategies

Transplantation of embryonic brain tissue into a damaged adult brain was one of the first strategies developed for circuit repair. Generally, select tissue from the donor embryo brain that contains the neurons destined to provide a replacement for the damaged circuit is surgically implanted in the deafferented region. The most successful animal models have involved the initial surgical destruction of the dopaminergic innervation of caudate followed by the transplantation of fetal substantia nigra from a donor brain in the hopes of developing a therapy for Parkinson's disease. As early as the 1970s and 1980s, this strategy was demonstrated to be successful with respect to survival of the transplanted neurons, formation of the appropriate connections, and functional recovery of the animal (Bjorklund et al., 1981; Stromberg et al., 1985). Based on a large body of animal literature, the prospects for transplantation in such human neurodegenerative diseases as Parkinson's disease were considered in the 1980s, and there was limited success as a therapeutic intervention (see Lindvall, 1991, for a review).

However, in recent years the success of this strategy has improved, and in fact, there are now clinical trials with relatively long-term evaluation that demonstrate success with respect to the survival of the transplant, a degree of functional recovery, and even demonstrated release of dopamine from the transplanted axons into the newly innervated striatum (Olanow et al., 1996; Hauser et al., 1999; Piccini et al., 1999). The strategy of transplanting fetal tissue has been modified and improved through the use of genetically modified cells that secrete dopamine into the striatum, and these cells can be injected directly into the striatum (Martinez-Serrano et al., 1995; Kordower et al., 1994, 1995). In addition, a gene delivery system employing a viral vector to deliver a growth factor into the septum successfully protected experimentally damaged cholinergic neurons innervating the hippocampus (Blomer et al., 1998).

While these approaches are potentially very promising for certain neurodegenerative disorders such as Parkinson's disease, such transplant approaches will clearly be most successful with a target circuit that has relatively little synaptic specificity in its target region, which is the case with the nigrostriatal dopaminergic circuit. For example, such a strategy would seem to have very limited feasibility with respect to replacing complex, highly specific, corticocortical circuits.

Perhaps most relevant to aging are two recent primate studies that have employed gene therapy to reverse naturally occurring age-related compromise in two vulnerable circuits. One study targeted the cholinergic projection emanating from nucleus basalis that is known to be vulnerable in Alzheimer's disease (Smith et al., 1999a), and the other study used a viral vector approach to deliver a growth factor to reverse the natural age-related decline in dopamine function in the nigrostriatal projection (Kordower et al., 2000). Smith et al. demonstrated in primates that atrophic cell shrinkage and loss of cholinergic markers in nucleus basalis neurons could be reversed with human NGF (nerve growth factor) therapy. Interestingly, the neurons had not fully degenerated, and in that sense this is not analogous to late-stage Alzheimer's disease. The neurons had shrunk and their gene expression had shifted in a manner that impaired cholinergic function, but they had not degenerated. Both the morphologic and biochemical age-related shifts were reversible with NGF therapy.

In the analogous study of the dopamine neurons (Kordower et al., 2000), a viral vector was used to deliver GDNF, a growth factor that is known to be crucial for the sustained viability of the dopaminergic neurons that furnish the nigrostriatal projection. Several morphologic, neurochemical, and physiologic parameters of the nigrostriatal system were augmented in the GDNF-treated aged animals, and a healthy youthful phenotype of these neurons was restored.

The aspect of these two studies that is perhaps most interesting and relevant to the present discussion is that these circuits had not degenerated, they were simply in poor health and had lost their robust high-functioning phenotype. Thus, these experiments may be particularly relevant to the circumstances that occur in normal aging, in which circuits have suffered with respect to gene expression and subtle morphologic attributes that impact function, but they are still intact and still able to be rescued with no need to replace the circuit.

The Promise of Stem Cells

In all of the transplant approaches outlined above, it was crucial to provide either neurons, modified cells, or viral vectors that replaced a missing neurotransmitter or growth factor that was required at a high level in a particular target region. This approach will have limited application to many other kinds of age-related problems that involve more complex circuits with high synaptic specificity. While the recent discoveries regarding stem cells are still in their infancy with respect to relevance to brain aging, they may in fact have broad application to the brain in the near future.

Stem cells are cells within the body that continue to proliferate in a state that has not differentiated into any particular organ, and they therefore retain what is referred to as a "pluripotent" capacity. The fact that these cells can be coaxed into a particular path of differentiation has generated enormous excitement about their potential for restoration of damaged cells and related functions in multiple organ systems, including the brain. In fact, stem cells and their potential application was chosen as the breakthrough of the year for 1999 by the journal *Science*. The excitement in this area was fueled particularly by two reports in late 1998 that demonstrated the potential to keep undifferentiated embryonic stem cells alive for long periods of time, and then promote their differentiation into various target tissues after a sustained period of remaining undifferentiated (Thomson et al., 1998; Shamblott et al., 1998). However, reliance on human embryonic stem cells with an eye toward therapeutics presents both technical problems as well as political and ethical issues that revolve around the use of embryonic human tissue.

Soon after the initial discovery regarding embryonic stem cells it was shown that adult stem cells from one particular organ retained the capacity to survive, differentiate, and presumably function in a different organ; an example is the conversion of neural stem cells into a variety of blood cells that circulate and reside in the bone marrow (Bjornson et al., 1999; Scheffler et al., 1999). The reverse appears to be true as well, in that bone marrow stem cells can survive and migrate within the brain and differentiate into cells that developed a phenotype for astrocytes and, in some cases, neurons (Kopen et al., 1999). Also, embryonic and neural stem cells can replace oligodendrocytes in a brain deficient in such cells and the newly derived oligodendrocytes successfully myelinate axons (Brustle et al., 1999; Yandava et al., 1999).

These studies serve as a powerful animal model for testing potential therapies for such diseases as multiple sclerosis. It may also be possible to replace damaged neural circuits with such an approach. In such a study, neural embryonic stem cells from a healthy mouse were transplanted into a rat's spinal cord several days after traumatic injury (McDonald et al., 1999). Histological analysis showed that the transplant-derived cells from the mouse had not only survived but had differentiated into astrocytes as well as neurons, and the investigators were able to demonstrate some functional recovery in these animals. The potential of such approaches that utilize neural stem cells for therapies directed at age-related pathology and functional decline is profound, and while this research arena is still in its infancy, the progress that has already occurred is very impressive (see Shihabuddin et al., 1999, for a review).

The most likely limitation of the stem cell approaches will be the need for a high degree of circuit specificity in any devised therapy. The use of neural stem cells to achieve some recovery of function after spinal cord injury suggests that, at least in some cases, an adequate level of circuit specificity may emerge with little direct coaxing. However, it is not clear at this point whether or not this will occur in the key brain circuits affected in aging. For example, if we were to try and use stem cell therapy to replace the entorhinal neurons that provide the perforant path, how would we guide the neural stem cells and the differentiated neurons into becoming the particularly highly differentiated neurons that reside in layer II of entorhinal cortex with the appropriate afferents and efferents? Perhaps even more difficult, how would we replace the neurons that furnish the corticocortical circuits that interconnect frontal and temporal regions that are so damaged in Alzheimer's disease, while leaving the intact circuits unaffected? As described below, in some cases the brain may solve this problem itself by continuing to generate neurons that can replace certain circuits throughout life.

Neurogenesis in the Adult Hippocampus

The recent data on neurogenesis in the adult brain have demonstrated clearly that we need to reevaluate the accepted dogma that when neurons die they cannot be replaced by the generation of new neurons. While it has been known for a long time from work in rodents that some neurogenesis occurs in the adult dentate gyrus (Altman and Das, 1965), it was demonstrated only recently that this also occurs in the nonhuman primate (Gould et al., 1999b) and in humans as well (Eriksson et al., 1998). In addition, while the functional status of the new neurons in the dentate gyrus is unclear, it has been demonstrated that they project to CA3 and thus may form normal connections (Hastings and Gould, 1999). Furthermore, the prevailing notion that the hippocampus is the only telencephalic region in which neurogenesis occurs has now been challenged by a report that neurogenesis occurs in the nonhuman primate neocortex, particularly in cortical regions that would presumably play a dominant role in learning, memory, and cognition (Gould et al., 1999c); however, these data on neocortex are presently controversial and will need to be expanded and replicated.

How are we to integrate the notion of new neurons into our prevailing attitudes regarding age-related functional decline and neurodegenerative disorders? While much work lies ahead, several interesting recent reports demonstrate the potential importance of neurogenesis to aging, at least with respect to the dentate gyrus. For one thing, neurogenesis in the dentate gyrus is decreased in aging (Kuhn et al., 1996). There are also positive influences on neurogenesis that may be exploited in preventing the age-related decrease in neurogenesis. The simple process of training animals on a learning task that requires the hippocampus enhanced neurogenesis and the viability of the new neurons in the dentate gyrus of rats (Gould et al., 1999a). Similarly adult mice living in an enriched environment have increased neurogenesis in the hippocampus (Kempermann et al., 1997). Moreover, increased experience and social interaction led to an enhancement of neurogenesis in the dentate gyrus of aged animals (Kempermann et al., 1998). Finally, simple physical exercise (e.g., running) increased cell proliferation in the adult mouse dentate gyrus (van Praag et al., 1999).

The potential for hormonal impact on these processes makes this issue even more relevant to aging. For example, estrogen has been demonstrated to stimulate a transient increase in neurogenesis in the dentate gyrus of the adult female rat (Tanapat et al., 1999). Furthermore, it was recently demonstrated that the level of neurogenesis typical of a young animal could be restored in an aged animal by decreasing the high levels of circulating corticosteroids that commonly occur in aged animals (Cameron and McKay, 1999). Thus, while it is not yet possible to fit these data on neurogenesis into the present context of aging and the neurobiological substrate for age-related functional decline, it is clear that this will be an area of intense investigation in the future and an area of paramount importance in aging research. It will be especially important to determine the quantitative extent of neurogenesis and the functional implications of adding neurons to the aged brain. Do the new neurons participate in the appropriate circuits? To what degree does adult neurogenesis occur in areas other than the dentate gyrus? In a related fashion, to what degree can the natural process of neurogenesis in the hippocampus be used to replace neurons in a neurodegenerative disorder such as Alzheimer's disease? Obviously it will take time to obtain answers to these questions, but the field is moving rapidly, and we must now incorporate the potential for new neurons into our thinking about malfunctioning neurons and degenerating neurons in the aging brain.

CONCLUDING REMARKS

This report outlines a microscopic and neuroanatomic approach to understanding neurobiological events that underlie memory decline with aging. The available data suggest that the focus of such analyses should be the vulnerable circuit, and the delineation of phenotypic characteristics that render a cell class or circuit selectively vulnerable to aging. With respect to Alzheimer's disease, the key reflection of vulnerability is degeneration, whereas memory decline in the context of normal aging is likely due to subtle neurochemical and morphologic alterations that lead to functional impairment in the absence of frank neuronal degeneration. This differentiation is not absolute, however, in that degenerative events are clearly under way in the entorhinal cortex of neurologically normal elderly people. Many of these neurons appear as "transitional" with respect to degenerative profiles typical of Alzheimer's disease, and it will be critical to focus more attention on these transitional events if we are to adequately differentiate a stable, relatively high-functioning state from the early stages of a progression toward Alzheimer's disease. In addition, much of the work on animal models suggests that functional decline in the context of normal aging or senescence (e.g., age-related memory impairment) is unlikely to be due primarily to neuron loss and is more likely to be a reflection of shifts in gene expression or key neurochemical attributes that impair function in an intact circuit. This suggests that therapy targeted at restoring a youthful phenotype to vulnerable circuits may be particularly effective, and data exist demonstrating the rescue of age-impaired cholinergic and dopaminergic circuits. In addition, replacing dead neurons or impaired circuits through the use of stem cells may be more realistic than previously thought, although obtaining the requisite circuit specificity from such an approach may be problematic. Finally, naturally occurring neurogenesis, particularly in the adult dentate gyrus, offers another avenue for restoration of function, and data exist showing that the generation of new hippocampal neurons and their continued viability are responsive to behavioral and endocrine intervention.

Thus, while conditions such as Alzheimer's disease clearly involve devastating neuron loss, the scenario for normal aging is far more dynamic and adaptable than we once thought, and even neuron loss might not be as irreversible as we assumed just a few years ago. However, the development of helpful interventions will have to be carefully guided by a healthy respect for the specificity and heterogeneity of neural circuits, and the fact that even in regions considered vulnerable (e.g., the hippocampus), individual circuits vary enormously in their vulnerability to aging. Therapies that are not adequately specific with respect to targeting vulnerable circuits are likely to have unanticipated behavioral and functional consequences that will compromise their effectiveness.

ACKNOWLEDGMENTS

The author thanks Patrick Hof, Michelle Adams, Peter Rapp, and Bill Janssen for helpful discussions and comments regarding this manuscript.

REFERENCES

Abel, T.W., M.L. Voytko, and N.E. Rance
  1999   The effects of hormone replacement therapy on hypothalamic neuropeptide gene expression in a primate model of menopause. *Journal of Clinical Endocrinology and Metabolism* 84:2111-2118.
Adams, M.M., T.D. Smith, P.R. Rapp, M. Gallagher, and J.H. Morrison
  1999   Immunofluorescence intensity in CA3 of hippocampus predicts spatial learning in young and aged rats. *Society for Neuroscience Abstracts* 25:2163.
Altman, J., and G.D. Das
  1965   Autoradiographic and histological evidence of postnatal neurogenesis in rats. *Journal of Comparative Neurology* 124:319-335.
Barnes, C.A.
  1994   Normal aging: Regionally specific changes in hippocampal synaptic transmission. *Trends in Neurosciences* 17:13-18.
Barnes, C.A., G. Rao, and J. Shen
  1997a Age-related decrease in the N-methyl-D-aspartateR-mediated excitatory postsynaptic potential in hippocampal region CA1. *Neurobiology of Aging* 18:445-452.
Barnes, C.A., M.S. Suster, J. Shen, and B.L. McNaughton
  1997b Multistability of cognitive maps in the hippocampus of old rats. *Nature* 388:272-275.
Bjorklund, A., U. Stenevi, S.B. Dunnett, and S.D. Iversen
  1981   Functional reactivation of the deafferented neostriatum by nigral transplants. *Nature* 289:497-499.
Bjornson, C.R., R.L. Rietze, B.A. Reynolds, M.C. Magli, and A.L. Vescovi
  1999   Turning brain into blood: A hematopoietic fate adopted by adult neural stem cells in vivo. *Science* 283:534-537.
Blomer, U., T. Kafri, L. Randolph-Moore, I.M. Verma, and F.H. Gage
  1998   Bcl-xL protects adult septal cholinergic neurons from axotomized cell death. *Proceedings of the National Academy of Sciences of the United States of America* 95:2603-2608.

Bouras, C., P.R. Hof, P. Giannakopoulos, J. Michel, and J.H. Morrison
   1994   Regional distribution of neurofibrillary tangles and senile plaques in the cerebral cortex of elderly patients: A quantitative evaluation of a one-year autopsy population from a geriatric hospital. *Cerebral Cortex* 4:138-150.
Brustle, O., K.N. Jones, R.D. Learish, K. Karram, K. Choudhary, O.D. Wiestler, I.D. Duncan, and R.D. McKay
   1999   Embryonic stem cell-derived glial precursors: A source of myelinating transplants. *Science* 285:754-756.
Bussière, T., B. Wicinsky, G.I. Lin, D.P. Perl, P. Davies, R. Nixon, J.H. Morrison, and P.R. Hof
   1999   Early neurodegenerative alterations in the cerebral cortex during normal aging and Alzheimer's disease. *Society for Neuroscience Abstracts* 25:593.
Cameron, H.A., and R.D.G. McKay
   1999   Restoring production of hippocampal neurons in old age. *Nature Neuroscience* 2:894-897.
Caramanos, Z., and M.L. Shapiro
   1994   Spatial memory and N-methyl-D-aspartate receptor antagonists APV and MK-801: Memory impairments depend on familiarity with the environment, drug dose, and training duration. *Behavioral Neuroscience* 108:30-43.
Chaudhry, F.A., K.P. Lehre, M. van Lookeren Campagne, O.P. Ottersen, N.C. Danbolt, and J. Storm Mathisen
   1995   Glutamate transporters in glial plasma membranes: High differentiated localizations revealed by quantitative ultrastructual immunocytochemistry. *Neuron* 15:711-720.
Clark, A.S., K.R. Magnusson, and C.W. Cotman
   1992   In vitro autoradiography of hippocampal excitatory amino acid binding in aged Fischer 344 rats: relationship to performance on Morris water maze. *Behavioral Neuroscience* 106(2):324-335.
Coggeshall, R.E., and H.A. Lekan
   1996   Methods for determining numbers of cells and synapses: A case for more uniform standards of review. *Journal of Comparative Neurology* 364:6-15.
Coleman, P.D., and D.G. Flood
   1987   Neuron numbers and dendritic extent in normal aging and Alzheimer's disease. *Neurobiology of Aging* 8:521-545.
DeKosky, S.T., and S.W. Scheff
   1990   Synapse loss in frontal cortex biopsies in Alzheimer's disease: Correlation with cognitive severity. *Annals of Neurology* 27:457-464.
Duan, H., Y. He, B. Wicinsky, G. Yeung, T.L. Page, W.G.M. Janssen, J.H. Morrison, and P.R. Hof
   1999   Age-related changes in cortical projection neurons in macaque monkey: Dendrite morphology, spine density, and neurochemical features. *Society for Neuroscience Abstracts* 25:362.
Eberwine, J., H. Yeh, K. Miyashiro, Y. Cao, S. Nair, R. Finnell, M. Zettel, and P. Coleman
   1992   Analysis of gene expression in single live neurons. *Proceedings of the National Academy of Sciences of the United States of America* 89:3010-3014.
Eichenbaum, H., P. Dudchenko, E. Wood, M.L. Shapiro, and H. Tanila
   1999   The hippocampus, memory, and place cells: Is it spatial memory or memory space? *Neuron* 23:209-226.
Eriksson, P.S., E. Perfilieva, T. Bjork-Eriksson, A.M. Alborn, C. Nordborg, D.A. Peterson, and F.H. Gage
   1998   Neurogenesis in the adult human hippocampus. *Nature Medicine* 4:1313-1317.

Gallagher, M., and P.R. Rapp
    1997   The use of animal models to study the effects of aging on cognition. *Annual Review of Psychology* 48:339-370.
Gazzaley, A.H., S.J. Siegel, J.H. Kordower, E.J. Mufson, and J.H. Morrison
    1996a   Circuit-specific alterations of N-methyl-D-aspartate subunit 1 in the dentate gyrus of aged monkeys. *Proceedings of the National Academy of Sciences of the United States of America* 93(7):3121-3125.
Gazzaley, A.H., M.M. Thakker, P.R. Hof, and J.H. Morrison
    1997   Preserved number of entorhinal cortex layer II neurons in aged macaque monkeys. *Neurobiology of Aging* 18:549-553.
Gazzaley, A.H., N.G. Weiland, B.S. McEwen, and J.H. Morrison
    1996b   Differential regulation of NMDAR1 mRNA and protein by estradiol in the rat hippocampus. *Journal of Neuroscience* 16:6830-6838.
Geinisman, Y., L. Detoledo-Morrell, F. Morrell, and R.E. Heller
    1995   Hippocampal markers of age-related memory dysfunction: Behavioral, electrophysiological and morphological perspective. *Progress in Neurobiology* 45:223-252.
Geinisman, Y., H.J. Gunderson, E. van der Zee, and M.J. West
    1996   Unbiased stereological estimation of the total number of synapses in a brain region. *Journal of Neurocytology* 25:805-819.
Gimmel, D., J.H. Morrison, D.P. Perl, C. Bouras, and P.R. Hof
    1998   Development of stereologic indices of neurodegeneration in the cerebral cortex during normal aging and Alzheimer's disease. *Society for Neuroscience Abstracts* 24:960.
Gomez-Isla, T., J.L. Price, D.W. McKeel, Jr., J.C. Morris, J.H. Growdon, and B.T. Hyman
    1996   Profound loss of layer II entorhinal cortex neurons occurs in very mild Alzheimer's disease. *Journal of Neuroscience* 16:4491-4500.
Gould, E., A. Beylin, P. Tanapat, A. Reeves, and T.J. Shors
    1999a   Learning enhances adult neurogenesis in the hippocampal formation. *Nature Neuroscience* 2:260-265.
Gould, E., A.J. Reeves, M. Fallah, P. Tanapat, C.G. Gross, and E. Fuchs
    1999b   Hippocampal neurogenesis in adult Old World primates. *Proceedings of the National Academy of Sciences of the United States of America* 96:5263-5267.
Gould, E., A.J. Reeves, M.S. Graziano, and C.G. Gross
    1999c   Neurogenesis in the neocortex of adult primates. *Science* 286:548-552.
Hastings, N.B., and E. Gould
    1999   Rapid extension of axons into the CA3 region by adult-generated granule cells. *Journal of Comparative Neurology* 413:146-154.
Hauser, R.A., T.B. Freeman, B.J. Snow, M. Nauert, L. Gauger, J.H. Kordower, and C.W. Olanow
    1999   Long-term evaluation of bilateral fetal nigral transplantation in Parkinson's disease. *Archives of Neurology* 56:179-187.
He, Y., W.G.M. Janssen, J.D. Rothstein, and J.H. Morrison
    2000   Differential synaptic localization of the glutamate transporter EAAC1 and glutamate receptor subunit GluR2 in the rat hippocampus. *Journal of Comparative Neurology* 418:255-269.
Hof, P.R., C. Bouras, and J.H. Morrison
    1999   Cortical neuropathology in aging and dementing disorders: Neuronal typology, connectivity, and selective vulnerability. Pp. 175-311 in *Cerebral Cortex, Vol. 14, Neurodegenerative and Age-Related Changes in Structure and Function of Cerebral Cortex*, A. Peters and J.H. Morrison, eds. New York: Kluwer Academic/Plenum Publishers.

Hof, P.R., K. Cox, and J.H. Morrison
1990   Quantitative analysis of a vulnerable subset of pyramidal neurons in Alzheimer's disease: I. Superior frontal and inferior temporal cortex. *Journal of Comparative Neurology* 301:44-54.

Hof, P.R., and J.H. Morrison
1990   Quantitative analysis of a vulnerable subset of pyramidal neurons in Alzheimer's disease: II. Primary and secondary visual cortex. *Journal of Comparative Neurology* 301:55-64.

Hollmann, M., and S. Heinemann
1994   Cloned glutamate receptors. *Annual Review of Neuroscience* 17:31-108.

Hyman, B.T., A.R. Damasio, G.W. Van Hoesen, and C.L. Barnes
1984   Alzheimer's disease: Cell specific pathology isolates the hippocampal formation. *Science* 225:1168-1170.

Johnson, M., R.H. Perry, M.A. Piggott, J.A. Court, D. Spurden, S. Lloyd, P.G. Ince, and E.K. Perry
1996   Glutamate receptor binding in the human hippocampus and adjacent cortex during development and aging. *Neurobiology of Aging* 17:639-651.

Kacharmina, J.E., P.B. Crino, and J. Eberwine
1999   Preparation of cDNA from single cells and subcellular regions. *Methods in Enzymology* 303:3-18.

Kemper, T.L.
1999   Age-related changes in subcortical nuclei that project to the cerebral cortex. Pp. 365-397 in *Cerebral Cortex, Vol. 14, Neurodegenerative and Age-Related Changes in Sructure and Function of Cerebral Cortex*, A. Peters and J.H. Morrison, eds. New York: Kluwer Academic/Plenum Publishers.

Kempermann, G., H.G. Kuhn, and F.H. Gage
1997   More hippocampal neurons in adult mice living in an enriched environment. *Nature* 386:493-495.
1998   Experience-induced neurogenesis in the senescent dentate gyrus. *Journal of Neuroscience* 18:3206-3212.

Kopen, G.C., D.J. Prockop, and D.G. Phinney
1999   Marrow stromal cells migrate throughout forebrain and cerebellum, and they differentiate into astrocytes after injection into neonatal mouse brains. *Proceedings of the National Academy of Sciences of the United States of America* 96:10711-10716.

Kordower, J.H., J. Blich, M.E. Emborg, S.Y. Ma, Y. Chu, E.-Y. Chen, S. Palfi, L. Leventhal, B.Z. Roitberg, W.D. Brown, J.E. Holden, R. Pyzalski, M.D. Taylor, P. Carvey, D. Trono, P. Hantraye, N. Deglon, and P. Aebischer
2000   A lentivirus encoding for GDNF reverses dopamine insufficiency in an aged monkey model of progressive nigrostriatal degeneration. (Submitted)

Kordower, J.H., Y.T. Liu, S. Winn, and D.F. Emerich
1995   Encapsulated PC12 cell transplants into hemiparkinsonian monkeys: A behavioral, neuroanatomical, and neurochemical analysis. *Cell Transplant* 4:155-171.

Kordower J.H., S.R. Winn, Y.T. Liu, E.J. Mufson, J.R. Sladek, Jr., J.P. Hammang, E.E. Baetge, and D.F. Emerich
1994   The aged monkey basal forebrain: Rescue and sprouting of axotomized basal forebrain neurons after grafts of encapsulated cells secreting human nerve growth factor. *Proceedings of the National Academy of Sciences of the United States of America* 91:10898-10902.

Kuhn, H.G., H. Dickinson-Anson, and F.H. Gage
1996   Neurogenesis in the dentate gyrus of the adult rat: Age-related decrease of neuronal progenitor proliferation. *Journal of Neuroscience* 16:2027-2033.

Le Jeune, H., D. Cecyre, M.J. Meaney, and R. Quirion
    1996   Ionotropic glutamate receptor subtypes in the aged memory-impaired and unim-
            paired Long-Evans rat. *Neuroscience* 74:349-363.
Lewis, D.A., M.J. Campbell, R.D. Terry, and J.H. Morrison
    1987   Laminar and regional distributions of neurofibrillary tangles and neuritic plaques in
            Alzheimer's disease: A quantitative study of visual and auditory cortices. *Journal of
            Neuroscience* 7:1799-1808.
Lindvall, O.
    1991   Prospects of transplantation in human neurodegenerative diseases. *Trends in Neuro-
            sciences* 14:376-384.
Magnusson, K.R., and C.W. Cotman
    1993   Age-related changes in excitatory amino acid receptors in two mouse strains. *Neuro-
            biology of Aging* 14:197-206.
Martinez-Serrano, A., W. Fischer, and A. Bjorklund
    1995   Reversal of age-dependent cognitive impairments and cholinergic neuron atrophy
            by NGF-secreting neural progenitors grafted to the basal forebrain. *Neuron* 15:473-
            484.
McDonald, J.W., X.Z. Liu, Y. Qu, S. Liu, S.K. Mickey, D. Turetsky, D.I. Gottlieb, and D.W.
Choi
    1999   Transplanted embryonic stem cells survive, differentiate and promote recovery in
            injured rat spinal cord. *Nature Medicine* 5:1410-1412.
McEwen, B.S., and S.E. Alves
    1999   Estrogen actions in the central nervous system. *Endocrine Reviews* 20:279-307.
Morrison, J.H., and P.R. Hof
    1997   Life and death of neurons in the aging brain. *Science* 278:412-419.
Morrison, J.H., D.A. Lewis, M.J. Campbell, G.W. Huntley, D.L. Benson, and C. Bouras
    1987   A monoclonal antibody to non-phosphorylated neurofilament protein marks the
            vulnerable cortical neurons in Alzheimer's disease. *Brain Research* 416:331-336.
Moss, M.B., R.J. Killiany, and J.G. Herndon
    1999   Age-related cognitive decline in the rhesus monkey. Pp. 21-48 in *Cerebral Cortex,
            Vol. 14, Neurodegenerative and Age-Related Changes in Structure and Function of Ce-
            rebral Cortex*, A. Peters and J.H. Morrison, eds. New York: Kluwer Academic/Ple-
            num Publishers.
Nicolle, M.M., J.L. Bizon, and M. Gallagher
    1996   In vitro autoradiography of ionotropic glutamate receptors in hippocampus and
            striatum of aged Long-Evans rats: Relationship to spatial learning. *Neuroscience*
            74:741-756.
Olanow, C.W., J.H. Kordower, and T.B. Freeman
    1996   Fetal nigral transplantation as a therapy for Parkinson's disease. *Trends in Neuro-
            sciences* 19:102-109.
Pearson, R.C.A., M.M. Esiri, R.W. Hiorns, G.K. Wilcock, and T.P.S. Powell
    1985   Anatomical correlates of the distribution of the pathological changes in the neocor-
            tex in Alzheimer's disease. *Proceedings of the National Academy of Sciences of the
            United States of America* 82:4531-4534.
Peters, A., J.H. Morrison, D.L. Rosene, and B.T. Hyman
    1998a   Are neurons lost from the primate cerebral cortex during aging? *Cerebral Cortex*
            8:295-300.
Peters, A., D.L. Rosene, M.B. Moss, T.L. Kemper, C.R. Abraham, J. Tigges, and M.S. Albert
    1996   Neurobiological bases of age-related cognitive decline in the rhesus monkey. *Journal
            of Neuropathology and Experimental Neurology* 55:861-874.

Peters, A., C. Sethares, and M.B. Moss
  1998b The effects of aging on layer 1 in area 46 of prefrontal cortex in the rhesus monkey. *Cerebral Cortex* 8:671-684.
Piccini, P., D.J. Brooks, A. Bjorklund, R.N. Gunn, P.M. Grasby, O. Rimoldi, P. Brundin, P. Hagell, S. Rehncrona, H. Widner, and O. Lindvall
  1999 Dopamine release from nigral transplants visualized in vivo in a Parkinson's patient. *Nature Neuroscience* 2(12):1137-1140.
Rapp, P.R., and D.G. Amaral
  1992 Individual differences in the cognitive and neurobiological consequences of normal aging. *Trends in Neurosciences* 15:340-345.
Rapp, P.R., and M. Gallagher
  1996 Preserved neuron number in the hippocampus of aged rats with spatial learning deficits. *Proceedings of the National Academy of Sciences of the United States of America* 93:9926-9930.
Rogers, J., and J.H. Morrison
  1985 Quantitative morphology and regional and laminar distribution of senile plaques in Alzheimer's disease. *Journal of Neuroscience* 5:2801-2808.
Rosene, D.L., and G.W. Van Hoesen
  1987 The hippocampal formation of the primate brain—A review of some comparative aspects of cytoarchitecture and connections. Pp. 345-356 in *Cerebral Cortex, Vol. 6, Further Aspects of Cortical Function, Including Hippocampus,* E.G. Jones and A. Peters, eds. New York: Plenum Press.
Scheffler, B., M. Horn, I. Blumcke, E.D. Laywell, D. Coomes, V.G. Kukekov, and D.A. Steindler
  1999 Narrow-mindedness: A perspective on neuropoiesis. *Trends in Neurosciences* 22:348-357.
Shamblott, M.J., J. Axelman, S. Wang, E.M. Bugg, J.W. Littlefield, P.J. Donovan, P.D. Blumenthal, G.R. Huggins, and J.D. Gearhart
  1998 Derivation of pluripotent stem cells from cultured human primordial germ cells. *Proceedings of the National Academy of Sciences of the United States of America* 95(23):13726-13731.
Shapiro, M.L., and H. Eichenbaum
  1999 Hippocampus as a memory map: Synaptic plasticity and memory encoding by hippocampal neurons. *Hippocampus* 9(4):365-384.
Shihabuddin, L.S., T.D. Palmer, and F.H. Gage
  1999 The search for neural progenitor cells: Prospects for the therapy of neurodegenerative disease. *Molecular Medicine Today* 5:474-480.
Siegel, S.J., W.G.M. Janssen, J.W. Tullai, S.W. Rogers, T. Moran, S.F. Heinemann, and J.H. Morrison
  1995 Distribution of the excitatory amino acid receptor subunits GluR2(4) in monkey hippocampus and colocalization with subunits GluR5-7 and NMDAR1. *Journal of Neuroscience* 15:2707-2719.
Smith D.E., J. Roberts, F.H. Gage, and M.H. Tuszynski
  1999a Age-associated neuronal atrophy occurs in the primate brain and is reversible by growth factor gene therapy. *Proceedings of the National Academy of Sciences of the United States of America* 96:10893-10898.
Smith, T.D., M.M. Adams, J.H. Morrison, M. Gallagher, and P.R. Rapp
  1999b Alterations in hippocampal synaptophysin immunoreactivity predict spatial learning impairment in the aged rat. *Society for Neuroscience Abstracts* 25:2163.
Squire, L.R., and S. Zola-Morgan
  1991 The medial temporal lobe memory system. *Science* 253:1380-1386.

Stromberg, I., S. Johnson, B. Hoffer, and L. Olson
  1985   Reinnervation of dopamine-denervated striatum by substantia nigra transplants: Immunohistochemical and electrophysiological correlates. *Neuroscience* 14:981-990.
Tanapat, P., N.B. Hastings, A.J. Reeves, and E. Gould
  1999   Estrogen stimulates a transient increase in the number of new neurons in the dentate gyrus of the adult female rat. *Journal of Neuroscience* 19:5792-5801.
Tang, Y.P., E. Shimizu, G.R. Dube, C. Rampon, G.A. Kerchner, M. Zhuo, G. Liu, and J.Z. Tsien
  1999   Genetic enhancement of learning and memory in mice. *Nature* 401:63-69.
Terry, R.D., E. Masliah, D.P. Salmon, N. Butters, R. DeTeresa, R. Hill, L.A. Hansen, and R. Katzman
  1991   Physical basis of cognitive alterations in Alzheimer's disease: Synapse loss is the major correlate of cognitive impairment. *Annals of Neurology* 30:572-580.
Thomson, J.A., J. Itskovitz-Eldor, S.S. Shapiro, M.A. Waknitz, J.J. Swiergiel, V.S. Marshall, and J.M. Jones
  1998   Embryonic stem cell lines derived from human blastocysts. *Science* 282:1145-1147.
Tigges, J., J.G. Herndon, and D.L. Rosene
  1996   Preservation into old age of synaptic number and size in the supragranular layer of the dentate gyrus in rhesus monkeys. *Acta Anatomica* 157:63-72.
Toni, N., P.A. Buchs, I. Nikonenko, C.R. Bron, and D. Muller
  1999   LTP promotes formation of multiple spine synapses between a single axon terminal and a dendrite. *Nature* 402:421-425.
Tsien, J.Z., P.T. Herta, and S. Tonegawa
  1996   The essential role of hippocampal CA1 NMDA receptor-dependent synaptic plasticity in spatial memory. *Cell* 87:1327-1338.
Van Hoesen, G.W., and D.N. Pandya
  1975   Some connections of the entorhinal (area 28) and perirhinal (area 35) cortices of the rhesus monkey. III. Efferent connections. *Brain Research* 95:39-59.
van Praag, H., G. Kempermann, and F.H. Gage
  1999   Running increases cell proliferation and neurogenesis in the adult mouse dentate gyrus. *Nature Neuroscience* 2:266-270.
Vickers, J.C., A. Delacourte, and J.H. Morrison
  1992   Progressive transformation of the cytoskeleton associated with normal aging and Alzheimer's disease. *Brain Research* 594:273-278.
Wenk, G.W., and L.C. Walker
  1991   Loss of NMDA, but not GABA-A, binding in the brains of aged rats and monkeys. *Neurobiology of Aging* 12:93-98.
West, M.J.
  1993a   New stereological methods for counting neurons. *Neurobiology of Aging* 14:275-285.
  1993b   Regionally specific loss of neurons in the aging human hippocampus. *Neurobiology of Aging* 14:287-293.
  1999   Stereological methods for estimating the total number of neurons and synapses: Issues of precision and bias. *Trends in Neurosciences* 22:51-61.
Whitehouse, P.J., D.L. Price, R.G. Struble, A.W. Clark, J.T. Coyle, and M.R. DeLong
  1982   Alzheimer's disease and senile dementia: Loss of neurons in basal forebrain. *Science* 215:1237-1239.
Witter, M.P., and D.G. Amaral
  1991   Entorhinal cortex of the monkey: V. Projections to dentate gyrus, hippocampus, and subicular complex. *Journal of Comparative Neurology* 307:437-459.
Wood, E.R., P.A. Dudchenko, and H. Eichenbaum
  1999   The global record of memory in hippocampal neuronal activity. *Nature* 397:613-616.

Woolley, C.S.
   1999   Electrophysiological and cellular effects of estrogen on neuronal function. *Critical Reviews in Neurobiology* 13:1-20.
Yandava, B.D., L.L. Billinhurst, and E.Y. Snyder
   1999   "Global" cell replacement is feasible via neural stem cell transplantation: Evidence from the dysmyelinated shiverer mouse brain. *Proceedings of the National Academy of Sciences of the United States of America* 96:7029-7034.
Zola-Morgan, S., and L.R. Squire
   1993   Neuroanatomy of memory. *Annual Review of Neuroscience* 16:547-563.

B
Homeostatic Processes in Brain Aging: The Role of Apoptosis, Inflammation, and Oxidative Stress in Regulating Healthy Neural Circuitry in the Aging Brain

Carl W. Cotman

INTRODUCTION

Research over the past several years has shown that the brain regions most vulnerable to mechanisms of inflammation, apoptosis, and free radical generation are those that serve primary functions in cognition. This must mean that mechanisms serving cognition and plasticity leave these circuits more vulnerable to injury and dysfunction. Curiously, many of the same molecules and molecular pathways can serve either beneficial or detrimental functions, depending on the exact cell, level of the factor, and acute versus chronic state. The mechanism can be local or can spread from the very local cellular microenvironment to cellular units and to entire systems. The progressive nature of the challenge faced can increasingly compromise cognitive functions.

During brain aging, the brain accumulates a series of insults and injuries and therefore must compensate through the activation of homeostatic mechanisms. Some of these mechanisms, however, once activated, may become part of degenerative cascades. Thus, the aging brain must accomplish homeostatic maintenance without the engagement of unregulated degenerative mechanisms. Over time, the compromising of circuitry integrity and function will take an inevitable toll on cognitive function. This paper presents the hypothesis that brain aging at a mechanistic level is resolvable into a series of distinct phases. These phases are associated with discrete molecular events that evolve into cascades, and, importantly, each phase may require different intervention strategies and certainly must be resolved in order to understand the overall aging process. The literature discussed in support of this hypothesis has been limited due to space constraints and thus some citations may have been unintentionally omitted.

BRAIN AGING, A MULTIPHASE PROCESS: INITIATION AND PROPAGATION PHASES

Several investigators have suggested that Alzheimer's disease may represent an accelerated decline of the normal processes of brain aging. Thus, for example, the normal aged brain appears to accumulate plaques and tangles. This hypothesis suggests that Alzheimer's disease then is simply a further progression in the accumulation of these hallmarks and that relative risk factors would determine the nature of when and how fast accumulation and cognitive decline occur. Hence, all individuals would be subject to the same basic mechanism, and only the rate constant would differ with aging. While this hypothesis is one possibility at a mechanistic level, it is imprecise and does not address the current body of data suggesting that Alzheimer's disease results from a series of mechanisms and cascades that, over time, drive progressive pathology.

I suggest that the aging process can be resolved into a series of distinct states (Figure B-1). Let us assume that under the arbitrary age of 120 it is

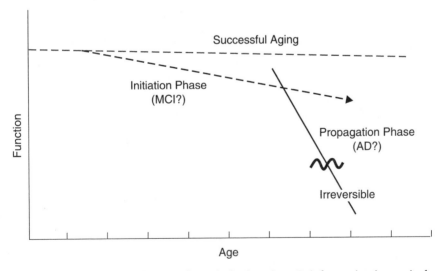

FIGURE B-1 Model for distinct phases in brain aging. It is becoming increasingly clear that at a mechanistic level, the primary driving mechanisms leading to progressive loss are multiphasic. The implication is that different therapeutic strategies will be needed at different phases of the processes.

possible to maintain normal brain function. This must be true, since some individuals maintain function for this period of time. Indeed, it appears that cognitive function can be preserved in some individuals even though some sensory functions may be compromised. Thus, as illustrated in Figure B-1, the successful aging line can be relatively flat.

Let us further postulate that the mechanism of decline can be divided into two general phases: initiation and propagation (Johnson et al., 1998). The initiation phase is distinct in terms of relative risk factors (e.g., *APOE* genotype) and protective factors. According to this hypothesis, the phase is relatively reversible and very amenable to interventions; it is relatively stable even though decline does occur. This idea is consistent with epidemiology data (e.g., Breitner, 1996) and histochemical data on factors affecting the accumulation of β-amyloid (see Johnson et al., 1998). For example, *APOE* at low levels of amyloid accumulation can determine the average age of decline onset. Once amyloid accumulation (or a similar process) reaches a certain level, however, the propagation phase is set in motion.

The propagation phase is distinct in that self-reinforcing molecular cascades are the net driving force; these cascades supersede contributing risk factors and accelerate pathogenesis. In terms of β-amyloid accumulation, this phase is largely independent of APOE-ε4, although it may have gender factors. Examples of possible autocatalytic cascades that could contribute to a propagation phase include the ability of amyloid to induce the amyloid precursor protein (APP) and chronic inflammation (see Cotman and Su, 1996). Such a propagation phase could be reversible up to a threshold point; however, once past this point, it may be irreversible.

This hypothetical model must also be considered in the context of the microenvironment. Thus, in the initiation phase, one would postulate that pathology is focused on vulnerable regions, but within those regions is largely confined to local domains, perhaps even individual cells. Subsequent transition/entry into the propagation phase results in the spread of pathology throughout the network. This propagation mechanism is unknown but may represent a breakdown of the local microenvironment. This is an important issue and is not addressed in the context of most current molecular mechanisms.

The progression of pathology is embodied in the Braak and Braak staging, in which the induction of tangles spreads through the limbic system network and is in essence the morphological equivalent of this set of events. Recently, my colleagues and I have established morphological evidence for transsynaptic propagation of neurofibrillary tangle pathology. We examined a series of neuropathologically staged cases and traced the temporal induction of AT8 and PHF staining in a well-established trisynaptic pathway: entorhinal stellate neurons, dentate gyrus granule cells, and CA4 pyramidal neurons. Cellular changes along this circuit appeared to initiate in the entorhinal cortex in early Alzheimer's disease and progress through the circuit as the disease progressed, suggestive of a transsynaptic mechanism of propagation. The stimulus/agent is, of course, unknown.

In summary, I suggest that a separation of mechanisms may occur in the evolution of Alzheimer's disease. These stages may parallel various clinical stages. The relatively flat progression has been referred to as successful aging, optimal aging, etc. The initiation phase may be similar to the phase called mild cognitive impairment. The propagation phase may be the entry into Alzheimer's disease and related dementias. Of course, the correlation between brain changes and functional state is challenging due in no small part to the reserves and functional plasticity of circuits, particularly in the successful aging and initiation phases. Thus, for example, it would be anticipated that changes that occur in the initiation phase are subclinical for many measures, even though from a mechanistic viewpoint these changes are signatures of progression.

The implication of this concept is that it suggests that different therapeutics will be necessary to abort or slow the mechanism, depending on the stage of progression. Thus the initiation phase may be amenable to such interventions as nonsteroidal anti-inflammatory drugs, estrogen, education, antioxidants, etc. The later propagation phase may be much less sensitive or even insensitive to such interventions, although there is evidence to suggest that antioxidants such as Vitamin E can modulate progression at this point.

THE INITIATION PHASE AND EARLY EVENTS IN A PATHOLOGICAL CASCADE

To study the initiation phase in vitro or in vivo, it is necessary to develop a model in which subthreshold insults occur that do not cause overt cell death but rather impair cellular function. An appropriate stimulus to promote cell dysfunction is $A\beta$, since this neurotoxic protein accumulates in the form of senile plaques in the aged human and canine brain. Exposing cell cultures to sufficient levels of $A\beta$ causes cell death in neurons and glia (see Cotman et al., 1999, for a review). Neurons die by initiating programmed cell death pathways, the up-regulation of pro-apoptotic proteins or the down-regulation of anti-apoptotic proteins (Paradis et al., 1996). To identify events associated with the initiation phase, we are now using subthreshold levels of $A\beta$ that do not cause overt neuronal death to determine the sequence of events that occur early in response to an injury. These events may be subtle indicators of neuron dysfunction that develops prior to the classic forms of pathology found in the aged brain, such as senile plaques, neurofibrillary tangles, and cell death. Once neurons are exposed to a potentially toxic stimulus, signal transduction pathways are activated that initiate a cascade of events leading to neuronal dysfunction. This hypothesis led us to examine the role of signal transduction pathways in neurons as early mediators of neuron dysfunction and subsequent death.

Signal Transduction Pathways May Be Compromised Much Sooner Than Degeneration Develops

One of the components that is critical in signal transduction is CREB (cyclic AMP response element binding protein), a molecule that mediates a plethora of responses involving gene transcription. Briefly, the pathway leading to the activation of CREB starts with an increase in Ca^{2+} or cAMP, which leads to the activation of calcium calmodulin-dependent (CAM) Kinase IV or cAMP-dependent protein kinase (protein kinase A). CAM Kinase IV or protein kinase A translocates into the nucleus and phosphorylates CREB, thereby activating this protein. Once CREB is phosphorylated, it can bind to cyclic AMP response element (CRE) in the promoter region of specific genes and increase transcription, leading to increased RNA and protein levels. One of these proteins is brain-derived neurotrophic factor (BDNF), which promotes neuron survival and plasticity (Cellerino et al., 1996; Galuske et al., 1996; Ma et al., 1998). As the actions of CREB become more elucidated, it is becoming apparent that CREB is functionally important for neuroplasticity (Ahn et al., 1999; Bailey et al., 1996; Glazewski et al., 1999; Schulz et al., 1999; Segal et al., 1998).

Recent data suggest that transgenic mice that do not express CREB or mice treated with antisense mRNA to CREB show impaired long-term potentiation, a physiological mechanism thought to underlie short-term memory (Glazewski et al., 1999; Schulz et al., 1999). A recent study also indicates that brains of humans diagnosed with Alzheimer's disease have decreased levels of phosphorylated CREB (pCREB) (Yamamoto-Sasaki et al., 1999), and it is hypothesized that this decline may have a role in memory decrements. While a direct mechanism or causal effect of declines in pCREB has not been established in normal aging in humans or animals, it is hypothesized that short-term memory deficits that occur as mild cognitive impairment in humans or as memory impairments in individual old canines may be a consequence of neuronal dysfunction associated with decreased phosphorylation of CREB signal transduction mechanisms or other transcription factors.

This leads to the question of whether a similar series of events occurs with sublethal exposures to Aβ, as would be expected in the early initiation phase. Depolarization of cells, as would occur in vivo with long-term potentiation, induces the phosphorylation of CREB. However, in the presence of subthreshold levels of Aβ, there is a significant reduction in pCREB (Tong et al., in press). One interpretation of these results is that transcriptional activation by CREB could be compromised in dysfunctional neurons prior to overt cell death. If the neuron can reverse dysfunction, such as a diminished CREB signaling pathway or an Aβ insult, then it can be returned to a functional state. Otherwise, apoptotic degenerative pathways may be initiated and the neuron removed from the system entirely.

Does the loss of pCREB regulation affect the encoding of proteins that are involved in neuroplasticity? The answer appears to be yes. CREB is involved with the transcription of BDNF, which is involved with learning and memory mechanisms, encoding long-term potentiation, cell health and survival, and protection from injury. In our culture model system, Aβ decreases depolarization-mediated induction of BDNF transcription (Tong et al., in press). Thus, subthreshold Aβ exposure can lead to some remarkable changes in neuron function, including decreased transcription of BDNF, a protein important for promoting neuron survival in the absence of any overt pathological change. In fact, BDNF is decreased in brains with Alzheimer's disease.

The proinflammatory cytokines are another illustration of the ability of the same molecule to support neuronal functions or contribute to dysfunction/degeneration. Experimentally, TNFα and IL-1β have been implicated in multiple examples of neurodegeneration (Feuerstein et al., 1998; Griffin et al., 1989; Martin et al., 1997). The engagement of these receptors can govern such diverse cellular responses as cellular proliferation, differentiation, and effector functions, or drive cells into apoptosis (Baker and Reddy, 1996, 1998). Therefore, the same signals that induce proliferation and differentiation can also induce cell death under different conditions, such as different activation states, developmental states, or cellular associations (Kang et al., 1992; Lenardo, 1991; Radvanyi et al., 1993). TNFα represents an excellent example of the pleiotrophic nature of these cytokines. TNFα can directly trigger apoptosis but has also been found to be neuroprotective in certain instances (Bruce et al., 1996). This difference in the response to TNFα may depend on the metabolic state of the cells and tissue being exposed to TNFα, because when TNFα is applied to a healthy brain, it typically does not induce neurodegeneration. However when TNFα is combined with an insult such as ischemia, TNF induces a robust increase in neuronal death (Rothwell and Hopkins, 1995).

In addition to having a direct effect on cellular physiology, TNFα has been shown to disrupt the signal transduction pathways induced by other physiological ligands, such as insulin (Peraldi et al., 1996; Paz et al., 1997). More recently, a new mechanism resulting in neurodegeneration involving TNFα has been proposed by Venters et al. (1999). They noted that in addition to an increase in TNFα during an inflammation in the central nervous system, there is also an increased expression of the hormone insulin-like growth factor (IGF-I). Activation of the IGF-I receptor on neurons is neuroprotective, inhibiting apoptosis (Dudek et al., 1997; Russell et al., 1998). Previous reports have shown that simply changing the ratio of IGF-I and TNFα can shift the balance between survival and neuronal death (Barone et al., 1997; Loddick et al., 1998). Venters et al. found that TNFα significantly reduces the ability of IGF-I to promote survival in cerebellar granule neurons. These investigators proceeded to show that TNFα inhibits the ability of IGF-I to initiate tyrosine phosphorylation of the insulin receptor substrate 2 (IRS-2), thereby blocking the activation of downstream PI3-kinase. Thus diseases of the central nervous system that have an inflammatory component involving TNFα, such as multiple sclerosis, AIDS-dementia complex, and Alzheimer's disease, may use intracellular cross-talk between TNFα and IGF-I receptors to inhibit survival signaling by IGF-I and perhaps other neurotrophic factors. Thus some molecules promote homeostasis by multiple mechanisms, and in diseases such as Alzheimer's disease, these mechanisms may be recruited into cascades that trigger disease progression.

In summary, neurons that experience pro-apoptotic insults appear to shut down key signal transduction pathways. At the single cell level, this is probably a wise strategy, because it potentially removes dysfunctional cells from the network. This would then, in turn, allow the fully functional cells to maintain brain function and possibly activate auxiliary use-dependent plasticity mechanisms (Figure B-2).

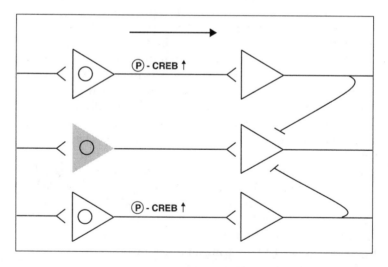

FIGURE B-2 Neurons subjected to sublethal pro-apoptotic insults may be deficient in their ability to regulate key signal transduction pathways serving functional plasticity. The presence of sublethal concentrations of B-amyloid results in an inability to phosphorylate CREB and thus control of essential transcriptional mechanisms. Thus these neurons are partially removed from the circuit (shaded cell).

Interventions During the Initiation Stage

What types of interventions could be implemented in the initiation stage of brain aging to promote successful aging? Clearly, the issue is to discover interventions that will in turn establish the validity of mechanistic predictions. One possibility is to regulate the expression of BDNF, a downstream product of the CREB signal transduction pathway. In general, behavioral modifications and exercise may have merit. Several years ago, we began to examine the possibility that simple behavioral interventions, such as voluntary running, could promote neuron function via increased expression of BDNF. The experimental design of these studies included providing rats with access to a running wheel and recording the distance traveled while allowing each animal to run voluntarily. Voluntary exercise increased BDNF mRNA in hippocampal areas after several hours (Oliff et al., 1998) or days (Neeper et al., 1995, 1996). Recently, we also have examined the possible involvement of CREB-mediated signal transduction and found that pCREB increased in response to the voluntary running paradigm during a period of seven days, while total levels of CREB were unchanged (Shen et al., in press). Recent data also suggest that exercise improves memory in aged humans (Binder et al., 1999; Grealy et al., 1999; Williams et al., 1997), but the cause of this improvement in cognition has not yet been determined. However, together these data suggest that exercise can be a driving force on plasticity mechanisms by enhancing the activation of factors that promote transcription of genes involved with neuron function and ultimate survival.

Other interventions may also increase the expression of BDNF and have functional consequences. Several studies have been examining this question; the work on environmental enrichment is particularly important (Kempermann et al., 1997, 1998). Three weeks of environmental enrichment significantly stimulated cell proliferation, BDNF expression and resistance to insults, and inhibited apoptotic cell death (Young et al., 1999). Proliferating cell nuclear antigen (PCNA) levels were increased and double-stranded DNA breaks (TUNEL) were decreased in the enrichment group relative to controls, suggesting that neurogenesis occurred in response to environmental enrichment. Furthermore, rats in the enriched environment were resistant to kainate-induced seizures, and neuron death in response to seizures was ameliorated (Young et al., 1999). Finally, the expression levels of BDNF were higher in the enrichment group relative to controls. Upstream of BDNF expression, the authors also showed that environmental enrichment increased the expression of CREB and pCREB, particularly in the proliferating zone of new neurons.

To summarize, many studies indicate that environmental enrichment and exercise, relatively modest interventions, can promote successful aging by modifying brain health at the single neuron level. Studies on behavioral interventions and brain aging are currently understudied in humans. Behavioral interventions in brain aging are popular at the community level, but clinical studies in patient populations are greatly lacking, as are mechanistic studies in animal models.

PROPAGATION PHASE: MANY INDUCERS OF APOPTOSIS ACCUMULATE IN THE AGING BRAIN

In the propagation phase, mechanisms including apoptosis, inflammation, and oxidation are activated either in combination or chronically beyond a certain level. Homeostatic balances are exceeded and dyshomeostasis prevails. This phase illustrates the importance of homeostasis in brain aging and the identification of mechanisms that can lead into dyshomeostasis. The discussion below illustrates the key principles. Apoptosis normally serves during development to remove excess cells, and in disease or injury it serves to destroy damaged cells. This is a well-accepted concept in all basic biological systems. With age, a variety of stimuli accumulate in the brain that may induce apoptotic pathways in neurons. In the aging and Alzheimer's-affected brain, β-amyloid, a 40-42 amino acid peptide, accumulates in the extracellular space as small deposits and senile plaques. Based on the observation that neurites surrounding β-amyloid deposits exhibit both sprouting and degenerative responses, we proposed that this peptide is not metabolically inert, but rather possesses biological activity. Our findings established two key principles: β-amyloid induces neurotoxicity in a conformation-specific manner, and apoptotic mechanisms underlie this toxicity (Cotman and Anderson, 1995; Anderson et al., 1995; Loo et al., 1995, 1993; Watt et al., 1994); these observations have since been confirmed by many others. Interestingly, prior to causing cell death, β-amyloid also induces the formation of dystrophic-like neurite morphology in cultured neurons (Pike et al., 1992; Fraser et al., 1994).

Oxidative insults also readily initiate apoptosis (Whittemore et al., 1994), and oxidative damage is known to occur in the aging and Alzheimer's-affected brain (Benzi and Moretti, 1995). Similarly, reductions in glucose metabolism have been suggested to contribute to neurodegeneration in Alzheimer's disease (Beal et al., 1993; Goto et al., 1993; Haxby and Rapoport, 1986; Hoyer et al., 1988; McGeer et al., 1986), and β-amyloid has been shown to exacerbate neurodegeneration in cultured neurons when glucose levels are reduced (Copani et al., 1991). Furthermore, excitotoxic damage can, under some conditions, initiate apoptosis, and many investigators have suggested that excitotoxic damage contributes to neurodegenerative diseases, including Alzheimer's disease (Dodd et al., 1994). Recent studies have also shown that glutamate transport proteins may be greatly reduced in the Alzheimer's-affected brain (Masliah et al., 1996; Simpson et al., 1994), which could exacerbate excitotoxic mechanisms. The profile of initiating factors strongly suggests that in the course of aging and age-related neurodegenerative disease, neurons are increasingly subjected to apoptosis inducers. In some cases, these factors may act synergistically. For example, neuronal apoptosis may be significantly potentiated by the addition of subthreshold doses of β-amyloid and either excitotoxic or oxidative insults (Dornan et al., 1993; Koh et al., 1990; Mattson et al., 1992; Pike et al., 1997). Finally, mitochondrial damage may contribute to apoptosis as an intracellular effector. Mitochondria are a major source of free radicals and the release of cytochrome c is a potent inducer of caspase activation. Indeed, this organelle may be a prime target of aging and thus a contributor to the apoptosis cascade.

Some genetic risk factors also increase the probability that cells will engage apoptotic mechanisms. Overexpression of presenilin (PS) 1 or 2 results in an increased susceptibility of cells to apoptotic insults. PS mutations sensitize neurons to apoptosis by trophic factor withdrawal, metabolic insults and β-amyloid (Deng et al., 1996; Wolozin et al., 1996; Kim et al., 1997). It has been suggested that PS mutations cause perturbed calcium release from the endoplasmic reticulum and increased levels of oxidative stress (Mattson et al., 1998). Indeed, introduction of PS-1 into oocytes results in enhanced release of intracellular calcium and this is further increased by the presence of a PS-1 mutation. The effect appears to be downstream from the inositol trisphosphate receptor, because inositol trisphosphate injected directly into the cell elicits the increased release. Thus, because calcium homeostasis contributes to apoptosis, these gene products increase the probably that neurons may degenerate via apoptosis. Thus, in patients carrying PS mutations, apoptosis is likely to be one of the mechanisms of neuronal degeneration. The amyloid precursor protein itself appears capable of initiating apoptosis. There is growing evidence that the amyloid precursor protein is a receptor resembling a polypeptide hormone receptor (Nishimoto et al., 1997). The cytoplasmic portion of the protein contains a G-protein activator sequence (H657-K676) and will bind and activate G_o. It has been suggested that the mutations result in a constitutively active G_o and that this causes apoptosis (Nishimoto et al., 1997; Yamatsuji et al., 1996).

Clearly then, there is ample potential for the induction of apoptosis mechanisms in the aging and Alzheimer's-affected brain. In this context, it is essential to determine if such pathways are activated in the Alzheimer's-affected brain. Indeed, a growing body of evidence supports this hypothesis (see Cotman et al., 1999).

In general, it appears as if brain aging acute phase responses often become chronic and escape the local microenvironment. The same mechanisms that are normally adaptive can become dysfunctional. This is "dysfunctional plasticity," in which the same adaptive mechanisms turn against the system as overcompensation evolves, safety margins decline, and redundancy is lost.

Multiple-level cascades can shift the balance between beneficial and nonbeneficial functions: The significance of cellular change to cognitive function evolves in a hierarchy from the cell, to cellular units, to systems.

• Each participating brain region in an overall system is selectively vulnerable to select genetic and/or environmental/disease-related conditions.
• Dysfunction in one part of the system can compromise the entire connectionist network.
• Dyshomeostasis is encoded into the network and alters input/output profiles, which may be optimal for the residual system, but the system now operates at another state function. Systems homeostasis/plasticity is understudied in aging, and that which is represented is largely limited to rodents.
• Progressively more network plasticity and more good cells are required to maintain even normal baseline functions. This further weakens the linkages. One process affects the others.

Inflammatory Mechanisms May Convert a Precarious State Into Net Degeneration

Acute injury initiates inflammatory mechanisms. Inflammatory mechanisms include the activation of complement pathways that lead to cell lysis and the up-regulation of death receptors and their respective ligands. These death receptors in the immune system serve to maintain homeostasis through selective cell death by way of apoptosis. In the brain, acute inflammatory responses are part of the natural repair process, but chronic inflammation probably drives degeneration, much like a chronic infection. Thus, inflammatory mechanisms are another example of the delicate balance. Clearly, inflammatory mechanisms suppress the initiation phase as anti-inflammatory medications delay the age of onset for Alzheimer's disease. It is, of course, unknown at the present time whether the same interventions will be effective during the propagation phase, but there are strong arguments to indicate they will probably be ineffective. Inflammation and beneficial actions have also been dramatically brought to the forefront by the discovery that antibodies developed against amyloid can activate the immune system to cause the remove of senile plaques (Schenk et al., 1999). Thus the balance of immune activity in the nervous system is highly critical.

Some age-related risk factors such as $A\beta$, oxidative damage, and imbalances in glutamate may contribute to the emergence of inflammation and place cells at further risk for degeneration. Recent evidence suggests that reactive oxygen intermediates (ROIs) are potent inducers of FasL and that antioxidants suppress this transcriptional dependent process. Inhibition of FasL expression appears associated with decreased binding of nuclear factor NF-kB, an important redox-controlled transcription factor (Bauer et al., 1998). In response to oxidative stress, there is an increase in FasL expression on microglia cells. Importantly, compared with classical mediators of microglia activation (e.g., TNFα, LPS), oxidative stress was the most potent. TNFα can render microglia sensitive to FasL apoptosis by inducing Fas expression and down-regulation of Bcl-2 and Bcl-xL (Spanaus et al., 1998). Further, hypoxia followed by re-oxygenation resulted in increased FasL expression (Vogt et al., 1998). Because the temporal and spatial patterns of microglia activation in injuries such as hypoxia coincides with the onset of DNA degradation and apoptosis in regions of selective neuronal loss, it has been suggested that microglia play a possible role in apoptosis.

Other risk factors can also induce FasL. In the Alzheimer's-affected brain, there is a reduction in the glutamate transporter (Masliah et al., 1996) that may contribute to neurodegeneration due to additional activation of glutamate receptors. Activation of NMDA receptors may also cause an increase in FasL. After a single injection of NMDA, there is an increase in FasL that begins after about 10 days and persists for up to 5 months. This increase may participate in long-term degeneration as part of a mechanism in the balance between repair and synaptic turnover/remodeling (Shin et al., 1998).

In summary, the gradual age-dependent increase of cytokines and their receptors capable of inducing apoptosis in the central nervous system could place neurons at increased risk for degeneration. It is possible that microglia and other cells in the brain also participate in the production of death ligands and thereby enhance the risk. Thus either autocrine or paracrine mechanisms may become active. Figure B-3 summarizes a model of the possible mechanism. At present a detailed study on the aging and Alzheimer's-affected brain has not been conducted, nor in fact has a detailed study at the anatomical level been reported in animal models. The development of many new reagents and the continued articulation of the mechanisms of Fas/caspase regulation provide a window of opportunity for the pursuit of this research direction.

Oxidative Stress is a Major Risk Factor for Brain Aging

Oxidative stress is a candidate for causing neuron dysfunction through a molecular cascade (Figure B-4). Oxidative stress is problematic for a number of reasons. Oxidation of proteins and enzymes within cells can interfere with their normal function (Stadtman, 1992). Free radicals can also damage DNA, and a 50 percent increase in DNA oxidative damage has been reported in the human brain (Lyras et al., 1997; Gabbita et al., 1998; Mecocci et al., 1994; Lovell et al., 1999). Indeed, extensive DNA damage appears to accumulate with age and is particularly prominent in the aged dog brain and in humans (Su et al., 1997; Anderson et al., in press). Lipids are also vulnerable to oxidative stress and the levels of lipid peroxidation are elevated in the human brain, which in turn may induce membrane disturbances and loss of homeostasis within cells (Balazs and Leon, 1994; Palmer and Burns, 1994). In fact,

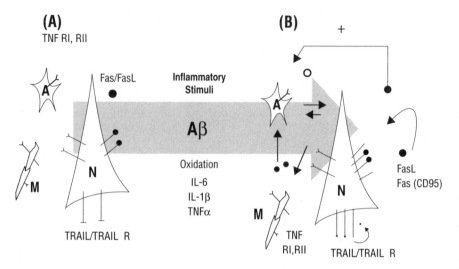

FIGURE B-3 The immune responses in the brain are a critical part of homeostasis but when chronically activated may contribute to the evolution of brain pathology. Neurons and glia express receptors and ligands in the TNF superfamily (A). In the presence of inflammatory stimuli such as Aβ, oxidation and select cytokines would be predicted to be up-regulated (B) and thus would make cells at risk for activating pro-apoptotic mechanisms similar to that reported in the aging immune system.

one lipid peroxidation product, 4-hydroxynonenal (HNE), is elevated in the brains and cerebrospinal fluids of cases of Alzheimer's disease (Lovell et al., 1997; Markesbery and Lovell, 1998), is toxic in vitro and in vivo, and impairs visuospatial memory in rats at physiological levels (Bruce-Keller et al., 1998). Isoprostane, a chemically stable peroxidation product of arachidonic acid, increases as well and is used as a marker for the extent of lipid peroxidation in vivo. In particular, Praticao et al. (1998) demonstrated that isoprostanes were elevated in the brains and cerebrospinal fluids of patients with Alzheimer's disease.

Oxidative stress can also lead to the misprocessing of APP to form amyloidogenic products. Several in vitro experiments suggest that energy-related metabolic stress leads to reduced levels of secreted APP mediated by β-secretase and in fact, may lead to increased production of amyloidogenic fragments (Gabuzda et al., 1994; Gasparini et al., 1997; Multhaup et al., 1997). Oxidative stress increases the production of both APP and β-amyloid (Frederikse et al., 1996). β-amyloid itself can lead to the generation of reactive oxygen species (ROS), superoxide radicals, hydroxynonenal (HNE), and membrane lipid peroxidation (Mark et al., 1997; Behl et al., 1992; Pereira et

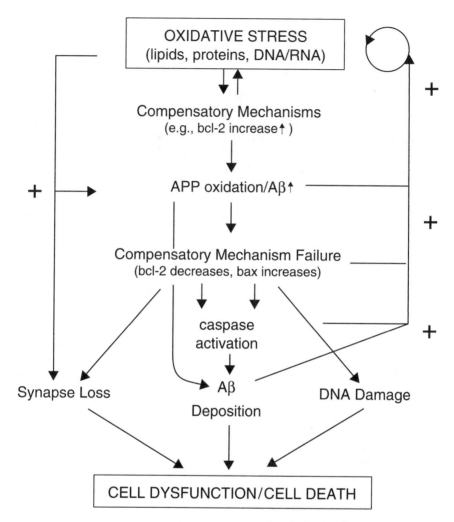

FIGURE B-4 Oxidative stress is an early and continued event in brain aging, leading to increases in expression of proteins involved with promoting cell survival (bcl-2). Oxidation causes damage to lipids, proteins, and DNA/RNA. Oxidative stress also induces the expression of APP and can contribute to the misprocessing of APP, leading to generation of amyloidogenic fragments. The production of Aβ fragments may lead to a loss of compensatory ability (decreased bcl-2, increased bax). All of these factors in turn contribute to more Aβ deposition, possibly synapse loss, and DNA damage. Ultimately the system converges and results in neuron dysfunction and/or in some neurons' death. At several points in this proposed framework, positive feedback loops exist such that the deposition of Aβ exacerbates oxidative stress and oxidative stress itself results in decreased levels of bcl-2 and increased levels of bax.

al., 1999; McDonald et al., 1997). There is also evidence that β-amyloid can itself be oxidized resulting in enhanced aggregation (Dyrks et al., 1992).

The accumulation of amyloidogenic fragments, in turn, accelerates existing molecular cascades associated with oxidative stress. β-amyloid also promotes cell dysfunction by increasing the expression levels of bax, decreasing levels of bcl-2 (Paradis et al., 1996), and, in many systems, activating caspases. Thus, decreases in bcl-2 from oxidative stress and Aβ insults can leave cells particularly vulnerable to oxidative stress (Hochman et al., 1998). Finally, activation of caspases cleaves APP, producing additional β-amyloid fragments (Gervais et al., 1999; Barnes et al., 1998; LeBlanc et al., 1999). These are exciting leads, as they suggest alternative mechanisms for the production of β-amyloid.

Oxidative stress may lead to an initial increase in cellular compensatory mechanisms mediated by the expression of pro- and anti-apoptotic proteins. One family of proteins, the bcl-2 family, serves as an intracellular checkpoint and determines whether or not a cell engages in an apoptotic program (Oltvai et al., 1993). Bcl-2 can be inactivated by the formation of heterodimers with a second highly homologous protein, bax. Bax promotes apoptotic cell death (Oltvai et al., 1993; Reed, 1994). Thus, the balance between levels of bcl-2 and bax can serve as an indicator of cellular state. Ultimately, we hypothesize, this compensatory mechanism is inadequate and eventually leads to decreased bcl-2 levels with a corresponding increase in bax, shifting the system to a neurodegenerative status. Exposing neuronal or endothelial cells to oxidative stress decreases levels of bcl-2 and increases the expression levels of bax (Longoni et al., 1999; Maroto and Perez-Polo, 1997).

Thus, we can hypothesize that oxidative stress causes a cascade of events in which there are multiple positive feedback loops that amplify the cascade. For example: (1) oxidative damage within mitochondria leads to further free radical production, (2) increased oxidation leads to additional Aβ, which in turn generates additional APP, (3) Aβ and accumulating oxidative damage activates caspases, which in turn cleaves APP and generates additional Aβ and oxidative damage, and (4) progressive oxidative damage and Aβ decreases bcl-2, leaving neurons more vulnerable to oxidative damage and other insults. Common to each of these events is oxidative damage. Thus, an antioxidant intervention should, in principle, suppress the progression of brain pathology at one or more steps in the cascade. This is consistent with a vast and somewhat unappreciated literature on the efficacy of antioxidants in the aging process.

Antioxidants Are Effective Interventions

There is a growing body of literature indicating that administration of antioxidants to aged animals and individuals can have dramatic effects on

TABLE B-1 Antioxidant Interventions and Improvements in Cognitive Function—A Summary of the Existing Literature

Antioxidant	Subjects	Duration of Study	Cognition
PBN	Gerbils	14 days	Improved spatial memory in radial arm maze
Blueberry spinach strawberry	19-month-old rats	8 weeks	Improved one-trial learning in the water maze Improved vitamin E levels in the hippocampus
PBN vitamin E	24-month-old rats	4-5 months	Improved memory retention on spatial memory task Improved learning of a spatial memory task
Strawberry spinach vitamin E	6-month-old rats	8 months	Enhanced retention in a spatial water maze task
PBN	24-month-old rats	9.5 months	Improved memory retention on spatial memory task Faster acquisition of a one-way activate avoidance task Improved learning of a spatial memory task
PBN	Senescence-accelerated mice	12 months	Significantly lengthened life span
Vitamin E	Rats receiving intraventricular Aβ	7 days	Reduced spatial memory impairments induced by Aβ
Vitamin E	Patients with Alzheimer's disease	2 years	Significantly delayed institutionalization

behavior and age-related brain oxidative status. Furthermore, in normal aging, reducing oxidative stress through the use of nutritional supplements including vitamin E is beneficial for cognition and immune system function (Fryer, 1998; Reidel and Jorissen, 1998; Blumberg and Halpner, 1999; Meydani et al., 1995; Perrig et al., 1997). Table B-1 summarizes the striking efficacy of antioxidant interventions.

Antioxidants can also significantly aid the human brain. Over 4 years ago, the inclusion of Vitamin E into a clinical trial of patients with mild to moderate Alzheimer's disease resulted in the finding that Vitamin E supplements given to patients significantly delayed the time to institutionalization (Sano et al., 1997). Antioxidants also enhance cognition in rat models, and antioxidant application or diet supplementation can improve spatial memory (Joseph et al., 1999; Socci et al., 1995). Currently, an Alzheimer's Disease Cooperative Study using a randomized, double-blind, placebo-controlled trial is evaluating the safety and efficacy of 2,000 IU of Vitamin E to delay the clinical progression of elderly populations from mild cognitive impairment to Alzheimer's disease. Thus, there is strong rationale for the further evaluation of this intervention in an aging model in which the time interval between cognitive assessment and biochemical/neuroanatomical study can be tightly controlled. We need to evaluate dietary interventions using both short-term and long-term clinical trials.

APOPTOSIS CHECKPOINT CASCADE IN THE ALZHEIMER'S-AFFECTED BRAIN: THE SEARCH FOR HOMEOSTASIS

The presence of a mechanism to hold degeneration in check may provide an explanation for one of the seeming controversies in the Alzheimer's disease literature. As we have described, TUNEL labeling provides evidence for active apoptosis in a large subset of neurons in the Alzheimer's-affected brain. However, many more Alzheimer's-affected neurons exhibit evidence for DNA damage in the absence of morphological changes, indicative of terminal apoptosis, for example, the formation of nuclear apoptotic bodies. In classical apoptosis, cells die within hours or days of the initial insult. If TUNEL labeling in the Alzheimer's-affected brain reflected the true initiation of classical apoptosis, then it follows that most TUNEL-positive neurons would die in a few days. However, in many mild cases of Alzheimer's disease (MMSE above 16), over 50 percent of the neurons exhibit TUNEL labeling. Thus, most neurons should have degenerated within a few days if apoptosis is actively in progress in these cells, a prediction that is inconsistent with the progression of neuronal loss in Alzheimer's disease. In addition, most TUNEL-positive neurons do not exhibit morphological markers of apoptosis, such as nuclear apoptotic bodies or other key molecular factors (Su et al., 1994; Lucassen et al., 1997) This apparent inconsistency has led some to the conclusion that neurons in the Alzheimer's-affected brain die primarily by necrosis (Stadelmann et al., 1998).

On the other hand, it is possible that neurons have developed a series of counteractive measures to repair damage and delay death, in other words, a kind of molecular counterattack in order to minimize unnecessary cell loss. This concept of an apoptosis checkpoint cascade may help to understand an apparent puzzle in the neuronal apoptosis literature: the prolonged presence of indices of DNA damage and apoptotic regulatory protein expression may be a result of a counteractive strategy that neurons mobilize to hold apoptosis in check, delay death, and attempt repair. In this context, it is possible that cell cycle proteins could contribute to cellular repair in neurons. Repair of DNA damage may be a particularly key example of such a mechanism. For example, many neurons in vulnerable regions of the Alzheimer's-affected brain show an up-regulation of GADD45, a protein that is associated with DNA checkpoint repair at the G1 transition. Alzheimer's-affected neurons that express GADD45 often also show DNA damage and increased levels of Bcl-2. In addition, in support of a role in promoting cell survival, GADD45 transfected cells show improved survival after DNA damage (Torp et al., 1998). Thus, Bcl-2, GADD45, and other protective molecules such as PCNA could serve to help repair DNA damage and assist in neuronal survival. Similarly, p16, p21, and other negative regulators of the cell cycle could participate in delaying degeneration. That is, many checkpoints in the cell death pathway may exist and perhaps prevent the unnecessary loss of irreplaceable cells. This possibility may make the study of signal transduction pathways particularly critical, because it may provide an opportunity for early interventions.

Taken together, this hypothesis may suggest that neurons could activate an "apoptosis checkpoint cascade," in which injured neurons may regulate the activation of pro-apoptotic proteins such as bax with anti-apoptotic proteins such as Bcl-2. In addition, it can be hypothesized that damaged neurons could activate the cell cycle and perhaps employ checkpoint molecules in a similar pro- and anti-apoptotic regulation point (Figure B-5).

CHANGES IN CYTOKINES AND THEIR RECEPTORS IN LYMPHOCYTES OCCUR IN AGING AND, SURPRISINGLY, MANY OF THE MOLECULAR PROFILES IN THE AGING BRAIN ARE SIMILAR TO THESE AND TO THE IMMUNE SYSTEM

Normal aging is associated with a decrease in the proportion of lymphocytes in the blood (lymphopenia) and a progressive decline in T-cell function, although the underlying mechanisms that cause these changes are largely unknown (Miller, 1996; Nagel et al., 1988; Proust et al., 1987; Thoman and Weigle, 1989). The reductions in T-cell functions include a decrease in response to mitogens and soluble antigens, as well as defects in signal transduction. The initial investigations in this area indicated that lymphocytes from elderly individuals were significantly more sensitive to activation-induced apoptosis (Phelouzat et al., 1996; Herndon et al., 1997). The relationships between increased cytokine expression, sensitivity to apoptosis, and lymphopenia led Gupta and colleagues to investigate whether there is an increased expression of death receptors and associated adapter and initiator proteins. An increased expression of Fas and FasL was accompanied by a decrease in Bcl-2 expression in memory cells of both CD4+ and CD8+ T-cells from aged versus younger individuals. In addition, FasL caused an increased

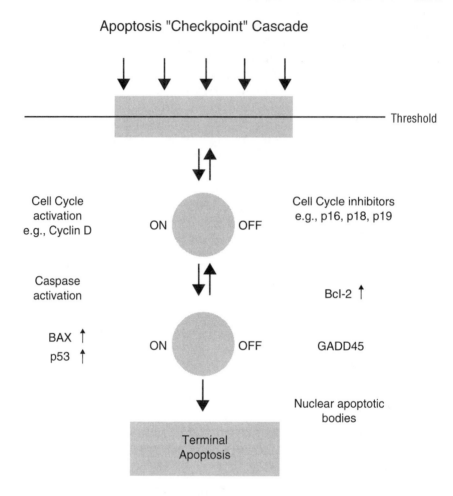

FIGURE B-5 Neurons as nondividing cells seem to delay or check the activation of apoptosis processes in order to attempt repair.

proportion of both T-cell subsets from older individuals to undergo apoptosis, indicating that the death receptors are functional in the aging immune system (Aggarwal and Gupta, 1998). In a follow-up study, two additional members of the Fas family of receptors, TNFRI and TNFRII, were examined in lymphocytes from aged individuals (Aggarwal et al., 1999). Once again, the investigators found increased sensitivity to undergo apoptosis, this time induced by TNFα. Moreover, they found that the TNFRI was expressed at elevated levels in aged lymphocytes and that the TNFRII was expressed at lower levels than in young individuals. Coinciding with the changes in the TNFRs was an increase in TNFR-associated death domain protein (TRADD) and a decrease in TNFR-associated factor 2 (TRAF-2). These changes mirror those previously reported by Ware et al. (1991) following T-cell activation. However, in the case of lymphocytes from aged individuals, there was no increase in the expression of activation antigens, thus indicating that the T-cells were not in an activated state but rather reflect changes associated with an aging immune system. The potential importance of the change in the ratio of the two TNF receptors becomes obvious when one considers that the TNFRI contains a death domain and, when oligomerized by TNFα binding, recruits TRADD and FADD, resulting in the activation one of the initiator caspases, caspase-8. The TNFRII and TRAF-2 are involved in activation of NFkB and JNK, which are believed to mediate the anti-apoptotic effects of TNFα (Baker and Reddy, 1996, 1998). Based on these observations, Gupta and colleagues have proposed that the cellular and subcellular basis of this age-related immunosenescence appears to at least partially involve increases in receptors linked with apoptosis and decreases in related compensatory receptors (Aggarwal and Gupta, 1998, 1999; Aggarwal et al., 1999).

Age-related changes may extend to other organs and may be displayed in the ratio of gene expression patterns. The recent introduction of gene chip technology into the field may have particular application to the field of aging. Thus, for example, the gene expression profile of aging in muscle tissue and the influence of caloric restriction have been described (Lee et al., 1999). In essence, using high-density oligonucleotide arrays representing 6,347 genes, it was shown that aging resulted in a differential gene expression pattern that reflected increased cellular stress and lower expression of metabolic and biosynthetic genes. Some of these, such as DNA repair enzymes, are the same as those induced in the nervous system with age and degeneration. An example of an up-regulated gene found in the muscle is GADD45, which as discussed above, we have found is also induced in Alzheimer's disease.

Importantly, caloric restriction, which is the only really true intervention known to retard aging in mammals, almost completely prevented the gene expression pattern changes that occur with aging. This is a technology that should find particular use in the study of brain aging and cognition but will probably be difficult to get funded through peer review panels because it will be considered just a "fishing expedition." These gene patterns summarize in one experiment the literature for the past 10 years of individual gene expression patterns. These expression patterns can be envisioned in essence as a fingerprint of homeostasis versus dyshomeostasis. In fact, this pattern of gene expression can be looked at as a view of the cells to engage homeostasis and plasticity mechanisms to compensate for age-related change.

CELLULAR PLASTICITY MECHANISMS AND
THE MAINTENANCE OF HOMEOSTASIS

As cells degenerate and their numbers are reduced in circuitry, other mechanisms become engaged at a cell and systems level beyond those of the molecular level. Examples include the sprouting of new synapses in response to nearby cell loss and the sprouting of dendrites in neighboring cells. In addition, whole networks respond in terms of altered processing using somewhat redundant, but maybe initially suboptimal strategies. These, oftentimes, can increase the time for cognitive processing, but will still accomplish the task. There is also a growing body of literature indicating that, in the course of brain aging, more of the brain has to be involved in a task that would normally require only minimal activation of circuits; thus, the circuits are working much harder to accomplish the same task. This would indicate that use-dependent change and practice effects, together with appropriate pharmaceuticals, might have a rational basis for cognitive rehabilitation.

STRATEGIES AND SOLUTIONS FOR THE FUTURE

In conclusion, there are several principles that appear to be evolving in the field that are in need of additional testing:

- Brain aging is not a linear process; the aging process passes through phases.
- The initiation phase can compromise neuronal function and is probably reversible as it represents functional homeostasis.
- Interventions include antioxidants, use-dependent plasticity (behavioral/physical/cognitive stimulation), regulation of inflammation, estrogen replacement therapy, etc., and are most effective in this phase.
- The propagation phase is initiated through a series of molecular cascades driven by accumulating failures and compensation mechanisms and is less readily reversible.
- Interventions may be phase-dependent, and effective interventions at one phase may be inappropriate/inadequate at others.

Strategies must and can be developed to identify weak molecular linkages and to assist cells in correcting them prior to irreversible losses and the development of cascades.

- There is a clear significant and major gap in supported research in the essential hierarchical areas, and circuit-based analyses at a systems level are needed.
- Transgenic animals offer great promise, but there is a great need for

aged animals and standard behavioral protocols. Other animal models should be supported.

- The single-variable approach inherent in most molecular studies at present is too limited; there is a great need to explore complex interactions at a molecular level.
- Many behavioral theories, particularly in the practice of neuropsychology, lack solid mechanistic foundations and quantitative support, handicapping the growth of the field.
- There is, in general, a gap between cognitive research and molecular mechanistic studies in brain aging. The National Institute on Aging should be encouraged continually to stimulate innovative approaches.

In summary, the key may very well be to create a shift in the intellectual environment in brain aging and cognition as well as pursue the leads already defined.

REFERENCES

Aggarwal, S., S. Gollapudi, and S. Gupta
    1999   Increased TNF-alpha-induced apoptosis in lymphocytes from aged humans: Changes in TNF-alpha receptor expression and activation of caspases. *Journal of Immunology* 162(4):2154-2161.
Aggarwal, S., and S. Gupta
    1998   Increased apoptosis of T cell subsets in aging humans: Altered expression of fas (CD95), fas ligand, Bcl-2, and bax. *Journal of Immunology* 160(4):1627-1637.
    1999   Increased activity of caspase 3 and caspase 8 in anti-fas-induced apoptosis in lymphocytes from ageing humans. *Clinical and Experimental Immunology* 117(2):285-290.
Ahn, S., et al.
    1999   A late phase of cerebellar long-term depression requires activation of CaMKIV and CREB. *Neuron* 23(3):559-568.
Anderson, A.J., C.J. Pike, and C.W. Cotman
    1995   Differential induction of immediate early gene proteins in cultured neurons by beta-amyloid (A beta): Association of c-jun with a beta-induced apoptosis. *Journal of Neurochemistry* 65(4):1487-1498.
Anderson, A.J., W.W. Ruehl, L.K. Fleischmann, K. Stenstrom, T.L. Entriken, and B.J. Cummings
    In   DNA damage is correlated with a beta deposition and unrelated to cytoskeletal neu-
    press   ropathology in the canine model of Alzheimer's disease. *Progress in Neuro-Pharmacology and Biological Psychiatry* 24.
Azizeh, B., F.L. Van Muiswinkel, D.H. Cribbs, A.J. Tenner, and C.W. Cotman
    1999   Non-filbrillar β-amyloid: Priming the respiratory burst of rat microglial cells and human monocytes. *Neurobiology of Aging* (submitted).
Bailey, C.H., et al.
    1996   Toward a molecular definition of long-term memory storage. *Proceedings of the National Academy of Sciences of the United States of America* 93(24):13445-13452.
Baker, S.J., and E.P. Reddy
    1996   Transducers of life and death: TNF receptor superfamily and associated proteins. *Oncogene* 12(1):1-9.

1998   Modulation of life and death by the TNF receptor superfamily. *Oncogene* 17(25):
        261-270.

Balazs, L., and M. Leon
1994   Evidence of an oxidative challenge in the Alzheimer's disease brain. *Neurochemical
        Research* 19(9):1131-1137.

Barnes, N.Y., L. Li, K. Yoshikawa, L.M. Schwartz, R.W. Oppenheim, and C.E. Milligram
1998   Increased production of amyloid precursor protein provides a substrate for caspase-
        3 cleavage in dying motoneurons. *Journal of Neuroscience* 18(15):5869-5880.

Barone, F.C., et al.
1997   Tumor necrosis factor-alpha. A mediator of focal ischemic brain injury. *Stroke*
        28(6):1233-1244.

Bauer, M.K.A., et al.
1998   Role of reactive oxygen intermediates in activation-induced CD95 (APO-1/fas) ligand
        expression. *Journal of Biological Chemistry* 273(14):8048-8055.

Beal, M.F., B.T. Hyman, and W. Koroshetz
1993   Do deficits in mitochendrial energy metabolism underlie the pathology of
        neurodegenerative diseases? *Trends in Neurosciences* 16(4):178-184.

Behl, C., J. Davis, G.M. Cole, and D. Schubert
1992   Vitamin E protects nerve cells from amyloid-beta protein toxicity. *Biochemical and
        Biophysical Research Communications* 186:944-950.

Benzi, G., and A. Moretti
1995   Are reactive oxygen species involved in Alzheimer's disease? *Neurobiology of Aging*
        16(4):661-674.

Binder, E.F., et al.
1999   The relation between psychometric test performance and physical performance in
        older adults. *Journal of Gerontology. Series A, Biological Sciences and Medical Sciences*
        54(8):M428-M432.

Blumberg, J., and A. Halpner
1999   Antioxidant status and function: Relationships to aging and exercise. Pp. 251-275 in
        Antioxidant Status, Diet, Nutrition and Health, A. Papas, ed. New York: CRC Press
        LLC.

Breitner, J.C.S.
1996   Inflammatory processes and anti-inflammatory drugs in Alzheimer's Disease: A cur-
        rent appraisal. *Neurobiology of Aging* 17:789-794.

Bruce, A.J., et al.
1996   Altered neuronal and microglial responses to excitotoxic and ischemic brain injury
        in mice lacking TNF receptors. *Nature Medicine* 2(7):788-794.

Bruce-Keller, A.J., Y.-J. Li, M.A. Lovell, P.J. Kraemer, D.S. Gary, R.R. Brown, W.R. Markesbery,
and M.P. Mattson
1998   4-hydroxynonenal, a product of lipid peroxidation, damages cholinergic neurons
        and impairs visuospatial memory in rats. *Journal of Neuropathology and Experimen-
        tal Neurology* 57(3):257-267.

Cellerino, A., et al.
1996   The action of neurotrophins in the development and plasticity of the visual cortex.
        Progress in Neurobiology 49(1):53-71. [Published erratum appears in *Progress in Neu-
        robiology* 50(2-3):333].

Copani, A., J.-Y. Koh, and C.W. Cotman
1991   ß-amyloid increases neuronal susceptibility to injury by glucose deprivation.
        NeuroReport 2(12):763-765.

Cotman, C.W., and A.J. Anderson
1995   A potential role for apoptosis in neurodegeneration and Alzheimer's disease. *Molecular Neurobiology* 10(1):19-45.
Cotman, C.W., K.J. Ivins, and A.J. Anderson
1999   Apoptosis in Alzheimer disease. Chapter 23 in *Alzheimer Disease*, 2nd ed., R.D. Terry, R. Katzman, K.L. Bick, and S.S. Sisodia, eds. Philadelphia: Lippincott, Williams & Wilkins.
Cotman, C.W., and J.H. Su
1996   Mechanisms of neuronal death in Alzheimer's disease. *Brain Pathology* 6:493-506.
Deng, G., J. Su, and C.W. Cotman
1996   Gene expression of Alzheimer's associated presenilin-2 in the frontal cortex of Alzheimer and aged control brain. *FEBS Letters* 3994:17-20.
Dodd, P.R., H.L. Scott, and R.I. Westphalen
1994   Excitotoxic mechanisms in the pathogenesis of dementia. *Neurochemistry International* 25(3):203-219.
Dornan, W.A., et al.
1993   Bilateral injections of ßA(25-35)+IBO into the hippocampus disrupts acquisition of spatial learning in the rat. *NeuroReport* 5:165-168.
Dudek, H., et al.
1997   Regulation of neuronal survival by the serine-threonine protein kinase akt. *Science* 275(5300):661-665.
Dyrks, T., E. Dyrks, T. Hartmann, C. Masters, and K. Beyreuther
1992   Amyloidogenicity of beta A4 and beta A4-bearing amyloid protein precursor fragments by metal-catalyzed oxidation. *Journal of Biological Chemistry* 267(25):18210-18217.
Feuerstein, G.Z., X. Wang, and F.C. Barone
1998   The role of cytokines in the neuropathology of stroke and neurotrauma. *Neuroimmunomodulation* 5(3-4):143-159.
Fraser, P.E., L. Levesque, and D.R. McLachlan
1994   Alzheimer Aß amyloid forms an inhibitory neuronal substrate. *Journal of Neurochemistry* 62(3):1227-1230.
Frederikse, P.H., D. Garland, J.S. Zigler, and J. Piatigorsky
1996   Oxidative stress increases production of β-amyloid precursor protein and b-amyloid (Aβ) in mammalian lenses, and Aβ has toxic effects on lens epithelial cells. *Journal of Biological Chemistry* 271(17):10169-10174.
Fryer, M.J.
1998   Vitamin E status and neurodegenerative disease. *Nutritional Neuroscience* 1:327-351.
Gabbita, S.P., M.A. Lovell, and W.R. Markesbery
1998   Increased nuclear DNA oxidation in the brain in Alzheimer's disease. *Journal of Neurochemistry* 71:2034-2040.
Gabuzda, D., J. Busciglio, L.B. Chen, P. Matsudaira, and B.A. Yankner
1994   Inhibition of energy metabolism alters the processing of amyloid precursor protein and induces a potentially amyloidogenic derivative. *Journal of Biological Chemistry* 269(18):13623-13628.
Galuske, R.A., et al.
1996   Brain-derived neurotrophic factor reversed experience-dependent synaptic modifications in kitten visual cortex. *European Journal of Neuroscience* 8(7): 1554-1559.
Gasparini, L., M. Racchi, L. Benussi, D. Curti, G. Binetti, A. Bianchetti, M. Trabucchi, and S. Govoni
1997   Effect energy shortage and oxidative stress on amyloid precursor protein metabolism in COS cells. *Neuroscience Letters* 231:113-117.

Gervais, F.G., et al.
1999	Involvement of caspases in proteolytic cleavage of Alzheimer's amyloid-beta precursor protein and amyloidogenic a beta peptide formation. *Cell* 97(3):395-406.
Glazewski, S., et al.
1999	Impaired experience-dependent plasticity in barrel cortex of mice lacking the alpha and delta isoforms of CREB. *Cerebral Cortex* 9(3):249-256.
Goto, I., et al.
1993	Positron emission tomographic (PET) studies in dementia. *Journal of the Neurological Sciences* 114(1):1-6.
Grealy, M.A., et al.
1999	Improving cognitive function after brain injury: The use of exercise and virtual reality. *Archives of Physical Medicine and Rehabilitation* 80(6):661-667.
Griffin, W.S., et al.
1989	Brain interleukin 1 and S-100 immunoreactivity are elevated in Down syndrome and Alzheimer disease. *Proceedings of the National Academy of Sciences of the United States of America* 86:7611-7615.
Haxby, J.V., and S.I. Rapoport
1986	Abnormalities of regional brain metabolism in Alzheimer's disease and their relation to functional impairment. *Progress in Neuro-Psychopharmacology and Biological Psychiatry* 10(3-5):427-438.
Herndon, F.J., H.C. Hsu, and J.D. Mountz
1997	Increased apoptosis of CD45RO- T cells with aging. *Mechanisms of Ageing and Development* 94(1-3):123-134.
Hochman, A., et al.
1998	Enhanced oxidative stress and altered antioxidants in brains of bcl-2-deficient mice. *Journal of Neurochemistry* 71(2):741-748.
Hoyer, S., K. Oesterreich, and O. Wagner
1988	Glucose metabolism as the site of the primary abnormality in early-onset dementia of Alzheimer type. *Journal of Neurology* 235:143-148.
Johnson, J.K., R. McCleary, M.H. Oshita, and C.W. Cotman
1998	Initiation and propagation stages of beta-amyloid are associated with distinctive apolipoprotein e, age, and gender profiles. *Brain Research* 798(1-2):18-24.
Joseph, J.A., B. Shukitt-Hale, N.A. Denisova, D. Bielinski, A. Martin, J.J. McEwen, and P.C. Bickford
1999	Reversals of age-related declines in neuronal signal transduction, cognitive and motor behavioral deficits with blueberry, spinach, or strawberry dietary supplementation. *Journal of Neuroscience* 19(18):8114-8121.
Kang, S.M., et al.
1992	Transactivation by AP-1 is a molecular target of T cell clonal anergy. *Science* 257(5073):1134-1138.
Kempermann, G., H.G. Kuhn, and F.H. Gage
1997	More hippocampal neurons in adult mice living in an enriched environment. *Nature* 386:493-495.
1998	Experience-induced neurogenesis in the senescent dentate gyrus. *Journal of Neuroscience* 18(9):3206-3212.
Kim, T.W., et al.
1997	Alternative cleavage of Alzheimer-associated presenilins during apoptosis by a caspase-3 family protease. *Science* 277(5324):373-376.
Koh, J.Y., L.L. Yang, and C.W. Cotman
1990	ß-amyloid protein increases the vulnerability of cultured cortical neurons to excitotoxic damage. *Brain Research* 533(2):315-320.

Korotzer, A.R., et al.
1993   Beta-amyloid peptides induce degeneration of cultured rat microglia. *Brain Research* 624(1-2):121-125.

LeBlanc, A., H. Liu, C. Goodyer, C. Bergeron, and J. Hammond
1999   Caspase-6 role in apoptosis of human neurons, amyloidgenesis, and Alzheimer's disease. *Journal of Biological Chemistry* 274 (33):23426-23436.

Lee, C.K., R.G. Klopp, R. Weindruch, and T.A. Prolla
1999   Gene expression profile of aging and its retardation by caloric restriction. *Science* 285:1390-1393.

Lenardo, M.J.
1991   Interleukin-2 programs mouse alpha beta t lymphocytes for apoptosis. *Nature* 353(6347):858-861.

Loddick, S.A., et al.
1998   Displacement of insulin-like growth factors from their binding proteins as a potential treatment for stroke. *Proceedings of the National Academy of Sciences of the United States of America* 95(4):1894-1898.

Longoni, B., E. Boschi, G.C. Demontis, P.L. Marchiafava, and F. Mosca
1999   Regulation of bcl-2 protein expression during oxidative stress in neuronal and endothelial cells. *Biochemical and Biophysical Research Communications* 260:522-526.

Loo, D.T., M.C. Althoen, and C.W. Cotman
1995   Differentiation of serum-free mouse embryo cells into astrocytes is accompanied by induction of glutamine synthetase activity. *Journal of Neuroscience Research* 42:184-191.

Loo, D., A. Copani, C.J. Pike, E. Whittemore, A.J. Walencewicz, and C.W. Cotman
1993   Apoptosis is induced by beta-amyloid in cultured central nervous system neurons. *Proceedings of the National Academy of Sciences of the United States of America* 90(17):7951-7955.

Lovell, M.A., W.D. Ehmann, M.P. Mattson, and W.R. Markesbery
1997   Elevated 4-hydroxynonenal in ventricular fluid in Alzheimer's disease. *Neurobiology of Aging* 18(5):457-461.

Lovell, M.A., S.P. Gabbita, and W.R. Markesbery
1999   Increased DNA oxidation and decreased levels of repair products in Alzheimer's disease ventricular CSF. *Journal of Neurochemistry* 72:771-776.

Lucassen, P.J., W.C. Chung, W. Kamphorst, and D.F. Swaab
1997   DNA damage distribution in the human brain as shown by in situ end labeling; Area-specific differences in aging and Alzheimer disease in the absence of apoptotic morphology. *Journal of Neuropathology and Experimental Neurology* 56:887-900.

Lyras, L., N.J. Cairns, A. Jenner, P. Jenner, and B. Halliwell
1997   An assessment of oxidative damage to proteins, lipids and DNA in brain from patients with Alzheimer's disease. *Journal of Neurochemistry* 68:2061-2069.

Ma, Y.L., et al.
1998   Brain-derived neurotrophic factor antisense oligonucleotide impairs memory retention and inhibits long-term potentiation in rats. *Neuroscience* 82(4):957-967.

Mark, R.J., Z. Pang, J.W. Geddes, K. Uchida, and M.P. Mattson
1997   Amyloid β peptide impairs glucose transport in hippocampal and cortical neurons: Involvement of membrane lipid peroxidation. *Journal of Neuroscience* 17(3):1046-1054.

Markesbery, W.R., and M.A. Lovell
1998   Four-hydroxynonenal, a product of lipid peroxidation, is increased in the brain in Alzheimer's disease. *Neurobiology of Aging* 19(1):33-36.

Maroto, R., and J.R. Perez-Polo
1997   BCL-2-related protein expression in apoptosis: Oxidative stress versus serum depri-
        vation in PC12 cells. *Journal of Neurochemistry* 69(2):514-523.
Martin, D., et al.
1997   Role of IL-1 in neurodegeneration: Preclinical findings with IL-1ra and ICE inhibi-
        tors. P. 392 in *Neuroinflammation: Mechanisms and Management*, P.L. Wood, ed.
        Totowa, NJ: Humana Press Inc.
Masliah, E., et al.
1996   Deficient glutamate transport is associated with neurodegeneration in Alzheimer's
        disease. *Annals of Neurology* 40(5):759-766.
Mattson, M.P., et al.
1992   B-amyloid peptides destabilize calcium homeostasis and render human cortical neu-
        rons vulnerable to excitotoxicity. *Journal of Neuroscience* 12(2):376-389.
1998   Presenilins, the endoplasmic reticulum, and neuronal apoptosis in Alzheimer's dis-
        ease. *Journal of Neurochemistry* 70(1):1-14.
McDonald, D.R., K.R. Brunden, and G.E. Landreth
1997   Amyloid fibrils activate tyrosine kinase-dependent signaling and superoxide produc-
        tion in microglia. *Journal of Neuroscience* 17(7):2284-2294.
McGeer, P.L., et al.
1986   Positron emission tomography in patients with clinically diagnosed Alzheimer's dis-
        ease. *Canadian Medical Association Journal* 134(6):597-607.
Mecocci, P., U. MacGarvey, et al.
1994   Oxidative damage to mitochondrial DNA is increased in Alzheimer's disease. *Annals
        of Neurology* 36(5):747-751.
Meydani, S., D. Wu, M. Santos, and M. Hayek
1995   Antioxidants and immune response in aged persons: Overview of present evidence.
        American Journal of Clinical Nutrition 62(Supplement):1462S-1476S.
Miller, R.A.
1996   The aging immune system: Primer and prospectus. *Science* 273(5271):70-74.
Multhaup, G., T. Ruppert, A. Schlicksupp, L. Hesse, D. Beher, C.L. Masters, and K. Beyreuther
1997   Reactive oxygen species and Alzheimer's disease. *Biochemical Pharmacology* 54:533-
        539.
Nagel, J.E., et al.
1988   Decreased proliferation, interleukin 2 synthesis, and interleukin 2 receptor expres-
        sion are accompanied by decreased mRNA expression in phytohemagglutinin-stimu-
        lated cells from elderly donors. *Journal of Clinical Investigation* 81(4):1096-1102.
Neeper, S.A., F. Gomez-Pinilla, J. Choi, and C.W. Cotman
1995   Exercise and brain neurotrophins. *Nature* 373:109.
1996   Physical activity increases mRNA for brain-derived neurotrophic factor and nerve
        growth factor in rat brain. *Brain Research* 726:49-56.
Nishimoto, I., et al.
1997   Apoptosis in neurodegenerative diseases. *Advances in Pharmacology* 41(5266):337-
        368.
Oliff, H.S., N.C. Berchtold, P. Isackson, and C.W. Cotman
1998   Exercise-induced regulation of brain-derived neurotrophic factor (BDNF) transcripts
        in the rat hippocampus. *Molecular Brain Research* 61:147-153.
Oltvai, Z.N., C.L. Milliman, and S.J. Korsmeyer
1993   Bcl-2 heterodimerizes in vivo with a conserved homolog, bax, that accelerates pro-
        grammed cell death. *Cell* 74(4):609-619.

Palmer, A.M., and M.A. Burns
1994   Selective increase in lipid peroxidation in the inferior temporal cortex in Alzheimer's disease. *Brain Research* 645(1-2):338-342.

Paradis, E., H. Douillard, M. Koutroumanis, C. Goodyer, and A. LeBlanc
1996   Amyloid beta peptide of Alzheimer's disease downregulates bcl-2 and upregulates bax expression in human neurons. *Journal of Neuroscience* 16(23):7533-7539.

Paz, K., et al.
1997   A molecular basis for insulin resistance. Elevated serine/threonine phosphorylation of IRS-1 and IRS-2 inhibits their binding to the juxtamembrane region of the insulin receptor and impairs their ability to undergo insulin-induced tyrosine phosphorylation. *Journal of Biological Chemistry* 272(47):29911-29918.

Peraldi, P., et al.
1996   Tumor necrosis factor (TNF)-alpha inhibits insulin signaling through stimulation of the p55 TNF receptor and activation of sphingomyelinase. *Journal of Biological Chemistry* 271(22):13018-13022.

Pereira, C., M.S. Santos, and C. Oliveira
1999   Involvement of oxidative stress on the impairment of energy metabolism induced by $A\beta$ peptides on PC12 cells: Protection by antioxidants. *Neurobiology of Disease* 6:209-219.

Perrig, W.J., P. Perrig, and H.B. Stahelin
1997   The relation between antioxidants and memory performance in the old and very old. *Journal of the American Geriatrics Society* 45:718-724.

Phelouzat, M.A., et al.
1996   Excessive apoptosis of mature T lymphocytes is a characteristic feature of human immune senescence. *Mechanisms of Ageing and Development* 88(1-2):25-38.

Pike, C.J., et al.
1994   Beta-amyloid-induced changes in cultured astrocytes parallel reactive astrocytosis associated with senile plaques in Alzheimer's disease. *Neuroscience* 63(2):517-531.

Pike, C.J., B.J. Cummings, and C.W. Cotman
1992   ß-amyloid induces neuritic dystrophy in vitro: similarities with Alzheimer pathology. *Neuroreport* 3:769-772.

Pike, C.J., N. RamezanArab, and C.W. Cotman
1997   Beta-amyloid neurotoxicity in vitro: Evidence of oxidative stress but not protection by antioxidants. *Journal of Neurochemistry* 69(4):1601-1611.

Praticáo, D., M.Y. Lee, J.Q. Trojanowski, J. Rokach, and G.A. Fitzgerald
1998   Increased F2-isoprostanes in Alzheimer's disease: evidence for enhanced lipidperoxidation in vivo. *FASEB Journal* 12(15):1777-1783.

Proust, J.J., et al.
1987   Age-related defect in signal transduction during lectin activation of murine T lymphocytes. *Journal of Immunology* 139(5):1472-1478.

Radvanyi, L.G., G.B. Mills, and R.G. Miller
1993   Relegation of the T cell receptor after primary activation of mature T cells inhibits proliferation and induces apoptotic cell death. *Journal of Immunology* 150(12):5704-5715.

Reed, J.C.
1994   Bcl-2 and the regulation of programmed cell death. *Journal of Cell Biology* 124(1):1-6.

Reidel, W.J., and B.L. Jorissen
1998   Nutrients, age and cognitive function. *Current Opinion in Clinical Nutrition and Metabolic Care* 1:579-585.

Rothwell, N.J., and S.J. Hopkins
    1995   Cytokines and the nervous system II: Actions and mechanisms of action. *Trends in Neurosciences* 18(3):130-136.
Russell, J.W., et al.
    1998   Insulin-like growth factor-I prevents apoptosis in neurons after nerve growth factor withdrawal. *Journal of Neurobiology* 36(4):455-467.
Sano, M., C. Ernesto, R.G. Thomas, M.R. Klauber, K. Schafer, M. Grundman, P. Woodbury, J. Growdon, C.W. Cotman, E. Pfeiffer, L.S. Schneider, and L.J. Thal
    1997   A controlled trial of selegiline, alpha-tocopherol, or both as treatment for Alzheimer's disease. *The New England Journal of Medicine* 336:1216-1222.
Schenk, D., R. Barbour, W. Dunn, G. Gordon, H. Grajeda, T. Guido, K. Hu, J. Huang, K. Johnson-Wood, K. Khan, D. Kholodenko, M. Lee, Z. Liao, I. Lieberburg, R. Motter, L. Mutter, F. Soriano, G. Shopp, N. Vasquez, C. Vandevert, S. Walker, M. Wogulis, T. Yednock, D. Games, and P. Seubert
    1999   Immunization with amyloid-β attenuates Alzheimer-disease-like pathology in the PDAPP mouse. *Nature* 400:173-177.
Schulz, S., et al.
    1999   Direct evidence for biphasic cAMP responsive element-binding protein phosphorylation during long-term potentiation in the rat dentate gyrus in vivo. *Journal of Neuroscience* 19(13):5683-5692.
Segal, M., et al.
    1998   CREB activation mediates plasticity in cultured hippocampal neurons. *Neural Plasticity* 6(3):1-7.
Shen, H., L. Tong, and C.W. Cotman
    In   Effects of exercise on CREB phosphorylation and CRE DNA-binding activity in the
    press   rat hippocampus.
Shin, S.W., et al.
    1998   Persistent expression of fas/fasL mRNA in the mouse hippocampus after a single NMDA injection. *Journal of Neurochemistry* 71(4):1773-1776.
Simpson, I.A., et al.
    1994   Decreased concentrations of GLUT1 and GLUT3 glucose transporters in the brains of patients with Alzheimer's disease. *Annals of Neurology* 35(5):546-551.
Socci, D.J.C., B.M. Crandall, and G.W. Arendash
    1995   Chronic antioxidant treatment improves the cognitive performance of aged rats. *Brain Research* 693(1-2):88-94.
Spanaus, K.S., R. Schlapbach, and A. Fontana
    1998   TNF-alpha and IFN-gamma render microglia sensitive to fas ligand-induced apoptosis by induction of fas expression and down-regulation of bcl-2 and bcl-xL. *European Journal of Immunology* 28(12):4398-4408.
Stadelmann, C., W. Bruck, C. Bancher, K. Jellinger, and H. Lassmann
    1998   Alzheimer disease: DNA fragmentation indicates increased neuronal vulnerability, but not apoptosis. *Journal of Neuropathology and Experimental Neurology* 57:456-464.
Stadtman, E.R.
    1992   Protein oxidation and aging. *Science* 257:1220-1224.
Su, J.H., A.J. Anderson, B.J. Cummings, and C.W. Cotman
    1994   Immunohistochemical evidence for apoptosis in Alzheimer's disease. *NeuroReport* 5:2529-2533.
Su, J.H., G. Deng, and C.W. Cotman
    1997   Neuronal DNA damage precedes tangle formation and is associated with up-regulation of nitrotyrosine in Alzheimer's disease brain. *Brain Research* 774:193-199.

Thoman, M.L., and W.O. Weigle
    1989   The cellular and subcellular bases of immunosenescence. *Advances in Immunology* 46(3):221-261.
Tong, L., P.L. Thornton, and C.W. Cotman
    In   β-amyloid (1-42) impairs neuronal activity-dependent CREB signaling.
    press
Torp, R., J.H. Su, G. Deng, and C.W. Cotman
    1998   GADD45 is induced in Alzheimer's disease, and protects against apoptosis in vitro. *Neurobiology of Disease* 5:245-252.
Venters, H.D., et al.
    1999   A new mechanism of neurodegeneration: A proinflammatory cytokine inhibits receptor signaling by a survival peptide. *Proceedings of the National Academy of Sciences of the United States of America* 96(17):9879-9884.
Vogt, M., et al.
    1998   Oxidative stress and hypoxia/reoxygenation trigger CD95 (APO-1/fas) ligand expression in microglial cells. *FEBS Letters* 429(1):67-72.
Ware, C.F., et al.
    1991   Tumor necrosis factor (TNF) receptor expression in T lymphocytes. Differential regulation of the type I TNF receptor during activation of resting and effector T cells. *Journal of Immunology* 147(12):4229-4238.
Watt, J.A., C.J. Pike, A.J. Walencewicz, and C.W. Cotman
    1994   Ultrastructural analysis of beta-amyloid-induced apoptosis in cultured hippocampal neurons. *Brain Research* 661:147-156.
Whittemore, E.R., D.T. Loo, and C.W. Cotman
    1994   Exposure to hydrogen peroxide induces cell death via apoptosis in cultured rat cortical neurons. *NeuroReport* 5(13):1585-1588.
Williams, P., et al.
    1997   Effects of group exercise on cognitive functioning and mood in older women. *Australia and New Zealand Journal of Public Health* 21(1):45-52.
Wolozin, B., et al.
    1996   Participation of presenilin 2 in apoptosis: enhanced basal activity conferred by an Alzheimer mutation. *Science* 274(5293):1710-1713.
Yamamoto-Sasaki, M., et al.
    1999   Impaired phosphorylation of cyclic AMP response element binding protein in the hippocampus of dementia of the Alzheimer type. *Brain Research* 824(2):300-303.
Yamatsuji, T., et al.
    1996   G protein-mediated neuronal DNA fragmentation induced by familial Alzheimer's disease-associated mutants of APP. *Science* 272(5266):1349-1352.
Young, D., et al.
    1999   Environmental enrichment inhibits spontaneous apoptosis, prevents seizures and is neuroprotective. *Nature Medicine* 5(4):448-453.

C
The Bearable Lightness of Aging: Judgment and Decision Processes in Older Adults

Ellen Peters, Melissa L. Finucane,
Donald G. MacGregor, and Paul Slovic

INTRODUCTION

The problems and challenges of aging have long been an important societal concern. Accompanying the physical changes of aging are psychological changes that have critical implications for the quality of life that people experience. Equally critical may be the fact that, as people age, their opportunities to recover or compensate for poor-quality judgments and decisions diminish. For example, poor financial decisions early in life may be remedied by learning from mistakes and making better decisions in the future. Less than careful health care choices in one's earlier years may be compensated for by resilience to disease or injury. However, as one ages, diminished physical capacity and less time can translate into reduced opportunities to recover from the "normal" ups and downs of everyday decision outcomes. As a result, understanding the psychological processes that underlie the judgments and decisions of older adults can help us to identify areas in which they may be most vulnerable and therefore can guide efforts to help them face the challenges of aging.

Importance of Judgment and Decision Making for Older Adults

The impact of age-related changes is magnified further by recent social trends that create a need for maintaining strong decision-making capabilities for a greater number of years. To begin with, advances in modern medicine allow people to live longer than ever before and enjoy more years beyond retirement. In addition, our society places a strong value on independence and self-determinacy; this is often interpreted as living with less reliance on the help and resources of others. The trend toward geographically dispersed families means that older individuals may have limited access to knowledgeable and supportive family members. As a result of these trends, responsibility for sound judgment and good decision making rests more on the individual than it has in the past.

The quality of judgment and decision making is of great import in the lives of older adults, as can be readily seen in three contexts central to the lives of most people: (1) motor vehicle operation, (2) health care, and (3) financial management.

Although many of us take it for granted, driving is a complex judgment and decision-making task that requires people to be perceptive and vigilant. Safe operation of a motor vehicle includes the ability not only to perform in a real-time environment, but also to assess and judge correctly the situations (e.g., traffic speeds and densities) and environmental conditions (e.g., weather, darkness) in which they are capable of driving. Older individuals, in particular, need to assess the point when they should discontinue driving altogether. The trend in society toward independent living and the importance of automobiles as the main source of personal mobility, however, makes decisions and trade-offs concerning driving difficult.

Judgments of personal health status (e.g., "Am I ill?" "Should I go to the doctor?") are particularly important for individuals living alone or with limited access to a social support network. Once one enters the health care system, decisions there are often quite complex due to the vast array of health care options provided in the marketplace and the volume of information available for consumers to consider. In addition, the historically paternalistic approach to medical treatment has shifted toward a more patient-directed one (Zwahr, 1999). Having to choose among many and complex treatment or health insurance options carries not only consequences for the quality of health care that an individual receives, but also strong financial implications.

Effective financial management draws heavily on one's judgment and decision-making abilities. More and more people are relying heavily on individual, self-directed financial plans in order to maintain their standard of living after retirement. Although some individuals call on professionals to develop a formal financial plan, even formal plans require investors to make critical decisions about when to withdraw or reallocate money in an environment of changing market conditions and tax laws. As individuals live longer, their financial assets must go farther, and high-quality financial decision making must be maintained. In an information-rich and risky environment, this task can be difficult even for those who are knowledgeable and capable. For those with decrements in information-processing capabilities, exercising good judgment and making wise financial decisions may be beyond their capacities.

Research on Judgment and Decision Making

The psychological study of decision making, which we present here in a necessarily abbreviated form, examines the mechanisms that underlie people's choices, preferences, and judgments and attempts to discover how to improve decision-making processes.[1] Two relevant overviews of research on decision making and aging are Yates and Patalano (1999) and Sanfey and Hastie (in press).

Decision research developed out of economic theory and, as a result of this rationalistic origin, has concentrated mostly on reason-based explanations for how people make decisions and form judgments. The implicit assumption that good decision making is a conscious, deliberative process has been one of the field's most enduring themes. Recent research, however, has begun to examine the role of emotion, affect, and intuition in decisions.

In this paper we cover research and theories that address some of the issues that older adults face in making everyday judgments and decisions. A decision, of course, is a choice between two or more options or alternatives (e.g., choosing a car). One of those options could be the status quo (e.g., doing nothing or making no change). A judgment, in contrast, is the psychological appraisal of information. It is an understanding of a situation or an individual (e.g., "I'm having some stomach distress. How likely is it to be due to my new medication?").

Some general themes have emerged during the past 40 years of research on judgment and decision making. The first major theme we consider is that people (both older and younger adults) have limited resources to deal with complex decisions and the great quantity of information with which they are faced. As a result, they rely on mental shortcuts, called heuristics, to deal with such complexity. The use of mental shortcuts is frequently adaptive (because they are efficient and the resulting judgments or decisions are generally good enough), but it can also be maladaptive (resulting in poorer decisions). We

---

[1]Space does not allow us to pursue all of the important topics in decision-making research that could be examined in older adults. Judgments and decisions are influenced by many factors. Social and political attitudes, or worldviews, for example, have been shown to influence risk perceptions (Peters and Slovic, 1996). Cultural backgrounds may influence the propensity to take risks as well as risk attitudes and decision-making strategies (Weber and Hsee, in press). Other important work has been done using younger adults as subjects on the use of narratives and other display formats in communicating information (e.g., Sanfey and Hastie, 1998; Satterfield et al., in press), on the impact of reasons on choice (e.g., Shafir et al., 1993), and on the status quo effect (Thaler, 1980). Errors of omission versus commission have been examined (e.g., Ritov and Baron, 1990) as have protected values (e.g., Baron and Spranca, 1997). Disproportionate sensitivity to loss (i.e., loss aversion) has been studied extensively, particularly within the context of prospect theory (Kahneman and Tversky, 1979). A small number of studies have examined individual differences in decision making (e.g., Lopes, 1987; Peters and Slovic, in press), a topic that may have even greater relevance among older adults.

describe below the traditional heuristics and biases approach in research on judgment and decision making as well as the more recent study of affective processes and decisions. We use research and theory derived from the aging and social psychological literatures to speculate that aging will increase reliance on heuristics and affect in judgment and decision making.

A second major theme emerging from research is that people frequently do not know their own "true" values for an object or situation (e.g., the importance of the quality of a health plan versus the importance of its cost). Instead they construct values and preferences "on the spot" when asked to form a particular judgment or to make a specific decision (Slovic, 1995:365):

> Preferences appear to be remarkably labile, sensitive to the way a choice problem is described or "framed" and to the mode of response used to express the preference.... These failures of invariance have contributed to a new conception of judgment and choice in which beliefs and preferences are often constructed—not merely revealed—in the elicitation process.

With human judgment being a constructive process, individual preferences can be unstable across different contexts, and situational influences can carry great impact. The extent of this lability, particularly if greater in older adults, has implications for their decision-making competence. We explore the notion of decision-making competence among older adults from a decision theoretic perspective, including suggestions for how to assess such competence.

Despite the importance of good judgment and decision making and a wealth of knowledge about these processes, current understanding of judgment and decision making in older adults is poor. Researchers, for the most part, have neglected to recognize the importance of sound judgment and decision processes in later life and have tended to use only younger adults in their studies. One result, however, is that there is a wealth of theories and methodologies that can now be applied to the study of decision-making processes and decision-making competence among older adults. This paper highlights what we see to be the most fruitful initial approaches to the study of age and decision making. We examine three main questions: (1) Does heuristic processing increase with age? (2) Does the salience of affective processes in decision making increase among older adults? and (3) Are older adults influenced by the contextual frame of the decision situation in ways that affect their decision competence?

AGE AND HEURISTIC PROCESSING

Aging may be marked by the increased salience of associative and automatic processes such as heuristics (Mutter and Pliske, 1994; Yates and Patalano, 1999). Although life-span theories (e.g., Fredrickson and

Carstensen, 1990; Labouvie-Vief, 1999) do not make predictions about the salience of automatic, associative, and intuitive processes versus controlled and analytical processes in older (compared with younger) adults, aging research nonetheless supports this distinction. For example, Jennings and Jacoby (1993) demonstrated that older adults performed less well than their younger counterparts on tasks that required conscious control of memory, but they performed equally well on tasks that relied on automatic memory processes (i.e., familiarity). Although younger adults appear more likely than older adults to interpret a story analytically, older adults appear likely to focus less on the story's details and more on the gist of the story and its underlying significance (Adams et al., 1997). Older adults also have shown similar or better abilities to represent, update, and recall more global and holistic levels of understanding (e.g., Radvansky, 1999). Finally, prior research has demonstrated that aging is associated with increased dependence on schematic knowledge (e.g., Hess, 1990).[2]

Age-Related Increases in Heuristic Processing

Heuristics and biases (the systematic and nonnormative deviations that can result from heuristic processing) are studied in research on judgment and decision making because they can reveal the psychological processes that underlie how people judge and decide. In addition, however, the use of heuristics and their resulting biases have many practical implications. For example, using the availability heuristic, an older person might estimate the number and frequency of his or her symptoms for a doctor "by the ease with which instances or occurrences can be brought to mind" (Tversky and Kahneman, 1974:1127). The resulting estimate will be more or less accurate depending on the actual symptoms, the individual's capacity to remember, and the vividness and emotional character of the situations in which the symptoms were both experienced and reported.

Traditionally, heuristics have been considered serious sources of error due to their overuse or inappropriate application (Kahneman and Tversky, 1973). From Epstein's (1994) dual process theory,[3] however, we see a different view of the adaptive nature and organization of heuristics. Heuristic processing is central to the experiential system's natural mode of operation as

---

[2]As suggested by one reviewer, although age-related decrements in controlled processing may be greater than the corresponding decrements in automatic (i.e., heuristic) processing, it does not necessarily follow that older adults will use heuristics more often (relative to young adults). However, consistent with our hypothesis, Johnson (1990) demonstrated that older adults used decision strategies associated with heuristic processing (i.e., noncompensatory strategies) more often than younger adults.

an intuitive, rapid, automatic, crudely differentiated system. The experiential mode of processing represents events in the form of concrete, context-specific, and holistic images. Importantly, Epstein characterizes these ways of processing information as highly adaptive under normal circumstances, when rapid assessment and immediate action are often necessary. He also suggests that the various heuristics identified in research on judgment and decision making (e.g., availability, representativeness), traditionally thought to be unrelated to one another and caused by a limited capacity for information processing, might instead be the product of the organized experiential system. If true, then conditions that facilitate or constrain the use of one heuristic should tend to simultaneously influence the use of other heuristics. The process of aging may be one of the conditions that increases the use of heuristics.

Research Directions in Heuristic Processing

We focus here on two heuristics—the representativeness heuristic and the availability heuristic—in order to examine the implications that an increased reliance on heuristic processing might have on the aging individual.

The Representativeness Heuristic

To begin with, the representativeness heuristic is said to be invoked when a probability or frequency is estimated by thinking about similarity with a stereotype, schema, or other preexisting knowledge structure. The estimate is based on "the degree of correspondence between a sample and a population, an instance and a category, an act and an actor, or, more generally, between an outcome and a model" (Tversky and Kahneman, 1983:295).

Older adults, themselves more reliant on schematic knowledge (Hess, 1990), may be particularly likely to use this heuristic. Although this approach to processing is both fast and efficient and allows older adults to take advantage of the vast store of knowledge they have accumulated, it also leaves them susceptible to a number of biases. For example, highly detailed descriptions of an individual or an event may influence the judgments of older adults more. An older adult may judge the side effects from a particular medical operation as less likely to occur than side effects from that same operation described as leaving the older adult dependent on family and friends for mo-

---

[3]Epstein (1994) posits that two information-processing systems exist—the experiential system and the rational system. Whereas the experiential system processes information quickly and automatically and is driven primarily by affect, the rational system processes information more slowly, deliberatively, and logically. See Hammond's (1998) Cognitive Continuum Theory for a related distinction between intuitive and analytic thinking.

bility. The latter account may appear more plausible due to its greater detail and, as a result, the older adult may refuse treatment. However, that account is statistically less probable due to this same detail.

An increased use of the representativeness heuristic could have other effects as well. It could lead older adults to a greater neglect of base rates. With base rate neglect, older adults may be more likely to base their judgments of the best hospital on the quality of the food in the cafeteria, the number of magazines in the waiting room, and the friendliness of the nursing staff (all of which may be stereotypical indicators of a "good" hospital), rather than on the hospital's proportion of successful outcomes in cases similar to theirs. In another context, older adults observing a run of extremely good returns in the stock market might conclude that the fluctuation is representative of the future market and may make risky investments that then decline rapidly if the market "regresses toward the mean," as it often does.

The Availability Heuristic

With another well-known heuristic—the availability heuristic—frequencies and probabilities are judged by thinking of examples. The easier it is to retrieve examples, the higher the estimated likelihood of occurrence. On one hand, older adults may be slower and have more difficulty than younger adults at retrieving examples due to age-related deficits in memory and speed of processing (e.g., Salthouse, 1996) so that they may judge the likelihood of being in a car accident as lower because they cannot retrieve as many instances of car crashes. On the other hand, older adults have a much broader network of memories from which to draw, so that they may have many more car crash memories to retrieve. In addition, availability also appears to be influenced by emotionally compelling and vivid information at the time of the occurrence as well as at the time of memory retrieval. Results of studies with younger adults show that a handful of vivid testimonials, for example, can outweigh comprehensive statistical summaries (Borgida and Nisbett, 1977). As we observe in the next section, older adults may be particularly susceptible to (and helped by) emotional influences on judgments and decisions. The implications for older adults who must use statistical information about health care options and financial plans to make good decisions are important. It may be that marketers and con artists can take greater advantage of older than younger adults through the use of vivid stories and vignettes about their products.

We have been struck by the lack of research examining age-related differences in heuristic processing. The only research of which we are aware are the studies by Mutter and Pliske (1994) on illusory correlation, often explained with reference to the availability heuristic. In traditional studies of illusory correlation (e.g., Chapman and Chapman, 1967), researchers have found that people often perceive associations between two variables that are consistent with their intuitive associations and expectations, but are not actually present in the data they are observing. Mutter and Pliske showed age-related increases in illusory correlations as would be expected if older adults relied more than younger adults on heuristic processing. In their studies, older and younger subjects judged whether and to what extent two variables (a patient's response to a Rorschach Ink Blot and a patient's behavior) were related to one another. As pointed out by Yates and Patalano (1999), judgments of relatedness are fundamental to good decision making. For instance, suppose an older individual incorrectly infers the effectiveness of some ineffective home remedies. Mutter and Pliske found that older subjects were even more inclined than younger subjects to exhibit such illusory correlations. They offer as an explanation that older adults may rely to a greater extent than younger adults on heuristics to simplify the selection, encoding, and retrieval of evidence for co-occurrence judgments.

AFFECT AND DECISION MAKING AMONG OLDER ADULTS

The importance of affect[4] and emotion is increasingly being acknowledged by decision researchers. A strong early proponent of the importance of affect in decision making was Zajonc (1980), who argued that affective reactions to stimuli are often the very first reactions, occurring automatically and subsequently guiding information processing and judgment. If Zajonc is correct, then affective reactions may serve as orienting mechanisms, helping people navigate quickly and efficiently through a complex, uncertain, and sometimes dangerous world (e.g., Finucane et al., 2000). Important work on affect and decision making also has been done by Isen (1993), Johnson and Tversky (1983), Janis and Mann (1977), Kahneman and Snell (1990), Mellers et al. (1997), Loewenstein (1996), Rozin et al. (1993), Wilson et al. (1993), and others.

Theorists such as Mowrer (1960a, b) and Epstein (1994) give affect a direct role in motivating behavior, asserting or implying that people integrate positive and negative feelings according to some sort of automatic, rapid "affective algebra," whose operations and rules remain to be discovered. Epstein's (1994:716) view on this is concise:

> The experiential system is assumed to be intimately associated with the experience of affect, . . . which refer[s] to subtle feelings of which people are often unaware. When a person responds to an emotionally significant

---

[4]Affect may be viewed as a feeling state that people experience, such as happiness or sadness. It may also be viewed as a quality (e.g., goodness or badness) assigned to a stimulus. These two conceptions tend to be related.

event . . . the experiential system automatically searches its memory banks for related events, including their emotional accompaniments. . . . If the activated feelings are pleasant, they motivate actions and thoughts anticipated to reproduce the feelings. If the feelings are unpleasant, they motivate actions and thoughts anticipated to avoid the feelings.

Damasio's Somatic Marker Hypothesis

One of the most comprehensive and dramatic theoretical accounts of the role of affect and emotion in decision making is presented by the neurologist, Antonio Damasio (1994). In seeking to determine "what in the brain allows humans to behave rationally," Damasio argues that thought is made largely from images, broadly construed to include perceptual and symbolic representations. A lifetime of learning leads these images to become "marked" by positive and negative feelings linked directly or indirectly to somatic or bodily states. When a negative somatic marker is linked to an image of a future outcome, it sounds an alarm. When a positive marker is associated with the outcome image, it becomes a beacon of incentive. Damasio hypothesized that somatic markers increase the accuracy and efficiency of the decision process, and their absence, observed in people with certain types of brain damage, degrades decision performance.

There are numerous reasons to expect that the relative importance and salience of affect may increase with age. First, older adults might strategically change preferred decision modes (from more deliberative to more affective) in order to compensate for cognitive declines in everyday functioning. Second, such changes may be an indicator of ego development and emotional maturity (Labouvie-Vief et al., 1989a, 1989b). Third, such shifts may result from changing motivations (Carstensen et al., 1999; Fredrickson and Carstensen, 1990). Fourth, with the greater experience that comes with age, older adults, like other experts, may tend to approach tasks using more automatic processing (e.g., Myles-Worsley et al., 1988). Finally, an increased reliance on affect may be a relative change due to a decline in analytical processing. Although the evidence is somewhat mixed, in this section we examine whether affective processes may exert a greater influence on everyday choices in older adults.

Research Directions in Affect

At this point, little empirical support exists to demonstrate that affective processes carry greater weight in the decisions and behaviors of older adults. A wide range of tasks, however, has already been used successfully with younger adults and could be applied to older adults to examine age-induced changes in the relation between affect and behavior and in conflicts between emotional and analytical thinking.

Wisdom and Choice

A card-selection task was designed by Damasio and his colleagues (Bechara et al., 1994) to mimic the uncertainties of gains and losses in a real-world environment in order to test the idea that affective processing was related to good decision performance. The task may provide a unique method for testing changes in affective and analytical information-processing abilities through the life span. In it, subjects selected cards one at a time from four decks placed face-down in front of them. Each time they turned over a card (for 100 total cards), they were told how much play money they won or lost with that card. They were told to select from any deck as often or as seldom as they wished and in any order that they liked. They were given the goal to earn as much play money as possible. The decks were arranged so that two of the decks had low gains and low losses and, overall, would win money; the other two decks had high gains and high losses and, overall, would lose money. Damasio equated good judgment with more selections from the winning decks.

In her dissertation, Peters (1998) used a methodology identical to the above study from Damasio's group. However, participants in Peters's study chose about 10 fewer cards from the "good" decks relative to the nonclinical participants in the experiment reported by Bechara et al. (1994). Peters's participants were all college students; those in Bechara et al.'s study were older (age range = 20-79 years compared with 17-25 years in Peters' Experiment 1). It is possible that the older participants had more experience with card playing and that this factor improved their performance. However, the cards used in both of these studies were not ordinary cards, nor was the task an ordinary card game. It seems unlikely that experience playing poker or gin rummy would help individuals to learn in this unfamiliar task.

The most interesting possibility is that affect becomes more salient and/ or that the ability to integrate affective and analytical information processing improves with age (e.g., Blanchard-Fields et al., 1987; Labouvie-Vief et al., 1989a, 1989b). No direct evidence has been found, however, to support the notion that individuals become more sensitive to gains and/or to losses as they age or that older adults are better able to integrate the meaning of re-warding and punishing feedback when making subsequent responses to the same stimulus.

Affective reactions may play a bigger role in the construction of older (versus younger) adults' choices. It has been demonstrated that older adults generate fewer potential solutions to a given problem (McCrae et al., 1987). In general, this difference has been characterized as yet another inevitable decline. However, if affect is more salient to older adults, it may be that they simply are better at rejecting not-so-good options prior to consideration (Damasio, 1994:174):

[Affect] does not deliberate for us. [It] assists the deliberation by highlighting some options (either dangerous or favorable), and eliminating them rapidly from subsequent consideration. You may think of it as a system for automated qualification of predictions, which acts, whether you want it or not, to evaluate the extremely diverse scenarios of the anticipated future before you. Think of it as a biasing device.

As pointed out by Yates and Patalano (1999), real-world decision makers, such as firefighters, do not "wade through large numbers of alternatives. Instead, they want to zero in immediately on the best option, or at least one that is 'good enough'" (p. 41). The experience that comes with age may allow people to do just that. Indeed, at least one study has indicated that younger adults may tend to waste their energy generating excessive numbers of options that do not ultimately yield better decisions (Streufert et al., 1990).

Affect and Behavior

Affect has been shown to guide and orient choices and intended behaviors in college student as well as nationally representative samples (e.g., Frijda et al., 1989). No studies could be found, however, that examined whether age might induce a stronger correlation between affect and behavior. In a re-analysis of our own data (Peters and Slovic, 1996, $N = 1,512$), we found that the correlations between people's affect and their intended support or opposition toward nuclear power appeared to increase from young to middle ages and then decreased in older populations ($r = .49, .55$, and $.42$ for groups ages 18-39, 40-59, and 60+ with corresponding sample sizes N = 725, 485, and 246).[5] Although we expected the correlations to be highest in the older group, it may be that the particular affective technique used (which involved the production of images prior to the affective evaluation) imposed a cognitive burden that led to a reduction in the number and quality of images in the older respondents. Other affective techniques that do not impose as great a cognitive load may show the hypothesized age-related increases throughout the life span.

Affect and Time

It is also important to examine how increases in affect and experience relate to time phenomena, such as impulsive consumption, in different age

---

[5]In addition, the same pattern of correlations held in a second unpublished study in which subjects free-associated to the concept of eating beef. The subsequent affective ratings were correlated with perceived risks to the American public of eating red meat ($r = .24, .48$, and $.14$ for groups ages 18-39, 40-59, and 60+, respectively, with corresponding sample sizes N = 110, 68, and 37).

groups. We might expect that older adults would be less likely to delay positive outcomes and would have a preference for immediate consumption of goods if affective influences carried greater weight. In decision theoretic terms, older subjects might show high discount rates, so that they would prefer a much smaller amount of money (or other positive event) now rather than a larger amount of money at some specified time in the future. Although immediate consumption may be wise for an around-the-world cruise while the older adult is still in good health, impulsive consumption could be quite detrimental with respect to financial planning.

In fact, older subjects have been shown to have greater emotional control (Lawton et al., 1992) so that impulsive consumption should be less likely in an older age group. In addition, Loewenstein (1992; Loewenstein and Prelec, 1992) reports that for goods for which consumption is fleeting and easily imaginable, individuals prefer to delay the consumption of goods (and speed up the consumption of bads). He attributes this behavior to the existence of "anticipatory" affect—the savoring or dread that occurs while anticipating an event, separate from any affect experienced during actual consumption. On the basis of this analysis, older adults might be expected to delay their consumption of goods (and speed up their consumption of bads) more than younger adults, since this time preference should maximize the overall hedonic value of the affect anticipated *and* experienced.

Conflicts Between Emotional and Analytical Modes of Thought

It is also possible to explicitly assess reliance on affective reactions versus analytical considerations. Denes-Raj and Epstein (1994) did this by giving college-aged subjects an opportunity to win $1 by drawing a red jelly bean from a bowl.[6] They found that many subjects chose to draw from a bowl containing 5 red beans out of 100 beans (5 percent chance of winning; see Figure C-1), even though they knew analytically that the winning odds were better in the smaller bowl that contained 1 red bean out of 10 (10 percent chance of winning). Apparently the greater number of winning beans was more appealing to some subjects than the proportion of winning beans. This result was interpreted as indicating that intuitive, affective processes dominated their rational processing systems. A number of subjects indicated, for example, that the larger bowl "looked more inviting." If older adults rely more on affective processing, they would be expected to draw from the nonoptimal larger bowl more often.

A less frivolous example of how the balance between affective and analytic processing can be assessed arises from the different responses people

---

[6]The beans were spread in a single layer in the bottom of the bowl.

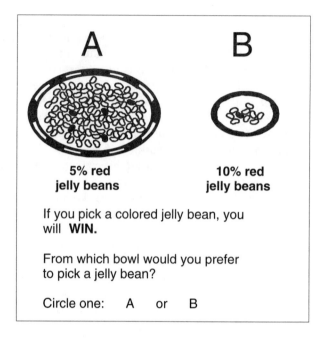

FIGURE C-1 Win condition trial.

make to likelihood assessments portrayed as percentages or probabilities (e.g., "persons like Joe are assessed as having a 10 percent chance of committing a violent act during the next 6 months") and assessments portrayed as relative frequencies (e.g. "of 100 persons like Joe, 10 would be expected to commit a violent act during the next 6 months"). Slovic et al. (in press) found that the frequentistic portrayal evoked more violent imagery and negative affect, leading many people to judge the risk of releasing Joe from a psychiatric hospital as higher compared with the perceived risk evoked by the percentage probability frame. If affect is more salient to older adults, we might expect that the stronger reaction to relative frequency frames (compared with probability frames) would be more evident in older than in younger adults. If so, implications for risk communication would be evident (e.g., rare but important dangers might be better appreciated by older people when described in frequentistic terms).

AGING, DECISION-MAKING COMPETENCE, AND PREFERENCE CONSISTENCY

As people get older, their competence at everyday decision making seems to be questioned more often. While formal assessments of mental competence are sometimes required in general medical or legal settings (e.g., when patients' abilities to consent to or refuse treatment are suspect), implicit judgments by families or clinicians are more common. In either respect, judging someone to be incompetent can have a dramatic effect on his or her life.

Competence Criteria

For the purpose of defining and measuring competence, five commonly cited criteria from research on adolescents and young adults include the ability to (1) structure a decision, (2) understand and remember relevant information, (3) appreciate the personal significance of the information, (4) temper impulsivity, and (5) rationally integrate the information and reason about it[7] (Appelbaum and Grisso, 1988; Parker and Fischhoff, 1999; Rosenfeld and Turkheimer, 1995; see also Sanfey and Hastie, in press, and Yates and Patalano, 1999, for alternative classifications).

Research Directions in Decision-Making Competence

Despite its importance, research on how to measure decision-making competence in the elderly is virtually nonexistent. However, the knowledge gathered by researchers in recent decades can be used to develop a behaviorally based measure of older adults' decision-making competence. In this section we focus on information integration and reasoning, with particular emphasis on consistency and the impact of preference reversals on decision-making competence. Information integration is the skill that has been most thoroughly examined by judgment and decision researchers to date, and is therefore an excellent starting point for the development of a decision-making competence scale.

Many professionals (physicians, lawyers, economists, psychologists) have much to say about how information should be integrated, because proper integration is a hallmark of rationality, from which good decisions are most likely to result. However, with the exception of a few studies (e.g., Malloy et al., 1992; Rosenfeld and Turkheimer, 1995), no studies of aging have focused on one of the aspects of information integration most relevant to competency in decision making—the ability to weigh attributes in a consistent manner.

Consistency is important because it both generates and reflects reliable preferences. For instance, an individual who weighs information in a way that results in a good decision will benefit from repeating that decision. If an individual integrates the same information in different ways, he or she may

---

[7]The ability to express a choice is also a common definition of decision competence, but is mainly of interest in severely impaired individuals.

end up with different decision outcomes, being unable to reap the same benefits more than once, or at least predictably. Moreover, some unscrupulous individuals may take advantage of others by maximizing conditions under which inconsistencies may arise. In studies with younger adults, Lichtenstein and Slovic (1971) demonstrated that inconsistencies in preferences could lead undergraduate subjects to becoming "money pumps," constantly giving more money to the experimenter as the experimenter manipulated the situation. Lichtenstein and Slovic (1973) replicated their findings using real money and real gamblers in a Las Vegas casino.

Earlier, we highlighted the constructive nature of judgment and decision processes as one of the main themes emerging from research on judgment and decision making. Preference construction often leads to inconsistency. Several decades of research have conclusively demonstrated that characteristics of the task (e.g., the way the stimulus information or question is framed, the number of options and attributes given) strongly influence people's preferences, in some cases resulting in complete reversals of preference.

Preference reversals due to framing effects have important implications for many life decisions, such as choosing which health care option to pursue. For instance, the impact of dying seems to be greater when it is framed as a mortality rate of 10 percent, than when it is framed as a survival rate of 90 percent. In terms of decision behavior, such as choosing between alternative treatments for lung cancer, McNeil et al. (1982) showed that surgery was relatively less attractive than radiation therapy when risk information was presented in terms of mortality rather than survival, despite surgery having better long-term prospects. The effect was demonstrated for naïve subjects (patients) as well as experts (physicians). Of course, for a 95-year-old, long-term survival prospects may not be important, but an otherwise healthy 65-year-old may not wish to be led astray by the framing effect and reduce his or her life span unintentionally.

Malloy et al. (1992) examined the influence of treatment descriptions on medical decisions by older adults. They presented 201 individuals (ages 65 to 94) with descriptions of three life-sustaining interventions. The interventions were described in three ways: positively (e.g., "device to help you breathe"), negatively (e.g., "machine that controls your breathing"), and exactly as they are worded in a widely used advance directive (e.g., "breathing by machine"). Results showed that for the three interventions presented in the three wordings, individuals were less likely to opt for an intervention when it was worded negatively than when it was framed positively or phrased as the directive already in use (12, 30, and 19 percent opted for the intervention with negative, positive, and current wordings, respectively). Moreover, most subjects appeared inconsistent from one moment to the next: 77 percent changed their minds at least once when given the same scenario but a different description of the intervention.

Malloy et al. (1992) concluded that their results highlight the need for older adults to get more decision-making help from their doctors. However, their study does not permit any conclusion to be made about whether elderly individuals are any worse at decision making than others, or whether they would in fact benefit from decision aiding by a doctor. In short, we do not know whether Malloy et al.'s elderly sample was any more inconsistent than young adults (or physicians for that matter) faced with the same decision tasks. Weber et al. (1995), however, do provide evidence that short-term memory limitations can lead to some preference reversals as the result of simplification in the encoding of presented information. Given the strong evidence of age-related declines in working memory found in the aging literature and the role of memory in the use of such judgmental heuristics as the availability heuristic, older adults may be more easily influenced by the decision context.

Age-related differences in decision consistency have been examined by Chasseigne et al. (1997) in a multiple-cue probability learning (MCPL) task. Learning probabilistic judgments is especially critical in the later stages of life, because major changes (such as retirement, loss of partner, and relocation) occur and individuals need to learn to cope with a new set of probabilistic relations in a new environment. For instance, coping with many illnesses simultaneously requires learning complex relations between the number of pills taken for each of several conditions and pain status.

In Chasseigne et al.'s study three groups of subjects (ages 20-30, 65-75, and 76-90) were asked to learn the relationships between three knobs on a boiler (the cues) and the boiler's water temperature (the criterion). The study tested and confirmed the hypothesis that due to their reduced working memory, older subjects have more difficulty remembering and processing the necessary information, resulting in more trial-to-trial variability or error variance (i.e., lower consistency). Providing task information that explicitly described the relation between each cue and the criterion improved the consistency of the two youngest groups, but not the 76-90-year-old group. Like other cognitive abilities, MCPL depends on information-processing speed and working-memory capacity, but reducing the working-memory load by simplifying the task did not help the very elderly. Chasseigne et al. suggest that the very elderly may have lost their flexibility of functioning, making them unable to modify their responses despite the external information. Assessing age-related differences in various MCPL tasks, as well as the extent to which the differences can or cannot be influenced by judgment aids, is an important direction for future research in order to accurately identify and augment the decision competence of elderly individuals.

Despite the above focus on internal consistency, equal attention should be paid to the other important aspects of competent decision making: the abilities to structure a decision, understand and remember information, appreciate the information's personal significance and temper impulsivity. Each of these skills taps functionally different areas, and choosing one over another to represent an individual's decision-making competence may result in discrepant conclusions. Individuals may perform adequately on a measure of information integration, for example, but display impaired performance on recall. Basing judgments of competence on one or several different abilities affects the identity and proportion of patients classified as incompetent (Fitten et al., 1990; Grisso and Appelbaum, 1995).

Developing a reliable and valid measure of decision-making competence is important because it is potentially very harmful to an individual's well-being if those who need decision assistance are not identified, and those who do not need assistance are denied their right to choose for themselves. In addition, a good measure of decision competence is important for identifying a baseline against which to compare special subgroups (e.g., persons with different diseases, medications, living arrangements). As such, future research should address how decision-making competence in older adults may improve, as well as how it might decline, so that decision situations can be improved for older adults, and individuals who require professional help can be identified (Birren and Schroots, 1996).

CONCLUSION

The quality of the judgments and decisions made by older persons will determine, to a large extent, the quality of their lives. In this brief review, we have attempted to sketch ways in which existing theories and methods may illuminate age-related changes in judgment and decision making. Although our initial thoughts on decision making among older adults centered on the inevitable declines of aging, further consideration suggests that improvements associated with experiential thinking may create a decision-making process that is much more bearable to older adults. By bearable, we mean that, despite age declines in cognitive functioning, older adults may adapt quite well to the judgments and decisions required of them in later years. The study of decision making in older adults will undoubtedly provide great practical benefits by pointing the way toward aiding and improving decisions as well as identifying those older adults who might need the most help. In addition to these practical benefits, coordinating decision-making research with studies of age-related changes in memory, attention, affect, and other psychological processes may produce important scientific insights into the mechanisms that underlie the judgments and decisions of older and younger adults.

ACKNOWLEDGMENTS

The authors thank Reid Hastie, Judy Hibbard, and an anonymous reviewer for comments on an earlier draft of this paper. The preparation of this paper was supported in part by a National Institute of Mental Health Emotion Research Training grant (No. MH18935) and a National Science Foundation grant (SES-9975347) to the first author and a National Science Foundation grant (SBR-9876587) and a contract from the Health Care Financing Administration (No. 500-97-0440: 2011) to the fourth author.

REFERENCES

Adams, C., M.C. Smith, L. Nyquist, and M. Perlmutter
  1997   Adult age-group differences in recall for the literal and interpretive meanings of narrative text. *Journals of Gerontology Series B Psychological Sciences and Social Sciences* 4:187.
Appelbaum, P.S., and T. Grisso
  1988   Assessing patients' capacities to consent to treatment. *New England Journal of Medicine* 319(25):1635-1638.
Baron, J., and M. Spranca
  1997   Protected values. *Organizational Behavior and Human Decision Processes* 70(1):1-16.
Bechara, A., A.R. Damasio, H. Damasio, and S.W. Anderson
  1994   Insensitivity to future consequences following damage to human prefrontal cortex. *Cognition* 50:7-15.
Birren, J.E., and J.J.F. Schroots
  1996   History, concepts, and theory in the psychology of aging. Pp. 3-23 in *Handbook of the Psychology of Aging, 4th ed. The Handbooks of Aging*, J.E. Birren, ed. San Diego: Academic Press, Inc.
Blanchard-Fields, F., J.R. Brannan, and C.J. Camp
  1987   Alternative conceptions of wisdom: An onion-peeling exercise. *Educational Gerontology* 13(6):497-503.
Borgida, E., and R.E. Nisbett
  1977   The differential impact of abstract vs. concrete information on decisions. *Journal of Applied Social Psychology* 7:258-271.
Carstensen, L.L., D.M. Isaacowitz, and S.T. Charles
  1999   Taking time seriously: A theory of socioemotional selectivity. *American Psychologist* 54(3):165-181.
Chapman, L.J., and J.P. Chapman
  1967   Genesis of popular but erroneous psychodiagnostic observations. *Journal of Abnormal Psychology* 72(3):193-204.
Chasseigne, G., E. Mullet, and T.R. Stewart
  1997   Aging and multiple cue probability learning: The case of inverse relationships. *Acta Psychologica* 97:235-252.
Damasio, A.R.
  1994   *Descartes' Error: Emotion, Reason, and the Human Brain.* New York: G.P. Putnam's Sons.
Denes-Raj, V., and S. Epstein
  1994   Conflict between intuitive and rational processing: When people behave against their better judgment. *Journal of Personality and Social Psychology* 66(5):819-829.

Epstein, S.
  1994   Integration of the cognitive and the psychodynamic unconscious. *American Psychologist* 49(8):709-724.
Finucane, M.L., A. Alhakami, P. Slovic, and S.M. Johnson
  2000   The affect heuristic in judgments of risks and benefits. *Journal of Behavioral Decision Making* 13:1-17.
Fitten, L.J., R. Lusky, and C. Hamann
  1990   Assessing treatment decision-making capacity in elderly nursing home residents. *Journal of the American Geriatrics Society* 38(10):1097-1104.
Fredrickson, B.L., and L.L. Carstensen
  1990   Choosing social partners: How old age and anticipated endings make people more selective. *Psychology and Aging* 5(3):335-347.
Frijda, N.H., P. Kuipers, and E. ter Schure
  1989   Relations among emotion, appraisal, and emotional action readiness. *Journal of Personality and Social Psychology* 57(2):212-228.
Grisso, T., and P.S. Appelbaum
  1995   Comparison of standards for assessing patients' capacities to make treatment decisions. *American Journal of Psychiatry* 152(7):1033-1037.
Hammond, K.
  1998   *Human Judgment and Social Policy.* New York: Cambridge University.
Hess, T.M.
  1990   Aging and schematic influences on memory. Pp. 93-160 in *Aging and Cognition: Knowledge Organization and Utilization. Advances in Psychology, 71,* T.M. Hess, ed. Amsterdam, Netherlands: North-Holland.
Isen, A.M.
  1993   Positive affect and decision making. Pp. 261-277 in *Handbook of Emotions,* M. Lewis and J.M. Haviland, eds. New York: Guilford.
Janis, I.L., and L. Mann
  1977   *Decision Making.* New York: The Free Press.
Jennings, J.M., and L.L. Jacoby
  1993   Automatic versus intentional uses of memory: Aging, attention, and control. *Psychology and Aging* 8(2):283-293.
Johnson, E.J., and A. Tversky
  1983   Affect, generalization, and the perception of risk. *Journal of Personality and Social Psychology* 45:20-31.
Johnson, M.M.S.
  1990   Age differences in decision making: A process methodology for examining strategic information processing. *Journal of Gerontology: Psychological Sciences* 45(2):P75-P78.
Kahneman, D., and J. Snell
  1990   Predicting utility. Pp. 295-310 in *Insights in Decision Making,* R.M. Hogarth, ed. Chicago: University of Chicago.
Kahneman, D., and A. Tversky
  1973   On the psychology of prediction. *Psychological Review* 80:237-251.
  1979   Prospect theory: An analysis of decision under risk. *Econometrica* 47:263-291.
Labouvie-Vief, G.
  1999   Emotions in adulthood. Pp. 253-267 in *Handbook of Theories of Aging,* V.L.S.K.W. Bengtson, ed. New York: Springer Publishing Co., Inc.
Labouvie-Vief, G., M. DeVoe, and D. Bulka
  1989a Speaking about feelings: Conceptions of emotion across the life span. *Psychology and Aging* 4(4):425-437.

Labouvie-Vief, G., J. Hakim-Larson, M. DeVoe, and S. Schoeberlein
  1989b Emotions and self-regulation: A life span view. *Human Development* 32(5):279-299.
Lawton, M.P., M.H. Kleban, D. Rajagopal, and J. Dean
  1992 Dimensions of affective experience in three age groups. *Psychology and Aging* 7(2):171-184.
Lichtenstein, S., and P. Slovic
  1971 Reversals of preference between bids and choices in gambling decisions. *Journal of Experimental Psychology* 89:46-55.
  1973 Response-induced reversals of preference in gambling: An extended replication in Las Vegas. *Journal of Experimental Psychology* 101:16-20.
Loewenstein, G.
  1992 The fall and rise of psychological explanations in the economics of intertemporal choice. Pp. 3-34 in *Choice Over Time*, G.E.J. Loewenstein, ed. New York: Russell Sage Foundation.
  1996 Out of control: Visceral influences on behavior. *Organizational Behavior and Human Decision Processes* 65(3):272-292.
Loewenstein, G., and D. Prelec
  1992 Anomalies in interpersonal choice: Evidence and an interpretation. Pp. 119-145 in *Choice Over Time*, G. Loewenstein and J. Elster, eds. New York: Russell Sage Foundation.
Lopes, L.L.
  1987 Between hope and fear: The psychology of risk. Pp. 255-295 in *Advances in Experimental Social Psychology*, 20th vol., L. Berkowitz, ed. San Diego: Academic.
Malloy, T.R., R.S. Wigton, J. Meeske, and T.G. Tape
  1992 The influence of treatment descriptions on advance medical directive decisions. *Journal of the American Geriatrics Society* 40(12):1255-1260.
McCrae, R.R., D. Arenberg, and P.T. Costa
  1987 Declines in divergent thinking with age: Cross-sectional, longitudinal, and cross-sequential analyses. *Psychology and Aging* 2(2):130-137.
McNeil, B.J., S.G. Pauker, H.C. Sox, Jr., and A. Tversky
  1982 On the elicitation of preferences for alternative therapies. *New England Journal of Medicine* 306:1259-1262.
Mellers, B.A., A. Schwartz, K. Ho, and I. Ritov
  1997 Decision affect theory: Emotional reactions to the outcomes of risky options. *Psychological Science* 8(6):423-429.
Mowrer, O.H.
  1960a *Learning Theory and Behavior*. New York: John Wiley and Sons, Inc.
  1960b *Learning Theory and the Symbolic Processes*. New York: John Wiley and Sons, Inc.
Mutter, S.A., and R.M. Pliske
  1994 Aging and illusory correlation in judgments of co-occurrence. *Psychology and Aging* 9(1):53-63.
Myles-Worsley, J., W.A. Johnston, and M.A. Simons
  1988 The influence of expertise on X-ray image processing. *Journal of Experimental Psychology: Learning, Memory, and Cognition* 14(3):553-557.
Parker, A.M., and B. Fischhoff
  1999 Individual Differences in Decision-Making Competence. Paper presented at the Annual Meeting of the American Economic Association, New York.
Peters, E.
  1998 The Springs of Action: Affective and Analytical Information Processing in Choice. Unpublished doctoral dissertation. University of Oregon, Eugene.

Peters, E., and P. Slovic
    1996   The role of affect and worldviews as orienting dispositions in the perception and
            acceptance of nuclear power. *Journal of Applied Social Psychology* 26(16):1427-1453.
    In   The springs of action: Affective and analytical information processing in choice.
    press   *Personality and Social Psychology Bulletin*.
Radvansky, G.A.
    1999   Aging, memory, and comprehension. *Current Directions in Psychological Science*
            8(2):49-53.
Ritov, I., and J. Baron
    1990   Reluctance to vaccinate: Omission bias and ambiguity. *Journal of Behavioral Deci-
            sion Making* 3:263-277.
Rosenfeld, B.D., and E.N. Turkheimer
    1995   Modeling psychiatric patients' treatment decision making. *Law and Human Behav-
            ior* 19(4):389-405.
Rozin, P., J. Haidt, and C.R. McCauley
    1993   Disgust. Pp. 575-594 in *Handbook of Emotions*, M.H.J.M. Lewis, ed. New York:
            Guilford Press.
Salthouse, T.A.
    1996   The processing-speed theory of adult age differences in cognition. *Psychological Re-
            view* 103(3):403-428.
Sanfey, A.G., and R. Hastie
    1998   Does evidence presentation format affect judgment? An experimental evaluation of
            displays of data for judgments. *Psychological Science* 9(2):99-103.
    In   Judgment and decision making across the adult life span: A tutorial review of psy-
    press   chological research. In *Aging and Cognition: A Primer*, D. Park and N. Schwarz, eds.
            Philadelphia: Psychology Press.
Satterfield, T., P. Slovic, and R. Gregory
    In   Narrative valuation in a policy judgment context. *Ecological Economics*.
    press
Shafir, E., I. Simonson, and A. Tversky
    1993   Reason-based choice. *Cognition* 49:11-36.
Slovic, P.
    1995   The construction of preference. *American Psychologist* 50(5):364-371.
Slovic, P., J. Monahan, and D. MacGregor
    In   Violence risk assessment and risk communication: The effects of using actual cases,
    press   providing instruction, and employing probability versus frequency formats. *Law
            and Human Behavior*.
Streufert, S., R. Pogash, M. Piasecki, and G.M. Post
    1990   Age and management team performance. *Psychology and Aging* 5(4):551-559.
Thaler, R.
    1980   Toward a positive theory of consumer choice. *Journal of Economic Behavior and
            Organization* 1:39-60.
Tversky, A., and D. Kahneman
    1974   Judgment under uncertainty: Heuristics and biases. *Science* 185(4157):1124-1131.
    1983   Extensional versus intuitive reasoning: The conjunction fallacy in probability judg-
            ment. *Psychological Review* 90(4):293-315.
Weber, E.U., W.M. Goldstein, and S. Barlas
    1995   And let us not forget memory: The role of memory processes and techniques in the
            study of judgment and choice. Pp. 33-81 in *Decision Making from the Perspective of
            Cognitive Psychology*, 32d vol., J.R. Busemeyer, R. Hastie, and D.L. Medin, eds. San
            Diego: Academic Press, Inc.

Weber, E.U., and C. Hsee
  In   Models and mosaics: Investigating cross-cultural differences in risk perception and
  press   risk preference. *Psychonomic Bulletin and Review.*
Wilson, T.D., D.J. Lisle, J.W. Schooler, S.D. Hodges, K.J. Klaaren, and S.J. LaFleur
  1993   Introspecting about reasons can reduce post-choice satisfaction. *Personality and So-
           cial Psychology Bulletin* 19(3):331-339.
Yates, J.F., and A.L. Patalano
  1999   Decision making and aging. Pp. 31-54 in *Processing of Medical Information in Aging
           Patients*, D.C. Park and R.W. Morrell, eds. Mahwah, NJ: Lawrence Erlbaum Associ-
           ates Inc., Publisher.
Zajonc, R.B.
  1980   Feeling and thinking: Preferences need no inferences. *American Psychologist* 35:151-
           175.
Zwahr, M.D.
  1999   Cognitive processes and medical decisions. Pp. 55-68 in *Processing of Medical Infor-
           mation in Aging Patients*, D.C. Park and R.W. Morrell, eds. Mahwah, NJ: Lawrence
           Erlbaum Associates Inc., Publisher.

D

Cognitive Aging and Adaptive Technologies

Donald L. Fisher

INTRODUCTION

Adaptivity is an important aspect of human behavior, frequently determining those who will and will not perform a given task successfully. As adults grow older, they respond more slowly to simple stimuli and take longer to learn new material, thus potentially decreasing their ability to adapt. Their vision, speech, and hearing can become impaired. In addition, they often exhibit larger temporal variations in sensory, motor, and more abstract cognitive abilities than do younger and middle-aged adults. Until recently, technology could not address most of these decreases in potential adaptivity. However, as computers become smaller, more powerful, and more easily embedded in other objects and processes, they provide the opportunity to construct technology that can augment greatly the adaptivity and functionality of the older adult user.

Examples of current and future adaptive technologies include computers that can be worn—for example, eyeglasses that enhance the peripheral field of vision (Jebara et al., 1998)—and microelectromechanical systems, which can easily and unobtrusively be placed in objects that an individual might normally carry—for example, an ultrasound sensor embedded in a cane, which provides information about the nearby structures and terrain for older adults with vision impairments (Gao and Cai, 1998)—or with which an individual might normally interact—for example, head-up displays in an automobile (Tufano, 1997). Taking advantage of these advances will require a greatly expanded understanding of the effects of aging on cognition, since such effects are often dependent on the context, and the adaptive technologies will radically change this context.

Federal and private initiatives to advance adaptive technologies are extensive in the fields of biomedicine and bioengineering. They include everything from the support of the development of full-scale doctoral degree programs (the Whitaker Foundation) to the support of small projects to be undertaken by undergraduates in engineering with clients who have one or more disabilities (the National Science Foundation). However, no programs currently exist at the federal level that specifically target research that advances understanding of the basic cognitive behaviors in older adults that could serve as the foundation for the design of adaptive technologies.

The chapter is divided into four sections. The first section discusses the most promising of the new technologies (hardware and software) that have been developed for sensing environmental and behavioral information. The second section identifies a similarly promising group of new technologies that can be used to display information to individuals. The third section discusses powerful modeling tools that can be used to infer the behavior of individuals from the much more detailed record that the new sensing technologies provide. It also shows how these tools can lead directly to the development of a next generation of personalized, highly interactive interfaces that themselves increase the adaptivity of existing technologies. The final section discusses current and future applications of these technologies and identifies the basic research in cognitive aging that would be needed to carry forward the applications.

SENSING, INTEGRATING AND PLANNING

Advances in technologies are making it possible to put sensors and processors in locations that heretofore had been inaccessible. Advances in algorithms are making it possible to process intelligently and in real time the extraordinary amounts of data that can now be gathered by these devices. Increases in the raw speed of processing information are one major factor contributing to these advances. There is every likelihood that these increases will continue into the foreseeable future. Equally important in the domain of sensing is the development of microelectromechanical systems. They are defined as three-dimensional mechanical or electromechanical components/devices with sizes in the micrometer range, such as micro gears, beams, pumps, motors, hinges, and switches. These microscopic devices are designed to create controllable mechanical motions, which are the basis for a wide range of sensors, actuators, or mechanical structures that have been used in both industrial and commercial applications. Discussed below are new technologies for sensing environmental variables, integrating environmental information, and planning possible actions in order to make an older adults' behavior more broadly context sensitive and therefore more adaptive.

Driving

Sensors can now be placed in cars. Together with the associated image analysis algorithms and the necessary models of vehicle dynamics and traffic scenarios, they can provide selected, critical information to the driver about the roadway ahead (e.g., upcoming regulatory or warning signs). For example, existing systems have a range of 1 to 200 meters, can resolve detail as fine as 1 meter, and are about 150 mm in diameter and 100 mm in length. Each beam usually covers 5 to 8 degrees, leading typically to 3 or 4 beams in total for complete forward coverage. Doppler information can be read directly for the determination of velocity. Such sensors could potentially play a critical role in reducing the number of collisions for older adults. This is especially important given that older adults are more likely to be involved in a fatal crash than any other cohort (Barr, 1991). However, before sensor technology can be implemented, much must be learned about the basic visual search strategies of older adults, in order to know what information to present and when to present it, reducing to a minimum the number of false or useless warnings. And much must be learned about older adults' ability to handle successfully multiple forms of input when the load on the cognitive systems is especially high—as it will be during a potential collision.

Walking

For aided orientation and mobility, the majority of blind people use the long cane, which provides an extended spatial sensing of about 0.5 meter ahead of the user, within an arc of about 120 degrees. However, the use of a long cane does not provide protection for the body parts above the waist. Using microelectromechanical system technologies, miniaturized ultrasound sensors and on-board microelectronics have recently been developed that can be embedded in the shaft of the long cane, thereby providing added sensing capability for overhanging obstacle detection (Cai and Gao, in press). The ultrasound sensor has a detection range of 4-5 meters (or 12-15 feet), a distance resolution of about 20 mm (about an inch), and a scanning range that basically covers the user's body, roughly +15 to –15 degrees ahead. Improvements in the sensing capability of the long cane could have a large impact on older adults. More than 2 million Americans are blind or have severe visual impairments. Each year, around 35,000 adults become blind as a result of accidents, cataracts, glaucoma, diabetes, and other diseases. Many are older adults. Although the sensing technology is well developed, progress still needs to be made on the interface. A simple warning sound could be presented, but this would lack important location information. A synthesized voice could provide users with the azimuth, distance, and height of an object, but it is not yet clear how effective this would be. Of course, at some point, three-dimensional virtual auditory displays may make it possible to synthesize the warning at a point in virtual space coincident with its point in actual space (although see the section below on displays). More basic research is needed on sound localization in older adults in order to take full advantage of the blind cane with an ultrasound sensor.

Spatial Location

Global positioning systems (GPS), which consist of both a satellite network and a receiver, can now be used to give latitude and longitude positions to within 100 m without differential positioning and to within millimeters with differential positioning (referencing one GPS signal with the signal from a transmitter at a known location). GPS receivers have been miniaturized to just a few integrated circuits (Dye and Baylin, 1997). Such systems can be located in an automobile or carried on the person. Systems with the capability for differential positioning are relatively expensive; much cheaper systems exist that do not have this capability. The major disadvantage of using GPS to obtain location information while in transit is that the satellite transmissions can be blocked by tall structures and overhanging trees and other leafy vegetation. A minor disadvantage in most cases is that the accuracy of elevation information is considerably less, some 3-4 m, even with differential positioning.

GPS technologies have obvious applications to navigation systems in automobiles, and they may be especially useful for older adults. For example, older adults are overrepresented in crashes at signalized left turn intersections (Staplin and Fisk, 1991; Szymkowiak et al., 1997). Many older adults recognize this problem and so may take three right turns around a block rather than a single left turn. A GPS could let them know when this strategy is possible. Older adults would also prefer routes with less traffic and slower speeds. Again, a GPS, together with advances in intelligent transportation systems, could remedy this problem, at least in part. However, it still remains to be determined whether older adults can easily both drive and process input from an in-vehicle navigation system. Basic research on time sharing must be undertaken in order to make the best use of the GPS technologies.

GPS technologies may also have applications as reminder systems. Location can serve as a cue for helpful retrieval cues, which may assist an older adult who has difficulty remembering the names of people at particular locations (grocer, pharmacist, a neighbor). Basic research on the tip-of-the-tongue phenomenon and more general memory could prove especially helpful in this area (Burke and Harrold, 1988; Burke et al., 1988).

Eye Position

Eye trackers have existed for some time but have placed too many constraints on the individual to be useful in applied settings, requiring the individual either to remain motionless or to wear a bulky head-mounted device. However, such is no longer the case. The particular area of a scene or display at which an individual is looking can now be inferred from eye and head trackers that are totally removed from the individual. Many use a video-based technology and can sample the eye position at up to 240 Hz. The accuracy of the position so sampled is within a degree or so. Realistically, the head must remain in a relatively small volume of space. But at least in the cabin of an automobile, this is not a problem. Nor would it be a problem tracking someone using any of the various displays, computer or electromechanical, that now exist (e.g., ATMs).

Eye position information could be critical to the realization of the full potential of adaptive technologies, especially for older adults, since many difficulties that older adults have can only be remedied if more is known in real time about the behaviors of the individuals involved. For example, many older adults have great difficulty with automated teller machines (ATMs) (Rogers et al., 1996). We could better understand the problems if we knew where the older adult was focusing when the problems occurred. Older drivers also have particular difficulty negotiating left turns, as was noted above. We could better understand why this is the case if we knew when the older adult fixated each of the various sections of the roadway ahead and to the side. Basic research is needed that can be used to infer the behavior of the individual using an adaptive technology from the information on the position of the eyes, which is being gathered in real time. Such inferences have been possible when individuals are undertaking a relatively simple task, like reading (Rayner, 1998), and the extensions to adaptive technologies is a reasonable next step. Hidden Markov models may play a particularly important role in this context (Reichle et al., 1998).

DISPLAYS

Advances in miniaturization are not confined to sensor technologies. Such advances also alter greatly what can be displayed and when it can be displayed. These advances are being fueled by the same factors that are moving forward the development of sensor technologies. Increases in speed make it possible to expand the bandwidth of the channels that are processing the information displayed. Increases in miniaturization make it possible to produce displays so small that they can be mounted in the frames of eyeglasses.

Head-Up Displays

Head-up displays have been used for some time in aviation, and their benefits and disbenefits have been studied extensively in that context (Weintraub and Ensing, 1992). They make it possible for the pilot to keep his or her eyes focused on the outside world and simultaneously to monitor the critical instruments. Head-up displays can now be used in the automobile as well (Gish and Staplin, 1995). In such displays, images are projected onto the windshield in front of the driver. The driver then sees the image superimposed on the roadway outside the automobile. The images can be focused at optical infinity or at any point closer to the driver. Images are typically of the dials and gauges. Such displays are now available on the Corvette. It is also possible to project radar images of objects onto the window at the exact place they would appear were they truly visible. This is especially useful during poor weather or nighttime driving. The images could also be displayed in a separate window. For example, Cadillac now includes as an option a display of the roadway ahead at the bottom of the windshield. The roadway image is generated by infrared radar and can detect objects at night that might not otherwise be visible (e.g., deer crossing some distance in front of the driver). These displays may have the same benefits for drivers that they have for pilots. And they may benefit older adults most, since older adults take longer to scan for information on the standard dials and gauges of a car. However, the technology is being brought to market without extensive discussions in the open literature on the benefits and costs to all drivers, let alone to older drivers. Fundamental increases in understanding of the effects of aging on perception are needed before we can truly be confident that older adults will show a net benefit from these technologies (see the section below on future research areas).

Head-Mounted Displays

Head-mounted displays make it possible for a user to view a display while performing other tasks (Feiner et al., 1993). Typically, the display is located immediately in front of the eye, either overlaid (Starner et al., 1997) or not overlaid (Rhodes, 1997) on the real world. A relatively high resolution, 720 by 280, is possible. This produces an easily readable 80 by 25 character screen. One can imagine many uses for such technologies by older adults. For example, many older adults miss taking their medications (Park, 1992). This is of particular concern because the health needs of older adults are so much greater than those of younger adults (U.S. Department of Health and Human Services, 1991). A head-mounted display could alert an older adult that it was time to take a particular medication. The actual medication and location of the medication could be presented on the head-mounted display as well as any instructions relevant to the administration (e.g., take with water). Basic research is needed to identify the best format for presenting complex printed information to the older adult, one that conveys the various risks adequately as well. This research should build on the existing research in medical decision making (e.g., Cho et al., 1999; Miyamoto, 1999).

Variable Message Signs

Electronic variable message signs located over or by the side of the highway can be used to deliver to drivers in real time information about traffic, parking, weather, and other conditions (Kahn, 1992). Although such displays are not new, the technology used to implement the displays is changing rapidly. The displays are becoming much cheaper to produce and, as a consequence, are being implemented on a much broader basis. For example, variable message signs are now used to display the predicted travel time along a driver's current route and several alternative routes to a common destination. Research with younger adults suggests that the proportion diverting along the alternative route can be predicted and, more importantly (at least in the current context), the proportion diverting changes as the load on the driver increases (Katsikopoulos et al., 2000). The effect of load on the decision-making process is of some concern here, because older adults may have particular difficulty with the extra cognitive demands placed on them while driving (Sit and Fisk, 1999). Thus, these systems as proposed may be of little if any use to the older driver. And they could lead to more incidents (crashes, slowdowns) and therefore, ultimately, to more congestion, since it is such incidents that normally choke the progress of traffic. Clearly more needs to be known about how one can use intelligent transportation systems technologies without overwhelming the older driver (Kantowitz et al., 1997; Santiago, 1992; Sobbi, 1995; Walker et al., 1997). And this needs to build on the large body of work that already exists in transportation science (Ben-Akiva and Lerman, 1985).

Three-Dimensional Sound

Advanced digitizing capabilities and a greatly increased understanding of the exact interaural differences and spectral cues that help individuals localize a sound now make it possible to present a three-dimensional soundscape over headphones (Wightman and Kistler, 1989). Specifically, head-related transfer functions are computed for a particular individual (or group of individuals). These functions preserve both the pattern of interaural differences and the spectral cues that are needed to make location judgments. The use of three-dimensional virtual sound environments has been confined primarily to the military and, in particular, to the generation of auditory collision warnings for pilots. The auditory warning is located in virtual space at the same location as the object with which a collision is imminent. Such warnings can decrease greatly the time that it takes users to locate a potential threat, both when the warnings are generated externally (Perrott et al., 1990) and when the warnings are generated over headphones (Begault, 1993).

Three-dimensional audio displays may also have importance in the automobile for older drivers, both those with and without hearing impairments. It is now very difficult, even for drivers with good hearing, to localize in the saggital plane sounds that are either directly in front or directly in back of the driver (Caelli and Porter, 1980). For the hearing impaired, it is even more difficult. Wearable audio computing extends the range of applications (Roy et al., 1997), perhaps to collision warning systems for blind users of a long cane. Basic research on sound localization is needed in order to determine whether older adults can more quickly find a visual target and react appropriately when a sound is generated that occupies a position in virtual space identical to the target. This may be particularly problematic for older adults, who become less sensitive with time to high-frequency sounds; it is such frequencies that are important to localization. If this is the case, then perhaps basic research could identify other ways to cue location.

Digitized and Synthesized Voice

It is now possible to broadcast widely over the telephone personalized messages using either synthetic speech or digitized voice clips. Such a technology could have many different applications for older adults. One potential application is the automating of medical appointment information (Leirer et al., 1993). This is critical, since older adults frequently fail to attend their medical appointments (Deyo and Inui, 1980). Information about a medical appointment can be complex. Thus, it is not all that surprising that older adults have difficulty keeping track of their medical appointments. Early studies indicated that automated telephone reminders can help (Leirer et al., 1989). More recent studies have indicated that the format of the automated message (Morrow, 1997) and the number of repetitions (Morrow et al., 1999) have an effect on older adults' memory for automated messages. However, although both younger and older adults benefit from improvements in the format and increases in the number of message repetitions, the advantage that younger adults generally enjoy in such tasks is not reduced when the measure of message comprehension is free recall. Thus, room for improvement still exists and research is needed that identifies procedures that can increase further older adults' recall of medical appointments.

ADAPTIVE INTERFACES

Advances in sensors and display technologies can lead by themselves to increasingly adaptive interfaces. However, the adaptivity of an interface is not controlled by these technologies alone. Increases in adaptivity can be obtained by displaying to older adults an interface that is tailored to them as a group or to each individually. Increases in the adaptivity of an interface can also be achieved by predicting in real time the future behavior of an individual and adjusting the response of a system appropriately.

Personalized Interfaces

Increasingly personalized interfaces are made possible by rapid advances in wireless communication (to download a user's profile to an interface), much more sophisticated models of performance (for predicting response times and errors), and faster optimizing algorithms (for identifying the best interface). Most users of personal data assistants are familiar with at least one form of wireless communication. Specifically, infrared radiation is now used to send data from one device (e.g., computer or personal data assistant) to another at speeds that are fast enough to transmit easily tens of kilobytes of information in a second or less. With the advent of wearable computers and the recent development of flexible transistors (Markoff, 1999), this makes it possible to consider adaptive technologies that tune themselves to the individual at start-up. For example, as noted above, older adults generally have difficulty with ATMs. This might change greatly if the interface could be tailored to the user, which it could be if the relevant information on the user (say the relative duration of various cognitive processes) were beamed to the ATM from a user's wearable computer.

Quantitative models then make possible the individualization of the interface from the initialization data. Specifically, an analytic or computer model can be used to predict performance for any given design of an interface (e.g., the response time for that design). For example, consider the menu hierarchy that might be displayed to a user of an ATM. In this case, one can vary in each menu the option that is assigned to a key (assuming that a central display of options is surrounded by keys that point to each option). Suppose that the menu hierarchy has just two levels with six options in each menu (i.e., one menu with six options at the top level and six menus each with six options at the bottom level). The time on average that it takes an older adult to access an option in the bottom level will depend both on the time that it takes an individual to strike a pair of keys, one at the first level and one at the second, and on the frequency with which a given pair of options is used. Models exist that can predict the average access time for any given assignment (Rumelhart and Norman, 1982).

Finally, an optimal design of an interface needs to be established. Continuing with the example, note that there are 6! (six factorial) different assignments of options to keys in each menu, or a total of 720 different assignments for just the single menu in the top level of the hierarchy. Since there is one menu with 6 options in the highest level of the hierarchy and 6 menus with 6 options each in the next highest level, there are a total of 720^7 different assignments of options to keys in a simple ATM! Methods clearly are needed to identify the assignment that minimizes the average access time for an individual.

Point and click hierarchies also present the same opportunity for optimization (Fisher et al., 1990). A very, very large number of different organizations are possible, any one of which is semantically acceptable. The optimal organization in this case depends on the time that it takes an individual to analyze each option in a menu (or on a screen). A simple model can be used to predict the average terminal option access time. And then dynamic programming can be used to identify the hierarchy that minimizes the average terminal option access time. These are but a few of the many possible ways in which one can potentially individualize an interface for older adults and thereby adapt it to the user (Fisher, 1993).

Interactive Interfaces

Increasingly, interactive interfaces are made possible by many of the same improvements that are leading to the individualized interfaces described above: improvements in wireless communications, mathematical models of older adults' behavior, and real-time optimization algorithms. For example, older adults have difficulties maneuvering their vehicles that younger adults do not have (arthritis being one of the leading causes of these problems). This might change if the profile from an individual older adult could be beamed to devices in the vehicle that offered steering, braking, and throttle assistance. Models of the older adult can then be used both to initialize the interface and to predict the behavior of the older adult, intervening when it appears that assistance is needed, either passively (by providing information) or actively (by taking over the controls). These interventions can in many cases be optimized as well.

Passive interventions have been used for some time, at least on computers. For example, on the basis of the sequence of keystrokes that a user enters, help windows open at particular points to suggest possible actions the user might take. However, the range of assistance that can be provided is greatly expanded once we consider the new sensing technologies, especially the ability to track a user's eyes in real time (Byrne and Anderson, 1998; Salvucci and Anderson, 1998). For example, consider the potential assistance that might be provided were one to track the eyes of an older driver. Such information could be used to warn inattentive or sleepy drivers (Allen et al., 1994; Knipling and Wierwille, 1994; Wierwille, 1994; Wierwille et al., 1994). This information could also be used to alert drivers that attention should be paid to important warning or regulatory information. Specifically, knowing where an individual is fixating is critical to determining whether the individual sees a warning or regulatory sign. However, it is not the case that the fixation position can by itself be used to indicate just what has and has not been seen (Rayner, 1998). Information on the details of a stimulus that is not being fixated can also be identified, information such as the shape, color, and sometimes even the accompanying text and symbols. Thus, were one to warn drivers about signs to which attention must be paid immediately based solely on the fact that the sign had not yet been fixated, one would generate many false alarms. Soon, drivers would not heed the warning. What one needs in this case is a model of the visual scanning process that predicts at each point in time the likelihood a particular object has been identified given the prior sequence of fixations. Such models exist for simple scenes (Ranney, 1998). Basic research is needed to extend these models to the more complex scenes that confront the driver.

Consider now a more active intervention. Sensors can give to individuals important information about the environment around them. Sometimes, actions must be taken on that information very quickly, perhaps in order to avoid a collision. The sensor technology designed to yield such real-time information has great potential for older adults, aiding in nighttime driving, parallel parking maneuvers, intersection maneuvers, and steering and braking during potential collision scenarios. In order to assist efficiently the older driver, one must be able to predict the path of the vehicle (or vehicles) in a given scenario in real time. Sensor management systems that include real-time path planning and control algorithms for an automobile are likely soon. Such systems are available right now for indoor environments. They detect and model geometry in that environment and track other moving objects (Connolly and Grupen, 1993, 1994; Grupen et al., 1995; Stan et al., 1994). The major advances in technology that are needed at present are for sensor management systems operating in real time in the environment of an automobile that would detect and model the geometry in the roadway and track other vehicles on the roadway. One must also be able to predict the actions of the older driver. Hidden Markov models of lane changing have already been successfully developed and tested (Liu, 1998; Liu and Pentland, 1997). They can predict ahead when a driver is changing lanes. Models of braking are also available (Lee, 1976). The major advances in person-machine models needed at present are discrete state descriptions of a much wider range of driving behaviors, a better understanding of how to distribute control between the driver and the car, and a better appreciation for just what drivers will and will not accept as assistance in the car. Hidden Markov models and more general discrete state models have been used successfully to model a number of per-son-machine systems similar to the automobile (Miller, 1985; Rabiner, 1989; Wickens, 1982). Thus, there is reason to believe that the basic research will succeed.

FUTURE RESEARCH AREAS

It has been argued at length that the advances in adaptive technologies cannot be fully realized unless more is understood about the effects of aging on cognition. It is clear that we need to know more about perception, visual search, memory, decision making, learning and problem solving, and models of cognitive processing. Unfortunately, there is not the space needed to de-scribe all of the many research advances that are necessary. Below, the areas of basic research in cognitive aging that are likely to bear most critically on the implementation of adaptive technologies are discussed. An argument is made at the end that much of the research needs to be interdisciplinary in nature.

Sensors

The more one knows about the underlying behavior of an individual, the more one can potentially increase the individualization and interactivity of a given interface. The sensor technology most likely to yield this information in the future is the development of eye trackers that are transparent to the user. Currently, much is understood about both the components of visual search when the eyes remain stationary (or move little, if at all; e.g., Schneider and Shiffrin, 1977; Wolfe, 1994) and the effects of aging on these components (e.g., Plude and Doussard-Roosevelt, 1989). Much less is understood about the components of visual search when the eyes must move broadly across a static scene (Rayner and Pollatsek, 1992) or the effects of aging on these components (Whiteside, 1974). And even less is understood about the com-ponents of visual search and the effects of age on these components when the scenes being scanned are dynamic ones, as in driving (Szlyk et al., 1995) or when the observer is changing his or her point of view (Tarr, 1995). Interest-ingly, across all types of search, one observes a strong and consistent effect of aging: older adults take longer to find a target (e.g., Madden et al., 1996). This effect is not on the duration of the fixations, but instead the number of move-ments or saccades (Maltz and Shinar, 1999). We need to understand in much more detail how older adults scan both static and dynamic visual scenes. In order to make large advances in this understanding we will need to increase the ability to interpret patterns of eye movements, patterns that can reveal the underlying or latent cognitive processes (Rayner, 1998). And in order to make these advances, we will need to be able to model the behavior of the system so that we can better isolate the effect of aging on the individual components (processes) of the system (Reichle et al., 1998).

Displays

The advantages of head-up displays were initially thought to far outweigh their disadvantages. Indeed, early reports indicated that drivers more frequently identified distinctive stimuli in a traffic scenario when using a head-up display than when using a dashboard-mounted display (Sojourner and Antin, 1990). However, more recent tests with automobiles suggest that there may be problems with such devices, problems that need to be addressed right now as the first automotive head-up displays are coming to market (Tufano, 1997). These are problems with the very advantages that devices were supposed to provide.

First, there is now evidence that drivers do not focus at optical infinity when the image is collimated (Marran and Schor, 1997). Instead their misaccommodation is inward, tending by some accounts toward their accommodative resting position in the dark (Iavecchia et al., 1988) and by other accounts toward their vergence resting position (Weintraub and Ensing, 1992). In either case, the result is that objects in the outside world appear more distant and smaller than in fact they really are. In the aviation literature, it has been argued that this is the cause of many of the very hard landings that pilots make, the runway appearing farther away than it actually is when a head-up display is in use (Roscoe, 1987). However, it is still not known exactly what causes the objects in the real world to appear both more distant and smaller in size. Nor is it well known how aging affects misaccommodation.

Second, it is no longer universally believed that a head-up display will make it easier for drivers to attend to events in the outside world that require some action. In fact, Weintraub and Ensing (1992) have argued that the display images may actually capture the attention of the individual, making it more difficult to recognize unusual events in the real world. Attention to displays on the dashboard is associated with a multitude of cues (e.g., changes in accommodation, vergence, head position, ambient illumination) that alert the driver that he or she is paying attention to something other than the traffic in the outside world. A head-up display, in contrast, does not provide the user with these cues and therefore can cognitively capture the attention of the driver. Evidence is now accumulating suggesting that this may be a real problem (Wickens and Long, 1994). And given older adults' inability easily to switch attention and their greatly constricted useful field of view (Ball et al., 1990; Owsley et al., 1991; Sanders, 1970), a head-up display may capture the attention of an older adult much longer and more completely than it does that of a younger adult. Clearly, more research is needed before head-up displays are universally installed in automobiles.

Interfaces

The opportunity to individualize the design of an interface for a specific older adult is great. As noted above, it depends on our having for a given task both a quantitative model that can predict performance for each of the different possible interface designs and a mathematical or computer method that can be used to identify the optimal design. Such a capability depends on our having an understanding of the effects of aging on the structure and duration of the cognitive processes underlying the performance (Fisher and Glaser, 1996). The general statement that older adults are slower on speeded tasks is almost always true in practice. Many explanations for this slowing have been offered, including decreases in memory capacity (Salthouse, 1980) and increases in a failure to inhibit competing sources of information. But it is the slowing of the latent processes themselves that explains most of the overall slowing in response times (Salthouse, 1996a, 1996b). This slowing, at first thought to be proportional across all processes (Birren, 1965, 1974), is now known to vary across domains (Hale et al., 1987; Lima et al., 1991) and possibly within domains across individual processes (Fisk and Rogers, 1991; Fisk et al., 1992). This specificity requires much more systematic analyses. Quantitative models are now available that use standard additive factors techniques (Sternberg, 1969, 1975) to tease apart the structure of complex tasks (Schweickert, 1978; Schweickert and Townsend, 1989). And methods are available that can be used to predict response times with these more complex networks (Goldstein and Fisher, 1991, 1992). It is important to extend these methods to a great many more tasks than have been studied so far.

Interdisciplinary Research

The practical advances just described cannot be achieved solely by basic research within a single discipline. For example, consider the development of a collision avoidance system, which helps the older driver both notice and steer around obstacles without taking complete control of the vehicle. We need to know not only how to direct the driver's attention to a particular position ahead of the automobile where the collision is predicted to occur. We would also need to generalize our understanding of elementary motions, such as reaching (Berthier, 1996), and of the effects of various forms of visual and force feedback on operator performance learned from studies of teleoperation (Sheridan, 1991) to the fast-paced environment of the automobile. We then need to understand how to interface the driver's responses with the collision avoidance algorithms (Grupen et al., 1995; Stan et al., 1994), so that the assistance provided enhances (rather than detracts from) the driver's own steering efforts, an effort that requires a better understanding of control theory (Djaferis, 1995). Finally, we need to understand how best to implement the proposed assistive control system in hardware and software using the various micro-electromechanical miniaturization technologies (Holm-Hansen and Gao, 1997). In summary, basic research is needed that is at the interface of psychology (visual search and attention, psychomotor control), computer science (path planning algorithm development), electrical engineering (control theory), mechanical engineering (microelectromechanical systems), and human factors (person-machine systems models). Moreover, the basic research requires a fair degree of quantitative sophistication among all disciplines, a sophistication that is essential if the models of the person and the machine are ever going to be coordinated with one another.

SUMMARY AND IMPLICATIONS

As adults age, they lose their ability to lead their lives independently. Perhaps they can no longer drive, so shopping becomes a problem. Perhaps their own home becomes too difficult to navigate, so they must be moved to a retirement community. Perhaps they can no longer reliably remember when to take their medications or when to see a physician, so that their health is jeopardized. Or perhaps the rapid advances in the technologies they must master and with which they must interact (e.g., ATMs) leaves them behind. Any one of these conditions can lead to a loss of independence.

Advances in adaptive technologies have been identified in this paper that can potentially lead to a greater independence, advances in the sensing of environmental information, in the displaying of that information to the older adult, and in the individualization and interactivity of the interface. Many such advances will require models of the person (or person-machine system) that can be used to infer the behavior of the individual from the pattern of responses, models that may need to run in real time. Thus, advances have also been discussed in our ability to model the simple and complex behaviors that govern performance in discrete and continuous-control tasks. Some of the advances in adaptive technologies have already been implemented. Selective implementations were discussed, including those used in the car, the home, and more general commerce. Finally, the ongoing development of adaptive technologies suggests areas of research that will be critically important to future implementations of such technologies. Three areas in particular were identified, one most relevant to sensors (visual search), one most relevant to displays (perception and attention), and one most relevant to interfaces (mathematical modeling of cognitive tasks).

Four related implications follow from the review of adaptive technologies. First and foremost is the need to continue research in basic cognitive aging. Other areas of aging are receiving and should be receiving new emphasis, most notably cognitive neuroscience. But it is not the advances in cognitive neuroscience that will prepare the groundwork for the implementation of the first generation of adaptive technologies for older adults. The basic vocabulary is the elementary cognitive process, much as it was conceived by Donders (1868) over a century ago. Cognitive task analysis is at the center of the effort, and this level of abstraction is both necessary and sufficient at this point in time.

Second, and intimately related to the above, is the need to foster research and training that increases understanding not just of the effects of aging on performance, but also of the effects of aging on the structure and duration of the processes that underlie this performance. It is models of these processes, often quantitative, that will serve as the common language of the engineers and psychologists who try to bridge, through an adaptive technology, the worlds of cognition and control. Graduate training programs should be supported that emphasize modeling. Postdoctoral fellowships should be initiated that support individuals wanting to increase their understanding of cognitive models. And, to the extent possible, research initiatives should be encouraged that focus on both cognition and control.

Third, there is a clear need to support more multidisciplinary efforts. The National Science Foundation does this very successfully through vehicles such as the Science and Technology Centers, Engineering Research Centers, and major cross-disciplinary programs (e.g., Knowledge and Distributed Intelligence), which encourage collaboration across disciplines. The National Institutes of Health also have a mechanism in place for establishing centers. There is no obvious reason that the National Institute on Aging could not set out such programmatic initiatives, if not at the center level then certainly at the level of requests for proposals that are obviously multidisciplinary in focus.

Finally, there is a clear need to support the acquisition of adaptive technologies and the equipment that it takes to evaluate such technologies. For items that are relatively inexpensive, this would not seem to create a problem with the current funding mechanism. However, for more expensive items, a different mechanism may be needed, one that the National Institute on Aging is best positioned to detail.

ACKNOWLEDGMENTS

A number of individuals have read and commented on the chapter. I would particularly like to thank Robert Gao, Kathleen Hancock and Rod Grupen (all of the University of Massachusetts at Amherst), Richard Jagacinski (Ohio State University) and William Yost (Loyola University Chicago).

REFERENCES

Allen, R.W., Z. Parseghian, S. Kelly, and T. Rosenthal
  1994   An Experimental Study of Driver Alertness Monitoring (Paper 508). Hawthorne, CA: Systems Technology, Inc.
Ball, K., C. Wosley, and B. Beard
  1990   Clinical visual perimetry underestimates peripheral field problems in older adults. Clinical Visual Sciences 5:113-125.
Barr, R.A.
  1991   Recent changes in driving among older adults. Human Factors 33:597-600.
Begault, D.R.
  1993   Head-up auditory displays for traffic collision avoidance system advisories: A preliminary investigation. Human Factors 35:707-717.
Ben-Akiva, M., and S.R. Lerman
  1985   Discrete Choice Analysis. Cambridge, MA: MIT Press.
Berthier, N.E.
  1996   Learning to reach: A mathematical model. Developmental Psychology 32:811-823.
Birren, J.E.
  1965   Age-changes in speed of behavior: Its central nature and physiological correlates. Pp. 191-216 in Behavior, Aging and the Nervous System, A.T. Welford and J.E. Birren, eds. Springfield, IL.: Charles C. Thomas.
  1974   Translations in gerontology: From lab to life: Psychophysiology and speed of response. American Psychologist 29:808-815.
Burke, D.M., and R.M. Harrold
  1988   Automatic and effortful semantic processes in old age: Experimental and naturalistic approaches. Pp. 110-116 in Language, Memory and Aging, L.L. Light and D.M. Burke, eds. Cambridge, England: Cambridge University Press.
Burke, D.M., J. Worthley, and J. Martin
  1988   I'll never forget what's-her-name: Aging and the tip of the tongue experience. Pp. 113-118 in Practical Aspects of Memory: Current Research and Issues, 2d vol., M.M. Gruneberg, P. Morris, and R.N. Sykes, eds. Chichester, UK: Wiley.
Byrne, M.D., and J.R. Anderson
  1998   Perception and action. Chapter 6 in The Atomic Components of Thought, J.R. Anderson and C. Lebiere, eds. Mahway, NJ: Erlbaum.
Caelli, T., and D. Porter
  1980   On difficulties in localizing ambulance sirens. Human Factors 22:719-724.
Cai, X., and R. Gao
  In   Ultrasonic sensor placement strategy for a long cane. 1999 ASME IMECE, Sympo-
  press   sium on Dynamics, Control, and Design of Biomechanical Systems. Nashville, TN.
Cho, Y., R.L. Keller, and M.L. Cooper
  1999   Applying decision-making approaches to health risk-taking behaviors: Progress and remaining challenges. Journal of Mathematical Psychology 43:261-285.
Connolly, C.I., and R.A. Grupen
  1993   The applications of harmonic functions to robotics. Journal of Robotic Systems 10:931-946.
  1994   Nonholonomic Path Planning Using Harmonic Functions (Technical Report #94-50). Amherst, MA: University of Massachusetts Computer Science Department.
Deyo, R.A., and T.S. Inui
  1980   Dropouts and broken appointments: A literature review and agenda for future research. Medical Care 18:1146-1157.

Djaferis, T.E.
1995   *Robust Control Design: A Polynomial Approach.* Boston: Kluwer Academic Publishers.
Donders, F.C.
1868   Die Schnelligkeit Psychischer Processe. *Archiv fur Anatomic und Physiologie* 657-681. [On the speed of mental processes. Pp. 412-431 in *Attention and Performance II*, W.G. Koster, ed. and transl., 1969. Amsterdam: North Holland.]
Dye, S., and F. Baylin
1997   *The GPS Manual.* Boulder, CO: Baylin/Gale Productions.
Feiner, S., B. MacIntyre, M. Haupt, and E. Solomon
1993   Windows on the world: 2D windows for 3D augmented reality. Pp. 145-155 in *Proceedings of UIST 1993, ACM Symposium on User Interface Software and Technology.*
Fisher, D.L.
1993   Optimal performance engineering. *Human Factors* 35:115-140.
Fisher, D.L., and R. Glaser
1996   Molar and latent models of cognitive slowing: Implications for aging, dementia, depression, development and intelligence. *Psychonomic Bulletin and Review* 3:458-480.
Fisher, D.L., E. Yungkurth, and S. Moss
1990   Optimal menu hierarchy design: Syntax and semantics. *Human Factors* 32(6):665-683.
Fisk, A.D., D.L. Fisher, and W.A. Rogers
1992   General slowing alone cannot explain age-related search effects: A reply to Cerella. *Journal of Experimental Psychology: General* 121:73-78.
Fisk, A.D., and W.A. Rogers
1991   Towards an understanding of age-related visual search effects. *Journal of Experimental Psychology: General* 121:131-149.
Gao, R., and X. Cai
1998   Mechatronic long cane as a travel aid for the blind. Pp. 220-226 in *Proceedings of SPIE International Symposium on Sensors and Controls for Intelligent Machining, Agile Manufacturing, and Mechatronics*, 3518th vol. Boston, MA.
Gish, K.W., and L. Staplin
1995   *Human Factors Aspects of Using Head-Up Displays in Automobiles: A Review of the Literature.* Washington, D.C.: U.S. Department of Transportation.
Goldstein, W.M., and D.L. Fisher
1991   Stochastic networks as models of cognition: Derivation of response time distributions using the order-of-processing method. *Journal of Mathematical Psychology* 35(2):214-241.
1992   Stochastic networks as models of cognition: Deriving predictions for resource constrained mental processing. *Journal of Mathematical Psychology* 36:129-145.
Grupen, R.A., C.I. Connolly, K.X. Souccar, and W.P. Burleson
1995   Toward a path co-processor for automated vehicle control. *IEEE Symposium on Intelligent Vehicles.* Detroit, MI.
Hale, S., J. Myerson, and D. Wagstaff
1987   General slowing of nonverbal information processing: Evidence for a power law. *Journal of Gerontology* 34:553-560.
Holm-Hansen, B., and R. Gao
1997   Smart bearing utilizing embedded sensors: Design considerations. Pp. 602-610 in *SPIE 4th International Symposium on Smart Structures and Materials, The International Society for Optical Engineering, Vol. 3041.* San Diego, CA.

Iavecchia, J.H., H.P. Iavecchia, and S.N. Roscoe
    1988   Eye accommodation to head-up virtual images. *Human Factors* 30(6):689-702.
Jebara, T., B. Schiele, N. Oliver, and A. Pentland
    1998   DyPERS: Dynamic Personal Enhanced Reality System, Vision and Modeling (Technical Report #463). Cambridge, MA: Media Lab, MIT.
Kahn, A.M.
    1992   Technological response to urban traffic congestion. *Journal of Urban Technology* Fall:19-28.
Kantowitz, B.H., J.D. Lee, and S.C. Kantowitz
    1997   *Development of Human Factors Guidelines for Advanced Traveler Information Systems and Commercial Vehicle Operations: Definition and Prioritization of Research Studies.* Washington, D.C.: Federal Highway Administration, U.S. Department of Transportation.
Katsikopoulos, K.V., Y. Duse-Anthony, D.L. Fisher, and S.A. Duffy
    2000   Stated preference data for drivers' route choice in situations with varying degrees of cognitive load: The framing of route choices when travel time information is provided. *Human Factors.*
Knipling, R.R., and W.W. Wierwille
    1994   Vehicle-based drowsy driver detection: Current status and future prospects. Pp. 245-256 in *Proceedings of the IVHS America 1994 Annual Meeting.* Atlanta, GA.
Lee, D.N.
    1976   A theory of visual control of braking based on information about time-to-collision. *Perception* 5:437-459.
Leirer, V.O., D.G. Morrow, G. Pariante, and T. Doksum
    1989   Increasing influenza vaccination adherence through voice mail. *Journal of the American Geriatric Society* 17:1147-1150.
Leirer, V.O., E.D. Tanke, and D.G. Morrow
    1993   Commercial cognitive/memory systems: A case study. *Applied Cognitive Psychology* 7:675-689.
Lima, S.D., S. Hale, and J. Myerson
    1991   How general is general slowing? Evidence from the lexical domain. *Psychology and Aging* 6:416-425.
Liu, A.
    1998   What the driver's eye tells the car's brain. Pp. 431-452 in *Eye Guidance in Reading and Scene Perception,* G.J. Underwood, ed. Oxford, England: Elsevier.
Liu, A., and A. Pentland
    1997   Towards real-time recognition of driver intentions. Pp. 236-241 in *Proceedings of the 1997 IEEE Intelligent Transportation Systems Conference.* Boston, MA.
Madden, D.J., T.W. Pierce, and P.A. Allen
    1996   Adult age differences in the use of distractor homogeneity during visual search. *Psychology and Aging* 11:454-474.
Maltz, M., and D. Shinar
    1999   Eye movements of younger and older drivers. *Human Factors* 41:15-25.
Markoff, J.
    1999   I.B.M. to announce new, flexible transistors. *New York Times* October 29: C2.
Marran, L., and C. Schor
    1997   Multiaccommodative stimuli in VR systems: Problems and solutions. *Human Factors* 39:382-388.
Miller, R.A.
    1985   A systems approach to modeling discrete control performance. Pp. 177-248 in *Advances in Man-Machine Systems Research,* W.B. Rouse, ed. Greenwich, CT: JAI Press.

Miyamoto, J.M.
   1999   Quality-adjusted life years (QALY) utility models under expected utility and rank dependent utility assumptions. *Journal of Mathematical Psychology* 43:201-237.
Morrow, D.G.
   1997   Improving consultations between health professionals and clients: Implications for pharmacists. *International Journal of Aging and Human Development* 44:47-72.
Morrow, D.G., V.O. Leirer, L.M. Carver, E.D. Tanke, and A.D. McNally
   1999   Repetition improves older and younger adult memory for automated appointment messages. *Human Factors* 41:194-204.
Owsley, C., K. Ball, M.E. Sloane, D.L. Roenker, and J.R. Bruni
   1991   Visual perceptual/cognitive correlates of vehicle accidents in older drivers. *Psychology and Aging* 6:403-415.
Park, D.C.
   1992   Applied cognitive aging research. Pp. 449-493 in *The Handbook of Aging and Cognition*, F.I.M. Craik and T.A. Salthouse, eds. Hillsdale, NJ: Erlbaum.
Perrott, D.R., K. Saberi, K. Brown, and T.Z. Strybel
   1990   Auditory psychomotor coordination and visual search behavior. *Perception and Psychophysics* 48:214-226.
Plude, D.J., and J.A. Doussard-Roosevelt
   1989   Aging, selective attention, and feature integration. *Psychology and Aging* 4:98-105.
Rabiner, L.R.
   1989   A tutorial on hidden Markov models and selected applications in speech recognition. Pp. 257-286 in *Proceedings of the IEEE 77*.
Ranney, T.A.
   1998   Models of visual scanning for homogeneous displays: A test of two underlying assumptions. Unpublished doctoral dissertation. Amherst, MA: University of Massachusetts.
Rayner, K.
   1998   Eye movements in reading and information processing: 20 years of research. *Psychological Bulletin* 124:372-422.
Rayner, K., and A. Pollatsek
   1992   Eye movements and scene perception. *Canadian Journal of Psychology* 46:342-376.
Reichle, E.D., A. Pollatsek, D.L. Fisher, and K. Rayner
   1998   Towards a model of eye movement control in reading. *Psychological Review* 105:125-157.
Rhodes, B.J.
   1997   The wearable remembrance agent: A system for augmented memory. *Personal Technologies* 1:218-224.
Rogers, W.A., E.F. Cabrera, N. Walker, D.K. Gilbert, and A.D. Fisk
   1996   A survey of automatic teller machine usage across the adult life span. *Human Factors* 38:156-166.
Roscoe, S.N.
   1987   The trouble with HUDs and HMDs. *Human Factors Society Bulletin* 30:1-3.
Roy, D., N. Sawhney, C. Schmandt, and A. Pentland
   1997   *Wearable Audio Computing: A Survey of Interaction Techniques* (Perceptual Computing Technical Report #463). Cambridge, MA: MIT.
Rumelhart, D.E., and D.A. Norman
   1982   Simulating a skilled typist: A study of skilled cognitive-motor performance. *Cognitive Science* 6:1-36.

Salthouse, T.A.
   1980   Age and memory: Strategies for localizing loss. Pp. 47-65 in *New Directions in Memory and Aging: Proceedings of the George A. Talland Memorial Conference*, L.W. Poon, J.L. Fozard, L.S. Cermak, D. Arenberg, and L.W. Thompson, eds. Hillsdale, NJ: Erlbaum.
   1996a   Constraints on theories of cognitive aging. *Psychonomic Bulletin and Review* 3:287-299.
   1996b   The processing-speed theory of adult age differences in cognition. *Psychological Review* 103:403-428.
Salvucci, D.D., and J.R. Anderson
   1998   Tracing eye movement protocols with cognitive process models. Pp. 923-928 in *Proceedings of the Twentieth Annual Conference on Cognitive Science*. Hillsdale, NJ: Erlbaum.
Sanders, A.F.
   1970   Some aspects of the selective process in the functional field of view. *Ergonomics* 13:101-117.
Santiago, A.J.
   1992   ATMs technology—What we know and what we don't know. *Public Roads* 56:89-95.
Schneider, W., and R.M. Shiffrin
   1977   Controlled and automatic human information processing II: Perceptual learning, automatic attending, and a general theory. *Psychological Review* 84:127-190.
Schweickert, R.
   1978   A critical path generalization of the additive factor method: Analysis of a Stroop task. *Journal of Mathematical Psychology* 18:105-139.
Schweickert, R., and D.L. Fisher
   1987   Stochastic, network and deterministic models. Pp. 1171-1211 in *Handbook of Human Factors/Ergonomics*, G. Salvendy, ed. New York: Wiley.
Schweickert, R., D.L. Fisher, and W.M. Goldstein
   1992   *General Latent Network Theory: Structural and Quantitative Analysis of Networks of Cognitive Processes* (Technical Report 92-1). West Lafayette, IN: Purdue University Mathematical Psychology Program.
Schweickert, R., and J.T. Townsend
   1989   A trichotomy: Interactions of factors prolonging sequential and concurrent mental processes in stochastic discrete mental (PERT) networks. *Journal of Mathematical Psychology* 33:328-347.
Sheridan, T.B.
   1991   *Telerobotics, Automation, and Human Supervisory Control.* Cambridge, MA: MIT Press.
Sit, R.A., and A.D. Fisk
   1999   Age-related performance in a multiple task environment. *Human Factors* 41:26-34.
Sobbi, N.
   1995   Human factors in advanced parking management systems. *Public Roads* Winter:35-38.
Sojourner, R.J., and J.F. Antin
   1990   The effects of a simulated head-up display speedometer on perceptual task performance. *Human Factors* 32:329-339.
Stan, M.R., W.P. Burleson, C.I. Connolly, and R.A. Grupen
   1994   Analog VLSI for robot path planning. *Journal of VLSI Signal Processing* 8(1):61-73.
Staplin, L., and A.D. Fisk
   1991   A cognitive engineering approach to improving signalized left-turn intersections. *Human Factors* 33:559-572.

Starner, T., S. Mann, B. Rhodes, J. Levine, J. Healey, D. Kirsch, R.W. Picard, and A. Pentland
  1997   Augmented reality through wearable computing. *Presence: Teleoperators and Virtual Environments* 6(4):386-398.

Sternberg, S.
  1969   The discovery of processing stages: Extensions of Donder's method. *Acta Psychologica* 30:276-315.
  1975   Memory scanning: New findings and current controversies. *Quarterly Journal of Experimental Psychology* 27:1-32.

Szlyk, J.P., W. Seiple, and M. Viana
  1995   Relative effects of age and compromised vision on driving performance. *Human Factors* 37:430-436.

Szymkowiak, A., D.L. Fisher, and K.A. Connerny
  1997   False yield and false go decisions at signalized left-turn intersections: A driving simulator study. Pp. 226-235 in *Proceedings of the Europe Chapter of the Human Factors and Ergonomics Society Annual Conference*. Bochum, Germany.

Tarr, M.
  1995   Rotating objects to recognize them: A case study on the role of viewpoint dependency in the recognition of three-dimensional objects. *Psychological Bulletin and Review* 2:55-82.

Tufano, D.R.
  1997   Automotive HUDs: The overlooked safety issues. *Human Factors* 39:303-311.

U.S. Department of Health and Human Services
  1991   *Healthy People 2000: National Health Promotion and Disease Prevention Objectives.* Rockville, MD.

Walker, N., W.B. Fain, A.D. Fisk, and C.M. McGuire
  1997   Age and decision making: Driving-related problem solving. *Human Factors* 39:438-444.

Weintraub, D.J., and M. Ensing
  1992   *Human Factors Issues in Head-Up Display Design: The Book of HUD* (CSERIAC state of the art report). Wright-Patterson Air Force Base, OH: Crew Systems Ergonomics Information Analysis Center.

Whiteside, J.A.
  1974   Eye movements of children, adults, and elderly persons during inspection of dot patterns. *Journal of Experimental Child Psychology* 18:313-332.

Wickens, C.D., and J. Long
  1994   Conformal symbology, attention shifts, and the head-up display. Pp. 6-10 in *Proceedings of the Human Factors and Ergonomics Society 38th Annual Meeting*. Santa Monica, CA: Human Factors and Ergonomics Society.

Wickens, T.D.
  1982   *Models for Behaviors: Stochastic Processes in Psychology.* San Francisco: Freeman.

Wierwille, W.W.
  1994   Overview of research on driver drowsiness definition and driver drowsiness detection. Pp. 462-468 in *Proceedings of the Fourteenth International Technical Conference on the Enhanced Safety of Vehicles (ESV) Conference*, 1st vol. Washington, D.C.: National Highway Traffic Safety Administration, U.S. Department of Transportation.

Wierwille, W.W., S.S. Wreggit, and R.R. Knipling
  1994   Development of improved algorithms for on-line detection of driver drowsiness. Pp. 331-340 in *Proceedings of the International Congress on Transportation Electronics*. Detroit, MI: Society of Automotive Engineers.

Wightman, F.L., and D.J. Kistler
    1989   Headphone simulation of free-field listening: I. Stimulus synthesis. *Journal of the Acoustical Society of America* 85:858-867.
Wolfe, J.M.
    1994   Guided search 2.0: A revised model of guided search. *Psychonomic Bulletin and Review* 1:202-238.

E

Health Effects on Cognitive Aging

Shari R. Waldstein

Intact cognitive function is a critical dimension of quality of life. Cognitive difficulties can be disruptive to individuals' sense of well-being and to their everyday functioning. Age-related decrements in cognition are well documented (Salthouse, 1991; Wilson et al., 1997), but they are not thought to be entirely due to primary biological aging processes. In this regard, it has been suggested that age-related cognitive changes are attributable, at least in part, to systemic medical diseases (here defined as nonneurological diseases that affect one or more physiological systems) that are common in older adults (Fozard et al., 1990). Indeed, approximately four out of five Americans over the age of 65 have at least one or more chronic medical conditions (La Rue, 1992).

In recent years, the relation of systemic disease to cognition has received increasingly intensive investigation. Results of numerous available studies indicate that diseases of virtually any physiological system can have deleterious effects on cognitive function (Elias et al., 1989; Siegler and Costa, 1985; Tarter et al., in press, 1988). Although these influences may be particularly pertinent to older adults, who experience an increased incidence and prevalence of disease, systemic diseases have been shown to affect cognitive performance in persons of all ages in both cross-sectional and longitudinal investigations. Therefore disease-cognition relations should viewed from a life-span perspective. In this regard, degree of lifetime exposure to systemic illness(es) may be of critical importance in determining cognitive outcomes in older age.

The purpose of this paper is, first, to provide a brief overview of the types of systemic diseases and several associated lifestyle and biological factors that are known to affect the normal range of cognitive functioning (in the absence of dementia). Next, a more detailed description of the relation of hypertension and other cardiovascular diseases to cognition is provided. Methodological and conceptual challenges to this field of research are discussed, and future research directions are enumerated.

In general, the investigations described in this paper utilized clinical neuropsychological tests to measure cognitive functioning. These tests can be grouped according to the major domain of cognitive functioning assessed and include measures of attention, learning and memory, executive functions, visuospatial and visuoconstructional skills, psychomotor abilities, perceptual skills, and language functions. Screening tests such as mental status examinations and composite measures such as intelligence tests were also used. The interested reader is referred to Lezak (1995) for a detailed discussion of this particular taxonomy of tests. In addition, an appendix at the end of this paper lists brief descriptions of the major domains of cognitive functions and several representative tests that are commonly used in the literature described below.

HEALTH AND COGNITION

Numerous health-related factors have been demonstrated to influence cognition (with effect sizes ranging from small to large). Examples include lifestyle, endocrine, and genetic factors, systemic diseases, neurotoxic exposures, and medical and surgical treatments for disease. Each of these general areas is considered briefly below, with positive findings emphasized for illustrative purposes.

Lifestyle

A variety of lifestyle factors are known to affect cognitive function. Such factors may impact cognition by exerting direct biological influence on the brain or by promoting various systemic diseases (e.g., cardiovascular, pulmonary) that indirectly affect the brain. Less healthful lifestyles also tend to aggregate among individuals with lower levels of education and may, in part, explain previously noted associations between low education and/or socioeconomic status and poorer cognitive function (Kilander et al., 1997). Examples of such lifestyle factors include smoking, excessive alcohol consumption, illicit drug use, dietary factors, and physical inactivity.

With respect to health-compromising behaviors, several studies have revealed poorer cognitive performance among individuals who smoke tobacco products (M.F. Elias et al., in press; Galanis et al., 1997; Hill, 1989; Launer et al., 1996). Heavy alcohol consumption also has known deleterious effects on cognition (Rourke and Løberg, 1996; Tarter and Van Thiel, 1985). However, across a range of habitual drinking, several investigations have noted an inverted U- or J-shaped relation between alcohol consumption and cognitive function (Dufouil et al., 1997; M.F. Elias et al., in press; P.K. Elias et al., in press; Launer et al., 1996). Drugs of abuse (e.g., opiates, cocaine) have been associated with poorer cognitive performance (Carlin and O'Malley, 1996; Strickland and Stein, 1995). In addition, several dietary insufficiencies, such as vitamin B_6, vitamin B_{12}, thiamine, folate, and zinc, have been related to cognitive difficulties (Lester and Fishbein, 1988; Riggs et al., 1996; Whitehouse et al., 1993). Greater caloric consumption in middle age has been shown to predict poorer mental status in old age (Fraser et al., 1996), and a proportionally greater intake of dietary refined carbohydrates has predicted lower IQ scores in children (Lester et al., 1982).

Health-enhancing behaviors have been associated with better cognitive functioning. For example, greater intake of vitamin C, an antioxidant, has been related to enhanced cognitive test performance and/or a lower prevalence of cognitive impairment (Gale et al., 1996; Jama et al., 1996; Paleologos et al., 1998). Greater levels of physical fitness (or physical activity) have also been associated with higher levels of cognitive functioning (Dustman et al., 1994). In addition, several investigations have revealed improvements in cognitive performance with aerobic exercise training (Emery and Blumenthal, 1991; Kramer et al., 1998).

Endocrine and Genetic Factors

Various hormonal factors have been associated with cognitive functioning. Again, direct biological effects on the brain are likely, in addition to indirect effects via promotion of systemic diseases. Relevant examples include poorer cognitive function in individuals with low levels of estrogen (Gordon et al., 1988; Erlanger et al., 1999), both high and low levels of various thyroid and pituitary hormones (Beckwith and Tucker, 1988; Gordon et al., 1988; Whitehouse et al., 1993; Erlanger et al., 1999), and either high basal levels of cortisol or greater stress-induced cortisol responses (Kirschbaum et al., 1996; Lupien and McEwen, 1997; McEwen and Sapolsky, 1995; Seeman et al., 1997; Erlanger et al., 1999). Beneficial effects of estrogen replacement therapy have also been noted (Haskell et al., 1997; Erlanger et al., 1999).

Genetic factors may predispose individuals to systemic diseases and influence numerous biological variables that can affect cognitive performance. One such factor that has received much recent attention is apolipoprotein E (APOE) polymorphism. Although most commonly examined in relation to dementias, the presence of one or two APOE-ε4 alleles has also been associated with poorer cognitive function, particularly on tests of learning, memory, and psychomotor speed, among nondemented individuals across a wide range of ages (Bondi et al., 1995; Carmelli et al., 1998; Flory et al., 1999; Yaffe et al., 1997). Genetic influences may also modify the impact of disease on cognition. In this regard, Haan et al. (1999) found that individuals with carotid atherosclerosis, peripheral vascular disease, or diabetes mellitus, in addition to an APOE-ε4 allele, experienced a significantly greater rate of cognitive decline than individuals without an APOE-ε4 allele and or cardiovascular disease.

Neurotoxicity

Environmental or occupational exposure to chemicals, such as solvents and lead, exerts direct neurotoxic effects on the brain and is associated with diminished cognitive functioning (Hartmann, 1995; Morrow et al., in press). Both peak exposures and chronic low-level exposures are of concern. Individuals of lower socioeconomic status may be more likely to experience neurotoxic exposures.

Systemic Diseases

Numerous systemic diseases have been associated with poorer cognitive functioning. Examples include cardiovascular diseases, such as hypertension and myocardial infarction (Waldstein and Elias, in press; Waldstein et al., in press); pulmonary diseases, such as chronic obstructive pulmonary disease and asthma (Fitzpatrick et al., 1991; Hopkins and Bigler, in press; Grant et al., 1987; Prigatano et al., 1983); pancreatic diseases, such as diabetes mellitus (Reaven et al., 1990; Ryan, in press; Ryan et al., 1993); hepatic diseases, such as cirrhosis (Moss et al., 1995; Tarter and Van Thiel, in press); renal diseases (Hart et al., 1983; Pliskin et al., in press); autoimmune diseases, such as systemic lupus erythematosus (Beers, in press; Glanz et al., 1997); various cancers (Berg, 1988); sleep disorders, such as obstructive sleep apnea syndrome (Bédard et al., 1993; Kelly and Coppel, in press); and the human immunodeficiency virus and AIDS (Heaton et al., 1995; Kelly et al., 1996).

Disparities in health status among racial and ethnic minority groups and individuals of lower socioeconomic status or educational attainment are well documented (Haan and Kaplan, 1985; Haan et al., 1989; Kaplan and Keil, 1993). It is therefore possible that comorbidities may, in part, explain prior relations of race/ethnicity (e.g., for black Americans), lower education, and low socioeconomic status to poorer performance on cognitive tests. Health status should therefore be controlled in such investigations (Whitfield et al., 2000).

Medical and Surgical Treatments

A variety of medical and surgical treatments for disease have been shown to impact cognitive performance. Improvements, decrements, and absence of change have been noted in association with various medications, such as antihypertensive agents (Muldoon et al., 1991, 1995) and corticosteroid or theophylline treatment for asthma (Hopkins and Bigler, in press; Stein et al., 1996). Mixed findings are also apparent in association with surgical interventions, such as coronary artery bypass surgery (Newman et al., in press). Some improvements in cognitive performance have been associated with oxygen-related treatments for chronic obstructive pulmonary disease and obstructive sleep apnea syndrome (Hopkins and Bigler, in press) and chronic hemodialysis (Pliskin et al., in press).

Summary

Numerous lifestyle, biological, disease-related, and iatrogenic factors have been shown to influence cognitive function in persons of all ages. Research associated with each particular factor poses several common and unique sets of methodological and conceptual challenges, discussion of which is beyond the scope of this paper. Findings in each area are often mixed and may, in part, reflect these challenges. As mentioned above, positive results have generally been highlighted here to illustrate the striking range of potential health effects on cognition. In the following section, a more detailed description of the relation of hypertension and other cardiovascular diseases to cognitive function is presented as an example of research on health and cognition and its associated challenges.

CARDIOVASCULAR DISEASE AND COGNITION

Cardiovascular disease is the leading cause of death in the United States, affecting one in every five individuals (American Heart Association, 1998) and conferring substantially elevated risk for stroke and vascular dementia. However, prior to the development of cerebrovascular complications, even early manifestations of cardiovascular disease, such as hypertension, are associated with diminished cognitive function (Waldstein and Elias, in press; Waldstein et al., in press).

A deleterious impact of cardiovascular disease on the brain is not surprising when one considers the purpose of normal cardiovascular function. The cardiovascular system (i.e., the heart and vasculature) is responsible for supplying blood that transports oxygen, glucose, and other essential nutrients to all cells of the body. Because the brain is relatively unable to store nutrients, it is dependent on the cardiovascular system for a constant supply of blood and is highly vulnerable to interruptions of blood flow. Approximately one-fifth of the cardiac output is provided to the brain each minute, and even very brief cessation of this blood supply can damage the brain. Subtle reductions in cerebral blood flow that occur in association with cardiovascular disease (in addition to other mechanisms discussed below) can therefore have negative short- and long-term consequences for the brain.

When available studies to date are considered in aggregate, the relation of cardiovascular diseases to cognitive function has been one of the more extensively investigated of the research areas discussed above (Waldstein and Elias, in press; Waldstein et al., in press). Because hypertension is often one of the earliest manifestations of cardiovascular disease and can occur without substantial occult comorbidities, there is an opportunity to conduct tightly controlled investigations of hypertension and cognition. Perhaps for this reason, hypertension has been studied fairly intensively and thus is examined here as a pertinent illustration of health-cognition relations.

Hypertension

Hypertension—defined as a sustained systolic and diastolic blood pressure greater than or equal to 140 millimeters of mercury (mm Hg) and/or 90 mm Hg, respectively, as measured on at least two separate occasions (Joint National Committee on Prevention, Detection, Evaluation, and Treatment of High Blood Pressure, 1997)—affects one in four adults in the United States, or 50 million individuals (American Heart Association, 1998). Approximately 90 to 95 percent of all cases involve essential hypertension, a term that refers to a sustained blood pressure elevation of unknown cause. However, the etiology of essential hypertension actually involves a complex interplay of genetic and environmental factors (Kaplan, 1998). Elevated blood pressure that is attributable to a known medical disorder is called secondary hypertension.

Risk factors for hypertension include a positive family history, older age, male gender (until age 55, after which prevalence rates are greater among women), black race, and numerous lifestyle and behavioral factors such as excess body weight, physical inactivity, dietary factors including high sodium and low potassium or calcium intake, excessive alcohol consumption, oral contraceptive use, various psychosocial factors, and stress-related cardiovascular reactivity (American Heart Association, 1998; Joint National Committee, 1997; Kaplan, 1998). Hypertension is a major risk factor for atherosclerosis, coronary heart disease, and stroke (Stamler, 1992).

Hypertension and Cognitive Function

The relation of hypertension to cognitive function has been studied for over 50 years (for reviews see M.F. Elias et al., in press; Elias and Robbins, 1991; Waldstein, 1995; Waldstein and Katzel, in press; Waldstein et al., 1991a). Results of numerous case-control and cross-sectional, population-based studies indicate that hypertensives generally perform more poorly than normotensives across multiple domains of cognitive function, including learning and memory, attention, abstract reasoning and other executive functions, visuospatial, visuoconstructional, perceptual, and psychomotor abilities (e.g., Boller et al., 1977; Blumenthal et al., 1993; Elias et al., 1987, 1990b; Robbins et al., 1994; Shapiro et al., 1982; Waldstein et al., 1991b, 1996; Wallace et al., 1985). To date, hypertension typically has not predicted poorer performance on tests of general verbal intelligence or language abilities, although further investigation is necessary (e.g., Blumenthal et al., 1993; Boller et al., 1977; Waldstein et al., 1991b, 1996). Dose-response relations have been observed between progressive increments in blood pressure level and reduced cognitive performance (e.g., Elias et al., 1990b, Robbins et al., 1994). In addition, low levels of blood pressure have been associated with poorer cognitive function (Costa et al., 1998; Guo et al., 1997), and curvilinear (inverted U-shaped) relations of blood pressure to cognitive performance have also been noted (Glynn et al., 1999).

Although it is generally presumed that alterations in cognition occur as a result of pathological consequences of hypertension, lower levels of cognitive test performance have also been found to precede blood pressure elevation in individuals who are at risk for hypertension. More specifically, normotensive young adults who have a parental history of hypertension show lower levels of performance on tests of visuoperceptual, visuospatial, and visuoconstructional skill and speed of short-term memory search in comparison to the young adult offspring of normotensive parents (Pierce and Elias, 1993; Waldstein et al., 1994). These associations may thus reflect genetic and or environmental factors that predispose individuals to the development of hypertension.

Longitudinal or follow-up studies generally note the persistence of hypertensive-normotensive differences in cognitive performance over time, often with additional cognitive decline among hypertensives (e.g., Haan et al., 1999; Miller et al., 1984; Elias et al., 1986, 1996, 1998; Wilkie and Eisdorfer, 1971). Chronicity of hypertension has been identified as a critical variable in such investigations. Indeed, life-time exposure to elevated blood pressure may be a more potent predictor of poor cognitive outcome in older adults than cross-sectionally measured blood pressure (Elias et al., 1993; Swan et al., 1998).

Chronicity of hypertension was emphasized in several recent epidemiological studies in which persistent blood pressure elevation, measured across numerous examinations, predicted poorer cognitive functioning and/or greater rate of cognitive decline (Elias et al., 1993, 1998; Swan et al., 1998). Similarly, higher blood pressure during middle age has been shown to predict poorer cognitive outcomes in older age (Elias et al., 1993; Swan et al., 1996; Launer et al., 1995; Kilander et al., 1998).

Moderator Variables

Although many studies have revealed lower average levels of cognitive function in hypertensive groups, there is also pronounced interindividual variability within these groups with respect to performance (Waldstein, 1995). This variability may be explained, in part, by relevant moderators. In this regard, hypertension has been shown to interact with both age and education in studies of cognitive function.

Age as Moderator Several investigations have found interactions of age and hypertension such that young (less than 40 to 50 years of age) hypertensives performed more poorly than young normotensives on tests of attention, memory, executive functions, and psychomotor abilities, whereas middle-aged (upper limits ranging from 56 to 72 years) hypertensive and normotensive groups performed comparably (Elias et al., 1990b; Schultz et al., 1979; Waldstein et al., 1996). Madden and Blumenthal (1998) also noted that both young (ages 18 to 40) and middle-aged (ages 41 to 59) hypertensives displayed a slightly greater error rate on a test of visual selective attention than young or middle-aged normotensives, whereas older (ages 60 to 78) hypertensives and normotensives did not differ in performance. In contrast, such interactions were not noted among three age cohorts (55-64, 65-74, and 75-88 years) in a sample of 1,695 participants in the Framingham Heart Study on tests of memory, visual organization, attention, verbal comprehension, and concept formation (Elias et al., 1995).

In sum, when interactive effects of age and hypertension (or blood pressure) are noted, poorer performance tends to aggregate among the younger individuals in any particular investigation. Waldstein (1995) suggests that such trends may reflect survival effects and selective attrition from studies (see Feinleib and Pinsky, 1992), as individuals with early-onset hypertension develop cardiovascular and cerebrovascular complications and are thus excluded from investigations. Furthermore, it is possible that early-onset hypertension confers greater risk for cognitive impairment than late-onset hypertension. In general, interactions of age and hypertension may best be examined in longitudinal studies in order to address some of these methodological difficulties.

Other Moderators In one study, hypertensives having lower levels of educational attainment performed more poorly than comparably educated normotensives, whereas more highly educated hypertensives and normotensives did not differ in their performance (Elias et al., 1987). Relative preservation of cognitive function among more highly educated persons has also been noted in other contexts and may suggest protective effects associated with higher socioeconomic status and or an enhanced "cognitive reserve" (Katzman, 1993).

Another source of variability in cognitive performance among hypertensives relates to the heterogeneity of this disorder (Kaplan, 1998; Streeten et al., 1992). In this regard, it is possible that certain subgroups of hypertensives are more likely than others to experience diminished cognitive performance. For example, hyperinsulinemic hypertensives perform more poorly than either normoinsulinemic hypertensives or normotensives (Kuusisto et al., 1993). In addition, high levels of sympathetic nervous system arousal (as indicated by increased plasma renin activity) have been associated with diminished psychomotor performance among hypertensives (Light, 1975, 1978).

Mediation of Age-Related Variance

Continuous blood pressure levels have been found to partially mediate age-related variance in cognitive performance. In one investigation, systolic and diastolic blood pressure attenuated by almost 58 percent the age-related variance in performance of an attention-shift reaction time task (Madden and Blumenthal, 1998). Similarly, Elias et al. (1998) found that longitudinally assessed systolic blood pressure was associated with a 50 percent reduction in the relation between age and performance of Wechsler Adult Intelligence Scale (WAIS) subtests reflecting visualization-performance ability. These findings suggest that blood pressure is an important mediator of cognitive aging.

Methodological Issues

The study of hypertension and cognition faces a number of methodological challenges (Waldstein et al., 1998). For example, the accurate measurement of blood pressure is critical to any investigation of hypertension and cognition. Interpretation of a number of studies, particularly several population-based investigations, has been limited by the measurement of blood pressure on a single occasion. This methodology greatly limits measurement reliability (Llabre et al., 1988) and precludes hypertension classification (Joint National Committee, 1997). Other studies have relied on self-reported hypertensive status (Zelinski et al., 1998; Desmond et al., 1993). A sole reliance on self-reported health status should be avoided, if possible, due to limits in reliability and validity and likely underestimation of health-cognition relations.

Measurement of cognitive function, again particularly in certain population-based investigations, has been limited by use of brief screening measures (such as a mental status exam) or very few cognitive tests. Sampling of a broad range of cognitive functions is critical to understanding hypertension-cognition relations.

Investigations of hypertension and cognition typically control for numerous confounding variables by statistical adjustment (covariance), matching procedures, and/or study exclusions. Control variables often include age, education, alcohol consumption, anxiety, and depression, and they sometimes include smoking status, occupational status, race/ethnicity, socioeconomic status, and (if relevant) antihypertensive medications. Particularly in case-control studies, hypertensives are commonly either unmedicated or are removed from antihypertensive medication prior to the study. Individuals with medical, neurological, or psychiatric comorbidities are generally excluded from case-control studies. However, because of the resultant exclusion of hypertensives with major end-organ damage, the impact of hypertension on cognition may be underestimated, particularly among older adults.

Longitudinal studies of hypertension and cognition do not always control for comorbidities such as diabetes mellitus and coronary heart disease. This is an important consideration, because hypertension is highly prevalent among individuals having certain medical or psychiatric comorbidities (e.g, depression, diabetes mellitus). Furthermore, hypertension may bear relatively stronger or weaker relations to cognition in the presence of more severe cardiovascular or metabolic diseases. For example, Elias et al. (1997) have found synergistic effects of hypertension and noninsulin-dependent diabetes mellitus with respect to diminished cognitive function. However, Phillips and Mate-Kole (1997) did not find hypertension to be a predictor of cognitive performance in patients with peripheral vascular disease. In this group of patients, more potent manifestations of cardiovascular disease may have overshadowed any effects of hypertension.

Longitudinal investigations also have to contend with problems related to study attrition. It is often the least healthy or least motivated individuals who drop out of ongoing studies. Several available statistical methods for analyzing longitudinal datasets, such as two-stage growth curve analysis and survival analysis, will take such attrition into consideration (Collins and Horn, 1991; Dwyer and Feinleib, 1992; McCardle et al., 1991)

Clinical Significance

Although hypertensives generally should not be characterized as clinically impaired on cognitive tests (Elias et al., 1987), the impact of hypertension on cognition can be considered clinically significant at an individual level and significant at the population level. In this regard, although a full range of effect sizes is apparent (from $d < 0.1$ to $d > 1.0$), numerous case-control studies have found that hypertensive-normotensive differences in cognitive test scores are characterized by large effect sizes (Waldstein et al., 1991a). Indeed, several studies have found that the performance of hypertensives falls below that of normotensives by up to one standard deviation (Waldstein et al., 1991a, 1991b). At the individual level, this magnitude of difference could, for example, translate into a below-average versus average (or average versus above-average) test score. Among individuals, even subtle alterations in cognitive functioning can have negative consequences. Such changes can be distressing and may thus impact quality of life.

Lowering of cognitive performance associated with hypertension is also considered significant at the population level (M.F. Elias et al., in press). In this regard, a significantly increased risk for poor cognitive performance, both cross-sectionally and longitudinally, is associated with hypertension or progressive increments in blood pressure (M.F. Elias et al., in press). Data from the Framingham Heart Study indicate that chronic hypertensives displayed an increased risk of performing in the lowest quartile of the distribution of scores on several learning and memory tests, with odds ratios ranging from 1.29 to 1.62 (Elias et al., 1995).

Underlying Mechanisms

Numerous neurobiological mechanisms have been proposed to underlie the relation between hypertension and diminished cognitive function (see Elias and Robbins, 1991; Waldstein, 1995; Waldstein et al., 1991a; Waldstein and Katzel, in press). In this regard, studies have demonstrated that hypertensives exhibit reduced cerebral blood flow and/or metabolism, particularly in frontal, temporal, "watershed," and subcortical (e.g., basal ganglia) regions, autoregulatory disturbance, endothelial dysfunction, increased atherosclerosis in carotid and large cerebral arteries, increased cerebral white matter disease, silent infarction, cerebral atrophy, and cellular and neurochemical dysfunction (for a review, see Waldstein and Katzel, in press). However, it is rare that such mechanistic factors are considered in conjunction with cognitive performance. In this regard, both van Swieten et al. (1991) and Schmidt et al. (1993) found that hypertensives having significant white matter disease performed more poorly than either normotensives or hypertensives without notable white matter disease. However, because white matter lesions are generally not seen in young or middle-aged persons, it has been hypothesized that alterations in neurophysiology are more likely to account for the cognitive difficulties noted among hypertensives in these age groups (Waldstein, 1995).

Waldstein and Katzel (in press) have suggested that numerous factors may promote the neuropathological changes that can influence cognitive performance in hypertensives. These include the direct effects of elevated blood pressure, in addition to other factors that tend to co-occur with hypertension, such as the metabolic syndrome (e.g., hyperinsulinemia, dyslipidemia, central adiposity) and enhanced stress-induced cardiovascular and neuroendocrine (e.g., cortisol) reactivity. Furthermore, a variety of genetic and environmental factors may indirectly affect cognition by promoting hypertension, the metabolic syndrome, physiological reactivity, and associated neuropathology. This model therefore suggests that there are characteristics of hypertensives, other than elevated blood pressure per se, that are important to the development of diminished cognitive functioning.

Genetic and environmental influences may also exert direct effects on brain structure and function (and thereby cognition) or act as "third variables" that simultaneously influence both the development of hypertension and altered cognitive function, perhaps via similar neurobiological mechanisms. In this regard, findings indicating that the normotensive offspring of hypertensive parents display diminished cognitive performance are intriguing. It is important to note that the mechanisms underlying hypertension-cognition relations may vary over the course of the life span and among different subgroups of hypertensives (Waldstein, 1995).

Summary, Clinical Significance, and Future Directions

In sum, results of a large body of research indicate that hypertension is associated with poorer cognitive functioning across multiple domains of performance, and that chronic hypertension predicts cognitive decline over time. Although, to date, there has been fairly extensive investigation of hypertension-cognition relations, many questions remain. Further study of the patterns, predictors, and mechanisms of cognitive function (or dysfunction) among subgroup of hypertensives of differing ages remains critical.

Despite an overall increase in hypertension-related risk for poor cognitive function, the striking interindividual variability in performance noted within hypertensive groups suggests that it is important to continue to identify pertinent predictors of poor cognitive function among hypertensives. Identification of such factors could assist in determining potential areas for further prevention or intervention efforts. Thus far, age and education have been identified as important moderating variables. However, more research is needed with respect to these factors. Interactive effects of hypertension with many other sociodemographic (e.g., gender, race/ethnicity, socioeconomic status), lifestyle, genetic, and other biological factors are also possible, yet they remain virtually unexplored.

Further study of the relation of low blood pressure to cognitive performance (and associated mechanisms) is also necessary. Nonlinear statistics should be used to evaluate the potential presence of an inverted-U or a J-shaped cross-sectional relation between blood pressure and cognitive function. Further investigation of the performance of the normotensive offspring of hypertensive parents would also be useful. Both family history studies and hypertension studies could include some evaluation of the numerous candidate genes that have been implicated as determinants of interindividual variability in blood pressure (Krushkal et al., 1999).

Cross-sectional and longitudinal studies should determine the impact of hypertension on cognition in the presence of other cardiovascular risk factors and both cardiovascular and noncardiovascular diseases. Longitudinal studies should continue to consider chronicity of hypertension and the impact of long-term antihypertensive therapy and relative degree of blood pressure control with respect to cognitive outcomes. It would also be useful to determine whether hypertensives who display the lowest levels of cognitive performance are at greatest risk for future cerebrovascular events.

Further elucidation of the complicated mechanisms underlying hypertension-cognition relations is also necessary. As mentioned previously, predictors of cognitive functioning, and the mechanisms underlying these difficulties, may differ among subgroups of hypertensives and at distinct points in the life span. Future studies should sample numerous mechanistic variables in conjunction with measures of cognitive function and use statistical methods such as structural equation modeling to determine the interrelations among these variables.

Other Cardiovascular Diseases and Cognition

Hypertension is only one of several risk factors for later manifestations of cardiovascular disease that have been shown to impact cognitive function. Other cardiovascular risk factors that have been associated with poorer cognitive function include both high and low levels of total serum cholesterol (Benton, 1995; Desmond et al., 1993; Muldoon et al., 1997; Swan et al., 1992), insulin-dependent and noninsulin-dependent diabetes mellitus (Ryan, in press), and lifestyle factors such as smoking (discussed above, see M.F. Elias et al., in press). Epidemiological research indicates incrementally greater risk for cognitive impairment with increasing numbers of cardiovascular risk factors (M.F. Elias et al., in press).

Relatively few studies have examined the impact of later manifestations of cardiovascular disease (e.g., atherosclerosis, coronary heart disease, peripheral vascular disease) on cognition. Results of available research indicates that a greater extent of carotid atherosclerosis predicts poorer performance on various tests of cognitive function, such as memory, executive functions, psychomotor abilities, and mental status (Auperin et al., 1996; Breteler et al., 1994; Cerhan et al., 1998; Everson et al., in press). Because atherosclerosis tends to co-occur in carotid, coronary, and peripheral arteries, research has also examined cognitive function in peripheral vascular disease patients. Results indicate compromised performance on tests of attention, memory, and visuospatial, executive, and psychomotor functions in patients with peripheral vascular disease (Breteler et al., 1994; Phillips, in press), in comparison to both healthy control subjects (Phillips and Mate-Kole, 1997; Waldstein et al., 1999) and hypertensives (Waldstein et al., 1999). Phillips and Mate-Kole (1997) found that, in some instances, the performance of peripheral vascular disease patients was as poor as that of a control group of stroke patients.

Cognitive difficulties have also been noted in patients following myocardial infarction (Barclay et al., 1988; Breteler et al., 1994; Vingerhoets, in press) and in patients with cardiac arrhythmias such as atrial fibrillation (Kilander et al., 1998; Rockwood et al., 1992; Vingerhoets, in press). Studies of cognitive outcomes in patients who have been resuscitated following cardiac arrest also reveal cognitive (particularly memory) difficulties that range from mild to severe (Bertini et al., 1990; Roine et al., 1993; Vingerhoets, in press; Volpe et al., 1986). Results of the above studies indicate that numerous cognitive abilities are affected, including mental status, attention, memory, executive functions, and visuospatial and psychomotor abilities.   In contrast to the frequently mild to moderate cognitive difficulties associated with hypertension, cholesterol levels, and diabetes mellitus, studies of the cognitive concomitants of cardiac arrhythmias, cardiac arrest, myocardial infarction, and peripheral vascular disease sometimes identify more severe cognitive impairment or even dementia in a subgroup of patients (Phillips, in press; Vingerhoets, in press). This suggests the possibility of a continuum of cognitive impairment associated with increasingly severe manifestations of cardiovascular disease.

The cardiovascular diseases discussed above predispose to stroke (Kannel, 1992) and may be associated with diminished cognitive performance via many of the same neurobiological mechanisms as hypertension (see Vingerhoets, in press). Examples include increased atherosclerotic (macrovascular) disease, microvascular disease (e.g., white matter disease, silent infarction), and decreased cerebral perfusion. In addition, certain manifestations of cardiovascular disease, such as myocardial infarction and cardiac arrhythmias, often lead to diminished ventricular function that can result in a decreased cardiac output and perhaps decreased cerebral perfusion (or hypoxia). Cardiac arrhythmias are frequently associated with cardiogenic embolism. Furthermore, the cerebral consequences of cardiac arrest include hypoxia and complete anoxia.

Treatments for Cardiovascular Disease and Cognition

The degree to which cognitive difficulties associated with cardiovascular disease are reversible with treatment remains unclear. Insofar as cardiovascular disease leads to morphological changes in the brain, one may not necessarily expect treatment to be associated with cognitive improvements. However, it is possible that certain physiological mechanisms underlying cognitive dysfunction could be altered by various treatments. Furthermore, treatment for cardiovascular disease may avert further cognitive decline.

As discussed above, medical and surgical treatments for cardiovascular disease have been variously associated with cognitive improvements, further decrements, and no change. Studies of the short- and long-term effects of antihypertensive medications have yielded mixed findings (Jonas et al., in press; Muldoon et al., 1991, 1995), a conclusion that has not been clarified by examining studies according to class of medication or relative lipophilicity. Nonetheless, it is generally thought to be unlikely that hypertension-related cognitive deficits are completely reversed by antihypertensive agents and, on average, any direct treatment effects on cognition are believed to be small (Muldoon et al., 1991). However, long-term blood pressure control with antihypertensive therapy is likely to be critical for preservation of cognitive functioning over time.

The impact of coronary artery bypass surgery, a surgical treatment for coronary artery disease, on cognitive function is also inconclusive (Newman et al., in press). Whereas a number of studies have suggested a short-term (1-2 week) deterioration in cognitive function from preoperative status after surgery (Blumenthal et al., 1991; Hammeke and Hastings, 1988; Shaw et al., 1986; Townes et al., 1989), studies having longer-term follow-up (1-24 months) often suggest no change in the mean cognitive performance of patients from preoperative to postoperative periods (Hammeke and Hastings, 1988; Mattlar et al., 1991; Sellman et al., 1992; Townes et al., 1989; Waldstein et al., in press). However, the use of cutoff scores to characterize patients as deteriorated or improved from preoperative levels suggests that 7 to 57 percent of patients may exhibit impairments at approximately six months following coronary artery bypass surgery. It is thus likely that a subgroup of individuals experience negative cognitive consequences of coronary artery bypass surgery, possibly due to various mechanisms such as microemboli during surgery (Newman et al., in press).

With respect to other surgical procedures, studies generally find a lack of cognitive improvement in patients following heart transplantation (Bornstein, in press; Nussbaum and Goldstein, 1992) and carotid endarterectomy (Baird and Pieroth, in press). However, as in other medical and surgical literatures, it remains important to determine relevant predictors of good versus poor treatment outcomes with respect to cognitive functioning.

FUTURE DIRECTIONS FOR RESEARCH ON HEALTH AND COGNITION

The research presented in this paper strongly suggests a multitude of health (and illness) effects on cognitive function. Because of the greater incidence and prevalence of disease with increasing age, these findings are highly pertinent to the study of cognitive aging and indicate a need to characterize, and control for, health status in studies of "normal aging" (Fozard et al., 1990). Absence of control for health status may also partially explain mixed findings associated with research on neurological diseases and cognition. Most importantly, the promising findings emanating from the research reviewed here indicate a need for further investigation to enhance an understanding of health-cognition relations.

As illustrated by the example of hypertension-cognition relations, there are many avenues of research to pursue in terms of further characterizing the relation of health and illness to cognitive function. Discussion of the unique conceptual and methodological challenges associated with each specific subtopic in the broad field of health and cognition is beyond the scope of this paper. However, several common challenges can be identified.

Within any particular subtopic area, it remains critical to further identify, using comprehensive test batteries, what domains of cognitive function are most affected, and whether particular subgroups of individuals are most affected. In this regard, identification of pertinent moderating variables is critical. Examples include (but are not limited to) age, education, gender, race or ethnicity, socioeconomic status, genetic polymorphisms, and other biological variation.

It is important to define the magnitude of health effects on different types of cognitive processes. In this regard, it is helpful when individual studies provide an index of effect size. Determination of the clinical significance of these effects is necessary at an individual level and at a population level. With respect to individuals, it is important to determine whether daily functioning and quality of life are affected. In this regard, prior research has indicated that poor performance on certain cognitive tests predicts lower scores on self-reported quality of life in patients with chronic obstructive pulmonary disease (McSweeney and Labuhn, 1996) and poorer functional outcomes in peripheral vascular disease patients (Phillips, in press). In the instance of more severe disease-related cognitive difficulties, characterization of the magnitude and patterning of performance problems may be critical to medical management efforts, such as patients' ability to follow physicians' instructions and associated treatment (e.g., medication) regimens or to participate in rehabilitation programs (e.g., cardiac, exercise). As another example, Phillips (in press) highlights potential difficulties for peripheral vascular disease amputees in learning to use prosthetic devices.

Further characterization of the mechanisms underlying the relation of health effects to cognitive function is necessary using diverse methodologies such as neuroimaging, molecular biology, and psychophysiology. Identification of underlying mechanisms is necessary in order to further develop preventive strategies and methods of intervention geared toward preserving cognitive function. Relevant to the latter issue is the question of whether the impact of disease on cognition is, at least in part, modifiable. In this regard, further identification of the effects of medical and surgical treatments for disease on cognition is important, including a better understanding of the variables that predict treatment-related improvements versus decline.

It is critical to examine the impact of co-occurring medical diseases on cognition. To date, the cognitive consequences of various diseases have typically been studied in isolation. However, comorbidities are extremely common, particularly among older adults. Consider, as one example, that the coexistence of smoking, heavy alcohol consumption, physical inactivity, hypertension, dyslipidemia, diabetes mellitus, atherosclerosis, cardiac arrhythmias, myocardial infarction, and various medications in an individual patient is not unusual. As mentioned above, recent research has indicated that the presence of several cardiovascular risk factors (e.g., hypertension, diabetes, smoking) confers greater risk for poor cognitive performance than any single factor considered in isolation (M.F. Elias et al., in press). In addition, interactive effects of cardiovascular and metabolic disease have been noted (Elias et al., 1997).

Creative, multidisciplinary research is needed to address the research issues posed above. This exciting research area would benefit from collaborative work by individuals in such disciplines as neuropsychology, health psychology and behavioral medicine, aging and gerontology, medicine (e.g., internal medicine, cardiology, radiology, neurology), epidemiology, molecular biology, neuroscience, and genetics. Such collaboration is necessary to generate research on health-cognition relations that can effectively address issues that range from basic mechanisms to the real-life impact of cognitive problems.

APPENDIX

Commonly Assessed Domains of Cognitive Functioning and Representative Tests

Attention Basic attention involves the ability to selectively focus on, or perceive, specific incoming information while excluding other input; concentration refers to a heightened state of attention. Vigilance requires sustaining one's attention over time. Representative tests include Digit Span, Digit Vigilance, and the Continuous Performance Test.

Executive Function Executive functions are a series of self-regulatory processes, such as planning and organizational abilities, that are thought to be mediated largely by intact functioning of the frontal lobes. Mental flexibility, or the ability to shift one's cognitive or behavioral "set" in order to adapt to the current situation, is also considered to be a dimension of executive function. Representative tests include the Trail Making Test, the Stroop Color-Word Test, the Category Test, and the Wisconsin Card Sorting Test.

Learning and Memory Learning refers to the ability to acquire new information, whereas memory involves the storage and retrieval of information. Learning and memory tests are typically subclassified according to mode of acquisition (e.g., verbal, visual). Representative tests include Logical Memory, Visual Reproductions, Verbal Paired-Associate Learning, the Benton Visual Retention Test, the Tactual Performance Test, the Symbol-Digit Learning Test, and free recall of word lists.

Visuospatial/Visuoconstructional Ability Visuospatial ability involves the perception of spatial aspects of visual stimuli. Visuoconstructional skills, such as drawing, building, and assembling, typically require visuoperceptual ability, spatial skill, and a motor response. Hemiinattention, or neglect (spatial or personal), involves the failure to orient to, report, or respond to stimuli presented contralateral to a brain lesion. Representative tests include Block Design, Object Assembly, and the Rey-Osterreith Complex Figure.

Psychomotor Ability Psychomotor ability is a broad category that encompasses multiple areas of function. Examples include simple motor speed, perceptuomotor speed, and speed of information processing. Manual dexterity, another aspect of psychomotor function, refers to relative agility in manipulation. Representative tests include the Finger Tapping Test, the Grooved Pegboard, the Digit-Symbol Substitution Test, simple and choice reaction time, and speed of short-term memory search.

Perceptual Ability Perceptual abilities reflect the acquisition of simple sensory stimuli (e.g., visual, auditory, tactual) and/or their integration into meaningful information. Representative tests include the Critical Flicker Fusion test, determination of auditory thresholds, and time estimation.

Language Abilities Language abilities include skills such as comprehension, verbal expression, confrontation naming (ability to find a correct word on command), and fluency. Pronounced disorders of language are referred to as aphasias. Representative tests include the Boston Naming Test, the Controlled Oral Word Association Test, the Token Test, and subscales of the Boston Diagnostic Aphasia Examination.

Estimates of General Intelligence General intelligence involves multidimensional capabilities in addition to a general ability factor. Many unspeeded,

verbally based measures of general intelligence are thought to be greatly influenced by level of education, socioeconomic status, and acculturation. Representative tests include the Weschler Adult Intelligence Scale (WAIS) or WAIS-
Revised or its subscales. Estimates of general verbal intelligence are often
derived from the Information or Vocabulary subscales.

REFERENCES

American Heart Association
1998   *1999 Heart and Stroke Statistical Update.* Dallas, TX: American Heart Association.
Auperin, A., C. Berr, C. Bonithon-Kopp, P.J. Touboul, I. Ruelland, P. Ducimetiere, and A.
Alperovitch
1996   Ultrasonographic assessment of carotid wall characteristics and cognitive functions
        in a community sample of 59- to 71-year olds. The EVA Study Group. *Stroke*
        27:1290-1295.
Baird, A.D., and E.M. Pieroth
In   Tracking the cognitive effects of carotid endarterectomy. In *Neuropsychology of Car-*
press   *diovascular Disease*, S.R. Waldstein and M.F. Elias, eds. Mahwah, NJ: Lawrence
        Erlbaum Associates.
Barclay, L.L., E.M. Weiss, S. Mattis, O. Bond, and J.P. Blass
1988   Unrecognized cognitive impairment in cardiac rehabilitation patients. *Journal of the*
        American Geriatrics Society 36:22-28.
Beckwith, B.E., and D.M. Tucker
1988   Thyroid disorders. Pp. 197-222 in *Medical Neuropsychology*, R.E. Tarter, D.H. Van
        Thiel, and K.L. Edwards, eds. New York: Plenum Press.
Bédard, M.A., J. Montplaisir, J. Malo, R. Richer, and I. Rouleau
1993   Obstructive sleep apnea syndrome: Pathogenesis of neuropsychological deficits. *Jour-*
        nal of Clinical and Experimental Neuropsychology 13:950-964.
Beers, S.R.
In   Systemic autoimmune disease. In *Medical Neuropsychology*, 2nd ed., R.E. Tarter,
press   M.A. Butters, and S.R. Beers, eds. New York: Plenum Press.
Benton, D.
1995   Do low cholesterol levels slow mental processing? *Psychosomatic Medicine* 57:50-53.
Berg, R.A.
1988   Cancer. Pp. 265-290 in *Medical Neuropsychology*, R.E. Tarter, D.H. Van Thiel, and
        K.L. Edwards, eds. New York: Plenum Press.
Bertini, G., C. Giglioli, F. Giovannini, A. Bartoletti, F. Cricelli, M. Margheri, L. Russo, T. Taddei,
and A. Taiti
1990   Neuropsychological outcome of survivors of out-of-hospital cardiac arrest. *Journal*
        of Emergency Medicine 8:407-412.
Blumenthal, J.A., D.J. Madden, E.J. Burker, N. Croughwell, S. Schniebolk, R. Smith, W.D.
White, M. Hlatky, and J.G. Reves
1991   A preliminary study of the effects of cardiac procedures on cognitive performance.
        International Journal of Psychosomatics 38:13-16.
Blumenthal, J.A., D.J. Madden, T.W. Pierce, W.C. Siegel, and M. Appelbaum
1993   Hypertension affects neurobehavioral function. *Psychosomatic Medicine* 55:44-50.
Boller, F., P.B. Vrtunski, J.L. Mack, and Y. Kim
1977   Neuropsychological correlates of hypertension. *Archives of Neurology* 34:701-705.

Bondi, M.W., D.P. Salmon, A.U. Monsch, K. Galasko, N. Butters, M.R. Klauber, L.J. Thal, and T. Saitoh
1995   Episodic memory changes are associated with the APOE-ε4 allele in nondemented older adults. *Neurology* 45:2203-2206.

Bornstein, R.A.
In   Neuropsychological function before and after heart transplantation. In *Neuropsy-*
press   *chology of Cardiovascular Disease*, S.R. Waldstein and M.F. Elias, eds. Mahwah, NJ: Lawrence Erlbaum Associates.

Breteler, M.M.B., J.J. Claus, D.E. Grobbee, and A. Hofman
1994   Cardiovascular disease and distribution of cognitive function in elderly people: The Rotterdam study. *British Medical Journal* 308:1604-1608.

Carlin, A.S., and S. O'Malley
1996   Neuropsychological consequences of drug abuse. Pp. 486-503 in *Neuropsychological Assessment of Neuropsychiatric Disorders*, 2nd ed., I. Grant and K.M. Adams, eds. New York: Oxford.

Carmelli, D., G.E. Swan, T. Reed, B. Miller, P.A. Wolf, G.P. Jarvik, and G.D. Schellenberg
1998   Midlife cardiovascular risk factors, ApoE, and cognitive decline in elderly male twins. *American Academy of Neurology* 50:1580-1585.

Cerhan, J.R., A.R. Folsom, J.A. Mortimer, E. Shahar, D.S. Knopman, P.G. McGovern, M.A. Hays, L.D. Crum, and G. Heiss
1998   Correlates of cognitive function in middle-aged adults. Atherosclerosis Risk in Communities (ARIC) Study Investigators. *Gerontology* 44:95-105.

Collins, L.M., and J.M. Horn
1991   *Best Methods for the Analysis of Change. Future Directions.* Washington, DC: American Psychological Association.

Costa, M., L. Stegagno, R. Schandry, and P.E. Ricci Bitti
1998   Contingent negative variation and cognitive performance in hypotension. *Psychophysiology* 35:737-744.

Desmond, D.W., T.K. Tatemichi, M. Paik, and Y. Stern
1993   Risk factors for cerebrovascular disease as correlates of cognitive function in a stroke-free cohort. *Archives of Neurology* 50:162-166.

Dufouil, C., P. Ducimetiere, and A. Alperovitch
1997   Sex differences in the association between alcohol consumption and cognitive performance. *American Journal of Epidemiology* 146:405-412.

Dustman, R.E., R. Emmerson, and D. Shearer
1994   Physical activity, age, and cognitive-neuropsychological function. *Journal of Aging and Physical Activity* 2:143-181.

Dwyer, J., and M. Feinleib
1992   Introduction to statistical methods for longitudinal observation. Pp. 3-48 in *Statistical Models for Longitudinal Studies of Health*, J.H. Dwyer, M. Feinleib, et al., eds. New York: Oxford University Press.

Elias, M.F., R.B. D'Agostino, P.K. Elias, and P.A. Wolf
1995   Neuropsychological test performance, cognitive functioning, blood pressure, and age: The Framingham Study. *Experimental Aging Research* 21:369-391.

Elias, M.F., J.W. Elias, and P.K. Elias
1989   Biological and health influences on behavior. Pp. 79-102 in *Handbook on the Psychology of Aging*, 3rd ed., J.E. Birren and K.W. Schaie, eds. San Diego: Academic Press.

Elias, M.F., P.K. Elias, M.A. Robbins, P.A. Wolf, and R.B. D'Agostino
In   Cardiovascular risk factors and cognitive functioning: An epidemiological perspec-
press   tive. In *Neuropsychology of Cardiovascular Disease*, S.R. Waldstein and M.F. Elias, eds. Mahwah, NJ: Lawrence Erlbaum Associates.

Elias, M.F., and M.A. Robbins
1991   Cardiovascular disease, hypertension, and cognitive function. Pp. 249-285 in *Behavioral Aspects of Cardiovascular Disease*, A.P. Shapiro and A. Baum, eds. Hillsdale, NJ: Erlbaum.
Elias, M.F., M.A. Robbins, and P.K. Elias
1996   A 15-year longitudinal study of Halstead-Reitan neuropsychological test performance. *Journal of Gerontology: Psychological Sciences* 51B:P331-P334.
Elias, M.F., M.A. Robbins, P.K. Elias, and D.H.P. Streeten
1998   A longitudinal study of blood pressure in relation to performance on the Wechsler Adult Intelligence Scale. *Health Psychology* 17:486-493.
Elias, M.F., M.A. Robbins, N.R. Schultz, and T.W. Pierce
1990a   Is blood pressure an important variable in research on aging and neuropsychological test performance? *Journal of Gerontology: Psychological Sciences* 45:128-135.
Elias, M.F., M.A. Robbins, N.R. Schultz, and D.H.P. Streeten
1986   A longitudinal study of neuropsychological test performance for hypertensive and normotensive adults: Initial findings. *Journal of Gerontology* 41:503-505.
Elias, M.F., M.A. Robbins, N.R. Schultz, D.H.P. Streeten, and P.K. Elias
1987   Clinical significance of cognitive performance by hypertensive patients. *Hypertension* 9:192-197.
Elias, M.F., N.R. Schultz, M.A. Robbins, and P.K. Elias
1990b   A longitudinal study of neuropsychological performance by hypertensives and normotensives: A third measurement point. *Journal of Gerontology: Psychological Sciences* 44:25-28.
Elias, M.F., P.A. Wolf, R.B. D'Agostino, J. Cobb, and L.R. White
1993   Untreated blood pressure level is inversely related to cognitive functioning: The Framingham Study. *American Journal of Epidemiology* 138:353-364.
Elias, P.K., R.B. D'Agostino, M.F. Elias, and P.A. Wolf
1995   Blood pressure, hypertension, and age as risk factors for poor cognitive performance. *Experimental Aging Research* 21:393-417.
Elias, P.K., M.F. Elias, R.B. D'Agostino, L.A. Cupples, P.W. Wilson, H. Silbershatz, and P.A. Wolf
1997   NIDDM and blood pressure as risk factors for poor cognitive performance. *Diabetes Care* 20:1388-1395.
Elias, P.K., M.F. Elias, R.B. D'Agostino, H. Silbershatz, and P.A. Wolf
In   Alcohol consumption and cognitive performance in the Framingham Heart Study.
press   *American Journal of Epidemiology.*
Emery, C.F., and J.A. Blumenthal
1991   Effects of physical exercise on psychological and cognitive functioning of older adults. *Annals of Behavioral Medicine* 13:99-107.
Erlanger, D.M., K.C. Kutner, and A.R. Jacobs
1999   Hormones and cognition: Current concepts and issues in neuropsychology. *Neuropsychology Review* 9:175-207.
Everson, S.A., E.L. Helkala, G.A. Kaplan, and J.T. Salonen
In   Atherosclerosis and cognitive functioning. In *Neuropsychology of Cardiovascular Disease*, S.R. Waldstein and M.F. Elias, eds. Mahwah, NJ: Lawrence Erlbaum Associates.
press
Feinleib, M., and J. Pinsky
1992   Nonrandom attrition in the Framingham Heart Study. Pp. 261-276 in *Statistical Models for Longitudinal Studies of Health*, J.H. Dwyer, et al., eds. New York: Oxford University Press.

Fitzpatrick, M.R., H. Engleman, K.F. Whyte, I.J. Deary, C.M. Shapiro, and N.J. Douglas
    1991   Morbidity in nocturnal asthma: Sleep quality and daytime cognitive performance. *Thorax* 46:569-573.
Flory, J.D., S.B. Manuck, R.E. Ferrell, C.M. Ryan, and M.F. Muldoon
    1999   APOE-ε4 allele is associated with lower memory scores in middle-aged adults (Abstract). *Psychosomatic Medicine* 61:257.
Fozard, J.L., E.J. Metter, and L.J. Brant
    1990   Next steps in describing aging and disease in longitudinal studies. *Journal of Gerontology: Psychological Sciences* 45:P116-P127.
Fraser, G.E., R.N. Singh, and H. Bennett
    1996   Variables associated with cognitive function in elderly California Seventh-Day Adventists. *American Journal of Epidemiology* 143:1181-1190.
Galanis, D.J., H. Petrovich, L.J. Launer, T.B. Harris, D.J. Foley, and L.R. White
    1997   Smoking history in middle age and subsequent cognitive performance in elderly Japanese-American men. *American Journal of Epidemiology* 145:507-515.
Gale, C.R., C.N. Martyn, and C. Cooper
    1996   Cognitive impairment and mortality in a cohort of elderly people. *British Medical Journal* 312:608-611.
Glanz, B.I., D. Slonin, M.B. Urowitz, D.D. Gladman, J. Grough, M. Math, and A. MacKinnon
    1997   Pattern of neuropsychological dysfunction in inactive systemic lupus erythematosus. *Neuropsychiatry, Neuropsychology, and Behavioral Neurology* 10:232-238.
Glynn, R.J., L.A. Beckett, L.E. Hebert, M.C. Morris, P.A. Scherr, and D.A. Evans
    1999   Current and remote blood pressure and cognitive decline. *Journal of the American Medical Association* 281:438-445.
Gordon, H.W., P.A. Lee, and L.K. Tamres
    1988   The pituitary axis: Behavioral correlates. Pp. 159-196 in *Medical Neuropsychology*, R.E. Tarter, D.H. Van Thiel, and K.L. Edwards, eds. New York: Plenum Press.
Grant, I., G.P. Prigatano, R.K. Heaton, A.J. McSweeney, E.C. Wright, and D.M. Adams
    1987   Progressive neuropsychologic impairments and hypoxemia: Relationship in chronic obstructive pulmonary disease. *Archives of General Psychiatry* 44:999-1006.
Guo, Z., L. Fratiglioni, B. Winblad, and M. Viitanen
    1997   Blood pressure and performance on the Mini-Mental State Examination in the very old. Cross-sectional and longitudinal data from the Kungsholmen Project. *American Journal of Epidemiology* 145:1106-1113.
Haan, M.N., and G.A. Kaplan
    1985   The contribution of socioeconomic position to minority health. Pp. 69-103 in *Report of the Secretary's Task Force on Black and Minority Health*, 2d vol., M.M. Heckler, ed. Washington, DC: U.S. Department of Health and Human Services.
Haan, M.N., G.A. Kaplan, and S.L. Syme
    1989   Socioeconomic status and health: Old observations and new thoughts. Pp. 76-135 in *Pathways to Health: The Role of Social Factors*, J.P. Bunker, D.S. Gomby, and B.M. Kehrer, eds. Palo Alto, CA: Henry J. Kaiser Family Foundation.
Haan, M.N., L. Shemanski, W.J. Jagust, T.A. Manolio, and L. Kuller
    1999   The role of APOE-ε4 in modulating effects of other risk factors for cognitive decline in elderly persons. *Journal of the American Medical Association* 282:40-46.
Hammeke, T.A., and J.E. Hastings
    1988   Neuropsychologic alterations after cardiac operations. *Journal of Thoracic and Cardiovascular Surgery* 96:326-331.
Hart, R.P., J.A. Pederson, A.W. Czerwinski, and R.L. Adams
    1983   Chronic renal failure, dialysis, and neuropsychological function. *Journal of Neuropsychology* 4:301-312.

Hartmann, D.E.
1995   *Neuropsychological Toxicology: Identification and Assessment of Human Neurotoxic Syndromes*, 2nd ed. New York: Plenum Press.
Haskell, S., E. Richardson, and R. Horwitz
1997   The effect of estrogen replacement therapy on cognitive function in women: A critical review of the literature. *Journal of Clinical Epidemiology* 50:1249-1264.
Heaton, R.K, I. Grant, N. Butters, D.A. White, D. Kirson, J.H. Atkinson, J.A. McCutchan, M. Taylor, M.D. Kelly, R.J. Ellis, T. Wolfson, R. Velin, T.D. Marcotte, J.R. Hesselink, T.L. Jernigan, J. Chandler, M. Wallace, I. Abramson, and the HNRC Group
1995   The HNRC 500—Neuropsychology of HIV infection at different disease stages. *Journal of the International Neuropsychological Society* 1:231-251.
Hill, R.D.
1989   Residual effects of cigarette smoking on cognitive performance in normal aging. *Psychology and Aging* 4:251-254.
Hopkins, R.O., and E.D. Bigler
In   Pulmonary disorders. In *Medical Neuropsychology*, 2nd ed., R.E. Tarter, M.A.
press   Butters, and S.R. Beers, eds. New York: Plenum Press.
Jama, J.W., L.J. Launer, J.C. Witteman, et al.
1996   Dietary antioxidants and cognitive function in a population-based sample of older persons: The Rotterdam Study. *American Journal of Epidemiology* 144:275-280.
Joint National Committee on Prevention, Detection, Evaluation, and Treatment of High Blood Pressure
1997   The sixth report of the Joint National Committee on Prevention, Detection, Evaluation, and Treatment of High Blood Pressure. *Archives of Internal Medicine* 157:2413-2426.
Jonas, D.L., J.A. Blumenthal, D.J. Madden, and M. Serra
In   Cognitive consequences of antihypertensive medications. In *Neuropsychology of Car-*
press   *diovascular Disease*, S.R. Waldstein and M.F. Elias, eds. Mahwah, NJ: Lawrence Erlbaum Associates.
Kannel, W.B.
1992   The Framingham experience. Pp. 67-81 in *Coronary Heart Disease Epidemiology*, M. Marmot and P. Elliott, eds. New York: Oxford.
Kaplan, G.A., and J.E. Keil
1993   Socioeconomic factors and cardiovascular disease: A review of the literature. *Circulation* 88:1973-1998.
Kaplan, N.M.
1998   *Clinical Hypertension*, 7th ed. Baltimore, MD: Williams & Wilkens.
Katzman, R.
1993   Education and the prevalence of dementia and Alzheimer's disease. *Neurology* 43:13-20.
Kelly, D.A., and D.B. Coppel
In   Sleep disorders. In *Medical Neuropsychology*, 2nd ed., R.E. Tarter, M.A. Butters,
press   and S.R. Beers, eds. New York: Plenum Press.
Kelly, M.D., I. Grant, R.K. Heaton, T. Marcotte, and the HNRC Group
1996   Neuropsychological findings in HIV infection and AIDS. Pp. 403-422 in *Neuropsychological Assessment of Neuropsychiatric Disorders*, 2nd ed., I. Grant and K.M. Adams, eds. New York: Oxford.
Kennedy, G.J., M.A. Hofer, D. Cohen, R. Shindledecker, and J.D. Fisher
1987   Significance of depression and cognitive impairment in patients undergoing programmed stimulation of cardiac arrhythmias. *Psychosomatic Medicine* 49:410-421.

Kilander, L., B. Andren, H. Nyman, L. Lind, M. Boberg, and H. Lithell
1998   Atrial fibrillation is an independent determinant of low cognitive function. A cross-sectional study in elderly men. *Stroke* 29:1816-1820.
Kilander L., H. Nyman, M. Boberg, and H. Lithell
1997   Cognitive function, vascular risk factors and education. A cross-sectional study based on a cohort of 70-year-old men. *Journal of Internal Medicine* 242:313-321.
Kirschbaum, C., O.T. Wolf, M. May, W. Wippich, and D.H. Hellhammer
1996   Stress- and treatment-induced elevations of cortisol levels associated with impaired declarative memory in healthy adults. *Life Sciences* 58:1475-1483.
Kramer, A.R., S. Hahn, N.J. Cohen, M.T. Banich, E. McAuley, C.R. Harrison, J. Chason, E. Vakil, L. Bardell, R.A. Boileau, and A. Colcombe
1998   Ageing, fitness and neurocognitive function. *Nature* 400:418-419.
Krushkal, J., R. Ferrell, S.C. Mockrin, S.T. Turner, C.F. Sing, and E. Boerwinkle
1999   Genome-wide linkage analyses of systolic blood pressure using highly discordant siblings. *Circulation* 99:1407-1410.
Kuusisto, J., K. Koivisto, L. Mykkanen, E.L. Helkala, M. Vanhanen, T. Hanninen, K. Pyorala, P. Riekkinen, and M. Laakso
1993   Essential hypertension and cognitive function. The role of hyperinsulinemia. *Hypertension* 22:771-779.
La Rue, A.
1992   *Aging and Neuropsychological Assessment.* New York: Plenum Press.
La Rue, A., L. Bank, L. Jarvik, and M. Hetland
1979   Health in old age: How do physicians' ratings and self-ratings compare? *Journal of Gerontology* 34:687-691.
Launer, L.J., J.M. Feskens, S. Kalmijn, and D. Kromhout
1996   Smoking, drinking, and thinking. The Zutphen Elderly Study. *American Journal of Epidemiology* 143:219-227.
Launer, L.J., K. Masaki, H. Petrovitch, D. Foley, and R.J. Havlik
1995   The association between midlife blood pressure levels and late-life cognitive function. *Journal of the American Medical Association* 274:1846-1851.
Lester, M.L., and D.H. Fishbein
1988   Nutrition and childhood neuropsychological disorders. Pp. 291-335 *Medical Neuropsychology,* R.E. Tarter, D.H. Van Thiel, and K.L. Edwards, eds. New York: Plenum Press.
Lester, M.L., R.W. Thatcher, and L. Monroe-Lord
1982   Refined carbohydrate intake, hair cadmium levels and cognitive functioning in children. *Nutrition and Behavior* 1:1-14.
Lezak, M.D.
1995   *Neuropsychological Assessment,* 3rd ed. New York, Oxford University Press.
Light, K.C.
1975   Slowing of response time in young and middle-aged hypertensive patients. *Experimental Aging Research* 1:209-227.
1978   Effects of mild cardiovascular and cerebrovascular disorders on serial reaction time performance. *Experimental Aging Research* 4:3-22.
Llabre, M.M., G.H. Ironson, S.B. Spitzer, M.D. Gellman, D.J. Weidler, and N. Schneiderman
1988   How many blood pressure measurements are enough? An application of generalizability theory to the study of blood pressure reliability. *Psychophysiology* 25:97-106.
Lupien, S.J., and B.S. McEwen
1997   The acute effects of corticosteroids on cognition: Integration of animal and human model studies. *Brain Research Reviews* 24:1-27.

Madden, D.J., and J.A. Blumenthal
   1998   Interaction of hypertension and age in visual selective attention performance. *Health Psychology* 17:76-83.
Mattlar, C., E. Engblom, P. Vesala, E. Vanttinen, and L. Knuts
   1991   The proportion of patients with cognitive impairments after coronary artery bypass surgery: An 8-month follow-up study. *Psychotherapy and Psychosomatics* 55:145-150.
McCardle, J.J., F. Hamagami, M.F. Elias, and M.A. Robbins
   1991   Structural equation modeling of mixed longitudinal and cross-sectional data. *Experimental Aging Research* 17:29-52.
McEwen, B.S., and R.M. Sapolsky
   1995   Stress and cognitive function. *Current Opinion in Neurobiology* 5:205-216.
McSweeny, A.J., and K.T. Labuhn
   1996   The relationship of neuropsychological functioning to health-related quality of life in systemic medical disease: the example of chronic obstructive pulmonary disease. Pp. 577-602 in *Neuropsychological Assessment of Neuropsychiatric Disorders*, 2nd ed., I. Grant and K.M. Adams, eds. New York: Oxford.
Miller, R.E., A.P. Shapiro, H.E. King, E.H. Ginchereau, and J.A. Hosutt
   1984   Effect of antihypertensive treatment on the behavioral consequences of elevated blood pressure. *Hypertension* 6:202-208.
Morrow, L.A., S.B. Muldoon, and D.J. Sandstrom
   In   Neuropsychological sequelae associated with occupational and environmental expo-
   press   sure to chemicals. In *Medical Neuropsychology*, 2nd ed., R.E. Tarter, M.A. Butters, and S.R. Beers, eds. New York: Plenum Press.
Moss, H., R. Tarter, J. Yao, and D. Van Thiel
   1995   Subclinical hepatic encephalopathy: The determinants of neuropsychologic deficits as evaluated by standard laboratory tests assessing hepatic injury. *Archives of Clinical Neuropsychology* 7:419-429.
Muldoon, M.F., J.D. Flory, and C.M. Ryan
   In   Serum cholesterol, the brain, and cognitive functioning. In *Neuropsychology of Car-
   press   diovascular Disease*, S.R. Waldstein and M.F. Elias, eds. Mahwah, NJ: Lawrence Erlbaum Associates.
Muldoon, M.F., S.B. Manuck, A.P. Shapiro, and S.R. Waldstein
   1991   Neurobehavioral effects of antihypertensive medications. *Journal of Hypertension* 9:549-559.
Muldoon, M.F., C.M. Ryan, K.A. Matthews, and S.B. Manuck
   1997   Serum cholesterol and intellectual performance. *Psychosomatic Medicine* 59:382-387.
Muldoon, M.F., S.R. Waldstein, and J.R. Jennings
   1995   Neuropsychological consequences of antihypertensive medication use. *Experimental Aging Research* 21:353-368.
Newman, S.P., J. Stygall, and R. Kong
   In   Neuropsychological consequences of coronary artery bypass surgery. In *Neuropsy-
   press   chology of Cardiovascular Disease*, S.R. Waldstein and M.F. Elias, eds. Mahwah, NJ: Lawrence Erlbaum Associates.
Nussbaum, P.D., and G. Goldstein
   1992   Neuropsychological sequelae of heart transplantation: A preliminary review. *Clinical Psychology Review* 12:475-483.
Paleologos, M., R.G. Cumming, and R. Lazarus
   1998   Cohort study of vitamin C intake and cognitive impairment. *American Journal of Epidemiology* 148:45-50.

Phillips, N.A.
In   Thinking on your feet: A neuropsychological review of peripheral vascular disease.
press   In *Neuropsychology of Cardiovascular Disease*, S.R. Waldstein and M.F. Elias, eds.
          Mahwah, NJ: Lawrence Erlbaum Associates.
Phillips, N.A., and C.C. Mate-Kole
1997   Cognitive deficits in peripheral vascular disease. A comparison of mild stroke pa-
          tients and normal control subjects. *Stroke* 28:777-784.
Phillips, N.A., C.C. Mate-Kole, and R.L. Kirby
1993   Neuropsychological function in peripheral vascular amputees. *Archives of Physical
          Medicine and Rehabilitation* 74:1309-1314.
Pierce, T.W., and M.F. Elias
1993   Cognitive function and cardiovascular responsivity in subjects with a parental his-
          tory of hypertension. *Journal of Behavioral Medicine* 16:277-294.
Pliskin, N.H., T.A. Kiolbasa, R.P. Hart, and J.G. Umans
In   Neuropsychological function in renal disease and its treatments. In *Medical Neuro-
press   psychology*, 2nd ed., R.E. Tarter, M.A. Butters, and S.R. Beers, eds. New York: Ple-
          num Press.
Prigatano, G.P., O. Parsons, D.C. Levin, E. Wright, and G. Hawryluk
1983   Neuropsychological test performance in mildly hypoxemic patients with chronic ob-
          structive pulmonary disease. *Journal of Consulting and Clinical Psychology* 51:108-
          116.
Reaven, G.M., L.W. Thompson, D. Nahum, and E. Haskins
1990   Relationship between hyperglycemia and cognitive function in older NIDDM pa-
          tients. *Diabetes Care* 13:16-21.
Riggs, K.M., A. Spiro, K. Tucker, and D. Rusch
1996   Relation of vitamin, B-12, vitamin B-6, folate and homocysteine to cognitive perfor-
          mance in the Normative Aging Study. *American Journal of Clinical Nutrition* 63:306-
          314.
Robbins, M.A., M.F. Elias, S.H. Croog, and T. Colton
1994   Unmedicated blood pressure levels and quality of life in elderly hypertensive women.
          Psychosomatic Medicine 56:251-259.
Rockwood, K., A.R. Dobbs, B.G. Rule, S.E. Howlett, and W.R. Black
1992   The impact of pacemaker implantation on cognitive functioning in elderly patients.
          Journal of the American Geriatrics Society 40:142-146.
Roine, R.O., S. Kajaste, and M. Kaste
1993   Neuropsychological sequelae of cardiac arrest. *Journal of the American Medical Asso-
          ciation* 269:237-242.
Rourke, S.B., and T. Løberg
1996   The neurobehavioral correlates of alcoholism. Pp. 423-485 in *Neuropsychological
          Assessment of Neuropsychiatric Disorders*, 2nd ed., I. Grant and K.M. Adams, eds.
          New York: Oxford.
Ryan, C.M.
In   Diabetes-associated cognitive dysfunction. In *Neuropsychology of Cardiovascular Dis-
press   ease*, S.R. Waldstein and M.F. Elias, eds. Mahwah, NJ: Lawrence Erlbaum Associates.
Ryan, C.M., T.M. Williams, D.N. Finegold, and T.J. Orchard
1993   Cognitive dysfunction in adults with Type 1 (insulin-dependent) diabetes mellitus of
          long duration: effects of recurrent hypoglycemia and other chronic complications.
          Diabetologia 36:329-334.
Salthouse, T.A.
1991   Mediation of adult age differences in cognition by reductions in working memory
          and speed of processing. *Psychological Science* 2:179-183.

Schmidt, R., F. Fazekas, H. Offenbacher, T. Dusek, E. Zach, B. Reinhart, P. Grieshofer, W. Freidl, B. Eber, M. Schumacher, M. Koch, and H. Lechner
1993 Neuropsychologic correlates of MRI white matter hyperintensities: A study of 150 normal volunteers. *Neurology* 43:2490-2494.
Schultz, N.R., J.T. Dineen, M.F. Elias, C.A. Pentz, and W.G. Wood
1979 WAIS performance for different age groups of hypertensive and control subjects during the administration of a diuretic. *Journal of Gerontology* 34:246-253.
Schultz, N.R., M.F. Elias, M.A. Robbins, D.H.P. Streeten, and N. Blakeman
1986 A longitudinal comparison of hypertensives and normotensives on the Wechsler Adult Intelligence Scale: Initial findings. *Journal of Gerontology* 41:169-175.
Seeman, T.E., B.S. McEwen, M.S. Albert, and J.W. Rowe
1997 Urinary cortisol and decline in memory performance in older adults: MacArthur Studies of Successful Aging. *Journal of Clinical Endocrinology and Metabolism* 82:2458-2465.
Sellman, M., L. Holm, T. Ivert, and B.K.H. Semb
1993 A randomized study of neuropsychological function in patients undergoing coronary bypass surgery. *Thoracic and Cardiovascular Surgeon* 41:349-354.
Shapiro, A.P., R.E. Miller, H.E. King, E.H. Ginchereau, and K. Fitzgibbon
1982 Behavioral consequences of mild hypertension. *Hypertension* 4:355-360.
Shaw, P.J., D. Bates, N.E.F. Cartlidge, J.M. French, D. Heaviside, D.G. Julian, and D.A. Shaw
1986 Early intellectual dysfunction following coronary bypass surgery. *Quarterly Journal of Medicine* 225:59-68.
Siegler, I.C., and D.T. Costa
1985 Health behavior relationships. Pp. 144-166 in *Handbook on the Psychology of Aging*, 3rd ed., J.E. Birren and K.W. Schaie, eds. San Diego: Academic Press.
Stamler, J.
1992 Established major coronary risk factors. Pp. 35-65 in *Coronary Heart Disease Epidemiology*, M. Marmot and P. Elliott, eds. New York: Oxford.
Stein, M.A., M. Krasowski, B.L. Leventhal, W. Phillips, and B.G. Bender
1996 Behavioral and cognitive effects of methylxanthines: A meta-analysis of theophylline and caffeine. *Archives of Pediatric and Adolescent Medicine* 150:284-288.
Streeten, D.H.P., G.H. Anderson, Jr., and M.F. Elias
1992 Prevalence of secondary hypertension and unusual aspects of the treatment of hypertension in elderly individuals. *Geriatric Nephrology and Urology* 2:91-98.
Strickland, T.L., and R. Stein
1995 Cocaine-induced cerebrovascular impairment: Challenges to neuropsychological assessment. *Neuropsychology Reviews* 5:69-79.
Swan, G.E., D. Carmelli, and A. La Rue
1996 Relationship between blood pressure during middle age and cognitive impairment in old age: The Western Collaborative Group Study. *Aging, Neuropsychology, and Cognition* 3:241-250.
1998 Systolic blood pressure tracking over 25 to 30 years and cognitive performance in older adults. *Stroke* 29:2334-2340.
Swan, G.E., A. LaRue, D. Carmelli, T.E. Reed, and R.R. Fabsitz
1992 Decline in cognitive performance in aging twins. *Archives of Neurology* 49:476-481.
Tarter, R.E., M.A. Butters, and S.R. Beers, eds.
In press *Medical Neuropsychology*, 2nd ed. New York: Plenum Press.
Tarter, R.E., and D.H. Van Thiel
1985 *Alcohol and the Brain: Chronic Effects*. New York: Plenum Press.

In   Neuropsychological dysfunction due to liver disease. In *Medical Neuropsychology*,
press Press.   2nd ed., R.E. Tarter, M.A. Butters, and S.R. Beers, eds. New York: Plenum
R.E. Tarter, D.H. Van Thiel, and K.L. Edwards, eds.
1988   *Medical Neuropsychology*. New York: Plenum Press.
Townes, B.D., G. Bashein, T.F. Hornbein, D.B. Coppel, D.E. Goldstein, K.B. Davis, M.L. Nessly,
S.W. Bledsoe, R.C. Veith, T.D. Ivey, and M.A. Cohen
1989   Neurobehavioral outcomes in cardiac operations: A prospective controlled study.
       Journal of Thoracic and Cardiovascular Surgery 98:774-782.
van Swieten, J.C., G.G. Geyskes, M.M.A. Derix, B.M. Beeck, L.M.P. Ramos, J.C. van Latum, and
J. van Gijn
1991   Hypertension in the elderly is associated with white matter lesions and cognitive
       deficits. *Annals of Neurology* 30:825-830.
Vingerhoets, G.
In   Cognitive consequences of myocardial infarction, cardiac arrhythmias, and cardiac
press arrest. In *Neuropsychology of Cardiovascular Disease*, S.R. Waldstein and M.F. Elias,
       eds. Mahwah, NJ: Lawrence Erlbaum Associates.
Volpe, B.T., J.D. Holtzman, and W. Hirst
1986   Further characterization of patients with amnesia after cardiac arrest: Preserved
       recognition memory. *Neurology* 36:408-411.
Waldstein, S.R.
1995   Hypertension and neuropsychological function: A lifespan perspective. *Experimen-
       tal Aging Research* 21:321-352.
Waldstein, S.R., and M.F. Elias
In   *Neuropsychology of Cardiovascular Disease*. Mahwah, NJ: Lawrence Erlbaum Associ-
press ates.
Waldstein, S.R., J.R. Jennings, C.M. Ryan, M.F. Muldoon, A.P. Shapiro, J.M. Polefrone, T.V.
Fazzari, and S.B. Manuck
1996   Hypertension and neuropsychological performance in men: Interactive effects of age.
       Health Psychology 15:102-109.
Waldstein, S.R., and L.I. Katzel
In   Hypertension and cognitive function. In *Neuropsychology of Cardiovascular Disease*,
press S.R. Waldstein and M.F. Elias, eds. Mahwah, NJ: Lawrence Erlbaum Associates.
Waldstein, S.R., S.B. Manuck, C.M. Ryan, and M.F. Muldoon
1991a Neuropsychological correlates of hypertension: Review and methodologic consider-
       ations. *Psychological Bulletin* 110:451-468.
Waldstein, S.R., C.M. Ryan, S.B. Manuck, D.K. Parkinson, and E.J. Bromet
1991b Learning and memory function in men with untreated blood pressure elevation.
       Journal of Consulting and Clinical Psychology 59:513-517.
Waldstein, S.R., C.M. Ryan, J.M. Polefrone, and S.B. Manuck
1994   Neuropsychological performance of young men who vary in familial risk for hyper-
       tension. *Psychosomatic Medicine* 56:449-456.
Waldstein, S.R., J. Snow, and M.F. Muldoon
1998   Applications of neuropsychological assessment to the study of cardiovascular dis-
       ease. Pp. 69-94 in *Technology and Methods in Behavioral Medicine*, D.S. Krantz and
       A. Baum, eds. Mahwah, NJ: Lawrence Erlbaum Associates.
Waldstein, S.R., J. Snow, M.F. Muldoon, and L.I. Katzel
In   Neuropsychological consequences of cardiovascular disease. In *Medical Neuropsy-
press chology*, 2nd ed., R.E. Tarter, M.A. Butters, and S.R. Beers, eds. New York: Plenum
       Press.

Waldstein, S.R., J. Snow, C.F. Tankard, N. Tomoyasu, A.W. Gardner, and L.I. Katzel
   1999   Peripheral arterial disease and neuropsychological performance in older adults (Abstract). *Psychosomatic Medicine* 61:86.
Wallace, R.B., J.H. Lemke, M.C. Morris, M. Goodenberger, F. Kohout, and J.V. Hinrichs
   1985   Relationship of free-recall memory to hypertension in the elderly. The Iowa 65+ Rural Health Study. *Journal of Chronic Disease* 38:475-481.
Whitehouse, P.J., A. Lerner, and P. Hedera
   1993   Dementia. Pp. 603-645 in *Clinical Neuropsychology*, 3rd ed., K.M. Heilman and E. Valenstein, eds. New York: Oxford.
Whitfield, K.E., G. Fillenbaum, C. Peiper, T.E. Seeman, M.S. Albert, L.F. Berkman, D.G. Blazer, and J.W. Rowe
   2000   The effect of race and health related factors on naming and memory: The MacArthur Studies of Successful Aging. *Journal of Aging and Health* 12(1):69-89.
Wilkie, F., and C. Eisdorfer
   1971   Intelligence and blood pressure in the aged. *Science* 172:959-962.
Wilson, R.S., D.A. Bennett, and A. Swartzendruber
   1997   Age-related change in cognitive function. Pp. 7-14 in *Handbook of Neuropsychology and Aging*, P.D. Nussbaum, ed. New York: Plenum Press.
Yaffe, K., J. Cauley, L. Sands, and W. Browner
   1997   Apolipoprotein E phenotype and cognitive decline in a prospective study of elderly community women. *Archives of Neurology* 54:1110-1114.
Zelinski, E.M., E. Crimmins, S. Reynolds, and T. Seeman
   1998   Do medical conditions affect cognition in older adults? *Health Psychology* 17:504-512.

F

Cultural Variations in Cognition: Implications for Aging Research

Shinobu Kitayama

Cultural influence on cognitive aging has received renewed research interest in recent years (Baltes, 1997; Park et al., 1999). Many cognitive capacities decline as a function of age. For example, performance on psychometric intelligence tests, which often involve working memory, speed of information processing, and inhibitory efficacy, steadily declines after midlife, and it is reasonable to hypothesize that this decline reflects an age-related loss of biological potential (Lindenberger and Baltes, 1994). At the same time, however, many basic cognitive skills and processes, especially those that are "culturally saturated" (Park et al., 1999), may not show the same degree of functional decline. Such skills and processes are formed through cultural learning, and hence they are constituted primarily by learned knowledge structures and processing biases, which could compensate for the decline of biological potential. Furthermore, such knowledge structures and processing biases are likely to take cross-culturally divergent forms. It follows, then, that the undesirable effects of aging on many cognitive functions would be neither uniform across all cultures nor inevitable in any given culture.

Although the idea of biological decline in old age contains a kernel of truth and points to the fact that culture cannot change nature in any way it wants, it has to be supplemented with cultural considerations in order to obtain a more detailed and comprehensive account of cognitive aging. With this in mind, this paper highlights some issues and possibilities that could be illuminated by the perspective of cultural psychology. The purpose is not to review the existent literature, but to suggest potentially fruitful directions for research, thereby to encourage much-needed cross-cultural empirical work in this area.

CULTURAL PSYCHOLOGY

Cultural psychology is an approach to human and social sciences that has been inspired by the realization that "culture and the psyche make each other up" (Shweder, 1991). Culture is a package of meanings that are embodied in such human artifacts as icons, behavioral routines, conventions, social institutions, and political systems that as a whole constitute daily reality. These human artifacts and associated meanings are both inside and outside a person. On one hand, they are outside the person in that they, as a whole, define the external, "brutal" reality with which he or she has to cope, control, or adjust to. On the other hand, they are inside the person in that they are constantly reproduced and reconstituted by the collective actions of many individuals in the same society. Moreover, they are represented at least in part in both the declarative and the procedural knowledge of each individual. Psychological processes and structures are configured in such a way that the engagement of these processes and structures reproduces the cultural systems of artifacts. The primary mission of cultural psychology is to analyze the processes by which psyches and cultures construct each other, elucidating how cultures create and support psychological processes, and how these psychological tendencies in turn support, reproduce, and sometimes change the cultural systems (Fiske et al., 1998; Markus et al., 1996).

The cultural psychological perspective has been motivated by the emergence of findings and theories in the past decade that alert researchers in many behavioral and social science disciplines to the cultural specificity of some of the fundamental assumptions and phenomena of the respective fields. In social, personality, and developmental psychology, for example, a great many "anomalies" have been discovered in cultures outside North America: verbs are acquired before nouns by infants in Mandarin China (Tardif, 1996); Japanese self-criticize without any trace of depression (Kitayama et al., 1997); Chinese are often persuaded quite effectively by arguments that defy the fundamental premise of logical consistency (such as "losing is winning"; Peng and Nisbett, 1999); the fundamental attribution error fails to occur in India (Miller, 1984), China (Morris and Peng, 1994), and Japan (see below for detail); and the Japanese don't seem to engage in dissonance reduction (Heine and Lehman, 1997). Initial discoveries of such anomalies have prompted many theorists to raise questions about some of the assumptions hidden in the historical development of the field itself, not the least important of which is the assumption of a "bounded, independent person" as the "natural" unit of analysis in social, personality, cognitive, and developmental psychology (e.g., Cole, 1996; Geertz, 1973; Gergen, 1993; Markus and Kitayama, 1991;

Miller, 1994; Sampson, 1977, 1988; Shweder and Bourne, 1984; Shweder and Sullivan, 1993; Triandis, 1989, 1995).

The mutually constructed relation between culture and the psyche is formed through human development. We are born into a culture with its own set of practices and meanings, laid out by generations of people who have created, carried, maintained, and altered them. To engage in culturally patterned relationships and practices and to become a mature, well-functioning adult in society, new members of the culture must come to coordinate their responses with their particular social milieu. That is, people must come to think, feel, and act with reference to local practices, relationships, institutions, and artifacts; to do so they must use the local cultural models, which consequently become an integral part of their psychological systems. Each person actively seeks to behave adaptively in the attendant cultural context, and, in the process, different persons develop their own unique set of response tendencies, cognitive orientations, emotional preparedness, and structure of goals and values. This perspective, then, encompasses both cross-cultural divergence in psychological functions and intracultural variation in them (see *Culture and Psychology*, special issue, 1998).

Notably, different individuals have different biological propensities, potentials, and temperamental inclinations. Furthermore, humans as a species have important biological propensities that have made cultural adaptation possible (Brown, 1991; Durham, 1991; Fiske et al., 1998). Yet virtually none of these biological propensities is likely to determine in full the nature of the cognitive, emotional, and motivational organizations the person develops in the course of becoming a mature adult. The psychological structures and processes are one's characteristic ways of "handling" and "living with" an assortment of cultural affordances. Thus, the ways in which any given biological propensities are appropriated for use in this or that psychological structure (e.g., how cardiovascular systems are implicated in coping with stress), the meanings assigned to such propensities (e.g., facial musculature as a spontaneous expression of emotion or as a social mask), and which temperamental inclinations (e.g., "extroversion" as marked by contraction of zygomatic muscles in infants) are valued, fostered, and reinforced or despised, inhibited, and suspended are all closely intertwined with the attendant cultural pattern. And as we shall see, there exists a distinct possibility that sociopsychological consequences of aging are also culturally mediated to some significant extent.

The preceding analysis conceptualizes culture as an assortment of cultural resources. These resources may be symbolic or material; personal, interpersonal, or institutional; relatively specific to concrete social settings or more generally encompassing the entire cultural group. Each individual is assumed to actively engage in cultural resources, which in turn have *formative* influences on his or her psychological processes. Hence, culture not only provides cognitive content, but it may also shape cognitive processes, some of which can be reasonably called basic (see below). Another promising framework for conceptualizing culture is provided by Baltes and colleagues (e.g., Baltes, 1997), who assume that cultures vary in (1) what tasks or goals are made available (so that individuals can *select* what they do), (2) which of potentially usable means are presented (so that they can *optimize* their performance), and (3) what *compensatory* means are offered (in case they fail to adequately perform the task). Baltes and colleagues suggest that culture provides content for the fundamental architecture of the human mind that involves selection, optimization, and compensation. Furthermore, because of biological decline associated with aging, optimization becomes increasingly difficult and, as a consequence, selection and compensation become the key factors in modulating successful aging. Unlike the present view, then, Baltes and colleagues assume that culture is a source of cognitive content for a relatively fixed machinery of the mind. These two approaches, however, may highlight different facets of the culture-mind interface, and, as such, by no means are they mutually exclusive. Indeed, empirical work would benefit from insights from both.

CULTURALLY DIVERGENT IDEAS ABOUT AGING

Many, perhaps all known cultures have some classificatory schemas for a life course or cycle. These life schemas are often embedded in a larger framework used to understand the "entire universe" (Shweder, 1998). For example, Figure F-1 shows a symbolic representation of the life cycle that is inscribed on a wall in a Buddhist temple in Thailand. A glance at this picture reveals some significant elements in the Buddhist world view—and, more generally, Asian world views. Although diverse, many Asian ideologies, cosmologies, and philosophical commitments, including Hinduism, Confucianism, and Taoism, share some key elements with the Buddhist ideas revealed here. For the present purposes, two of them deserve a special emphasis.

First, life is conceptualized as perpetual cycle. Death is not the end of life, but the beginning of the next one. From this detached, encompassing, admittedly somewhat unworldly point of view, life is seen as a brief visit from the more fundamental process of the universe. Reincarnation, then, not only is a real possibility, but, in fact, life after death may be where we mortals truly belong; it is where one can have full freedom from a series of worldly toils, responsibilities, duties, and obligations. These ideas are relatively rare in European American cultures and, in fact, are in stark contrast with Judeo-Christian views that regard birth as the beginning and death as the end, at which point one is destined to either heaven or hell.

Second, Figure F-1 shows that in the Buddhist cosmology, the middle of

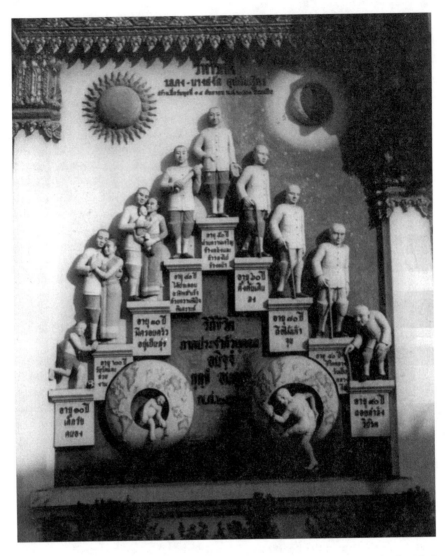

FIGURE F-1 A Buddhist image of the life cycle as inscribed in a wall of a Thai temple.

life, around the age of 50, is seen as its prime. The first half is brighter (under the sun) than the second half. Yet even the second part is lit up by the moon. The moon is darker, of course, but there is enough light to guide the person along the path toward reincarnation. Most notably, just as steps toward the prime of life are gradual, featured by age-graded events or attainments, such as mischievous youth, marriage, and attainment of fame or reputation, so are the steps toward death. Life then appears to be seen as a succession of different sorts of tasks, prescribed and acknowledged explicitly by the society or culture as a whole as both normal and normative. Each stage is associated with one's status in the family or in the larger social unit. One important consequence is that aging is seen as a task shared in a given cohort group rather than an exclusive function of biological chronology.

Evidence for the hypothesis that these ideas are socially shared and used to organize cultural practices comes from several ethnographies. These ideas can easily be seen in different forms for women in contemporary India (Seymour, 1999), contemporary Japanese individuals in midlife (Plath, 1980), and, to an even greater extent, in more traditional mythologies and teachings from the past. For example, according to Confucius, a person attains true freedom at the age of 70, when his or her natural desires coincide with demands of society. Life is seen as a pursuit of the path leading up to this stage of serenity—not unlike the Western conception of wisdom (Baltes and Staudinger, 1993).

Compare these Asian ideas with modern European American conceptions of life as unidirectional progress. Although there exists considerable overlap between them, the two sets of ideas also show some remarkable points of contrast. First, in culturally canonical discourses of the modern West, progress is often imagined to involve a series of age-graded tasks, such as growing up, becoming independent, getting a job, starting a family, and developing one's career (Cantor, 1994). These normative life tasks are usually reinforced and sustained by a variety of cultural conventions and practices. Encouragement and support come mostly from others in surrounding communities. The collectively held life tasks serve the significant sociopsychological function of keeping the person on track. Notably, however, the contemporary European American views rarely specify in any detail or in any future-oriented way any age-graded tasks in the post-prime half of life. This may not come as any surprise: if the goal of life is to live actively, events that occur after the prime of life may necessarily be considered to be a sequence of failures to act, to influence, and thus to live, culminating in eventual death.

Contrasts between Asian and European-American views provide an example of the ways in which culture may influence the aging process. Beliefs about life and death go beyond the imaginations of world-renouncing monks, philosophers, and historians of ideas. They organize life, in part because people necessarily live life not purely as a biologically prescribed event, but as a personally meaningful sequence of social and individual experiences. Cultural world views supply a system of meanings that are then appropriated by each and every one of the members of the culture to create personalized meanings for their life. These views also help organize each person's life, because they are often accompanied by corresponding collective practices and conventions that provide an overarching framework for activities. Hence, socially shared *ideas* about aging can cause changes in the psychological *realities* of aging. Ryan (1992) made this point with respect to memory. He noted that the expected decline of memory in the older age "[can] lead to poorer memory performance through their indirect impact on decreased effort, less use of adaptive strategies, avoidance of challenging situations, and failure to seek medical attention for disease-related symptoms of forgetfulness" (p. 41).

The hypothesis that social beliefs about aging have a causal impact on cognitive functioning in older age is provocative. Indeed, a promising lead for cross-cultural work on aging has begun to be made. We now turn to a review of this emerging literature, which suggests that culture's influence on cognitive aging is likely to exist, yet the form it takes is likely to be much more complicated than the foregoing hypothesis would suggest.

CULTURE AND BASIC COGNITIVE PROCESSES

In recent years, significant advances have been made in the cultural psychology of cognitive processes. This advance is fueled by a growing number of cross-cultural studies that have documented considerable cultural variations in biases in inference, reasoning, memory, and attention. So far, this literature is confined largely to a contrast between European American cultures and Asian cultures, although this presents two important limitations. First, there are many cultures outside the two regions. Second, each of the two cultural regions of European America and Asia is by itself diverse, composed of a variety of different subgroups.

Despite these limitations, this literature has begun to demonstrate the degree of cultural variation in cognition that raises significant doubt about the universalistic assumption that cognition is the hard-wired machinery of the psyche that exists independent of the cultural milieu. As we shall see, people in European American cultural contexts often exhibit a persistent tendency to focus on an object, along with a relatively lowered sensitivity toward contextual information. Their thought therefore tends to be object-centered, linear, logical in an Aristotelian sense, or, in short, *analytic*. In contrast, people in Asian cultural contexts tend to show a much-enhanced sensitivity to context. Their thought tends to be field-centered, dialectic, logical in a more inclusive sense, or, in short, *holistic* (Peng and Nisbett, 1999). These cognitive differences are deep and not just superficial variations in self-pretension or presentation. They are fundamental, rooted in correspondingly different systems of self, well-being, motivation, and emotion. And they are widespread and pervasive in the respective regions of the world.

Western and Eastern Naive Theories of Human Agency

Choi et al. (1999) have proposed that European American cultures share a strong dispositionist theory, which assumes that a person is a causal entity, consisting of a variety of internal attributes, such as attitude, personality traits, and motives, and that behavior is guided by pertinent ones of these internal attributes. These researchers have further argued that Asian cultures, in contrast, share a situationist theory, which explicitly acknowledges the role of situational constraints in addition to the role of each person's dispositions. As we shall see, there is enough evidence to suggest that in drawing inferences about another person, individuals often refer to these divergent naive theories.

As acknowledged by Choi and colleagues themselves, however, what is actually shared in Asian cultures may not be a situationist theory, but it may in fact be an idea about human agency that has already incorporated situational factors (Markus and Kitayama, 1991). What one wishes to do, for example, may be highly contingent on other people and on conditions that are available in the environment and that are waiting to unfold in response to one's willful engagement in them. From this perspective, which explicitly acknowledges the mutuality among people and between people and their surroundings, one's agency may be thought to derive from the social surroundings and, as such, be inseparable from them. The presumed antagonism between person and situation implicit in the formulation of Asian naive theories as situationist may be somewhat inaccurate. Instead, the Asian naive theories may be better conceptualized as more expanded or inclusive. They may regard a person as enabled by the social surroundings rather than as a force that is contrasted against the surroundings. Whereas human agency is imagined to be bounded and independent in the West, it may be imagined to be fundamentally relational, interdependent, and inclusive in Asia. In fact, Menon et al. (1999) have shown that Asians are more likely than Westerners to assign agency or dispositional characteristics to groups.

Memory of Contextual Information

Although the significance of culturally divergent naive theories in social inference is beyond any doubt, it is quite misleading to attribute all cultural differences to the differences in naive theories that are stored in individual memory and that are referred to when the person draws inferences about other people or events. Evidence suggests that there exist considerable cultural differences in the operation of processing systems themselves, especially the system of spontaneous allocation of attention. These biases in operating characteristics of the cognitive systems work in conjunction with culturally shared naive theories, often reinforcing each other.

Masuda and Nisbett (1999) presented both American and Japanese subjects with cartoons of fish and other underwater life. In each cartoon sequence there was a focal fish, which was larger and moved more rapidly than anything else in the cartoon. The researchers expected that Japanese subjects would spontaneously attend to the stimuli presented in context when observing the focal fish, and therefore that these stimuli should be incorporated into the memory representations of the focal fish. In contrast, American subjects were expected to be unlikely to spontaneously attend to the contextual stimuli, and therefore these stimuli would not be encoded along with the focal fish. To test these predictions, after the initial presentation of all the cartoon sequences, subjects were given a surprise recognition memory test under three different conditions. In the first condition, only the focal fish was presented along with filler fish. In the second, the focal fish was presented in the *correct* context—namely, in the context that had been paired with the focal fish in the initial presentation of the cartoon sequences. In the third, the focal fish was presented in the *incorrect* context—namely, in a context that had not been paired with the focal fish initially. The researchers' expectations were borne out by the data. Memory performance of the Japanese subjects was strongly influenced by the context manipulation: it was best in the correct-context condition, worst in the incorrect-context condition, and falling in between in the no-context condition. In contrast, there was no effect of the context manipulation for the American subjects. Importantly, the researchers have replicated the basic findings with another set of stimuli, this time with birds and mammals, so the demonstrated cross-cultural difference appears to have a degree of generality.

High- Versus Low-Context Forms of Communication

The relative significance of context in comprehension and communication in Asian cultures is hard-wired into the pragmatics of these cultures' languages. In his original formulation, Hall (1976) proposed that in some Western cultures/languages (e.g., North American/English), a greater proportion of information is conveyed by verbal content. Correspondingly, contextual cues, including nonverbal ones such as vocal tone, are likely to serve a relatively minor role. Hall referred to these cultures/languages as *low-context*. The low-context communicative practices appear to be grounded in a cultural assumption that the thoughts of each individual are unknowable in principle unless they are explicitly expressed in words. By contrast, in some East Asian cultures/languages (e.g., Japanese), the proportion of information conveyed by verbal content is relatively smaller and, correspondingly, contextual and nonverbal cues are likely to play a relatively greater role. These languages are thus called *high-context*. The high-context communicative practices appear to be grounded in a contrasting cultural assumption that the thoughts of each individual are knowable in principle once enough context is specified for an utterance.

Existent evidence is consistent with Hall's analysis. For example, Ambady et al. (1996) found that a choice of politeness strategies in social communication (see Brown and Levinson, 1987) is influenced more by the content of the communication in the United States, but it is influenced more by relational concerns (i.e., contextual information) in Korea. Focusing on Japanese communicative practices, several observers have noted that utterances in daily communications in Japan are often ambiguous when taken out of context (Barnlund, 1989; Borden, 1991; Ikegami, 1991). For example, "i-i" literally means "good." When this utterance is used in an actual, specific social context, however, it can mean praise ("It is good"), decline ("It is good that you don't do it," meaning "you don't have to do it"), or even rejection ("It is good that we are finished," meaning "go away!"). The intended meaning of a communication is dependent so much on the immediate social, relational context that it can diverge considerably from its literal verbal meaning. In a more systematic, cross-linguistic study, Kashima and Kashima (1998) have noted that in the languages of individualist cultures (e.g., English, German) it is often obligatory to include relevant pronouns in constructing grammatically permissible sentences. This structural feature of the languages lends itself to verbally explicit, low-context forms of communication. In contrast, the languages of collectivist cultures (e.g., Japanese, Chinese, Korean, and Spanish) tend to leave the use of pronouns largely optional, hence conducive to verbally ambiguous, high-context forms of communication.

The Role of Verbal Versus Vocal Information in Speech Comprehension

Recent work by Kitayama and Ishii (1999) has suggested that the high-versus low-context patterns of communicative practices and conventions are reflected in the nature of the processing systems that are brought to bear on the comprehension of emotional speech. Focusing on one low-context language, English, and one high-context language, Japanese, Kitayama and Ishii argued that in low-context cultures and languages, both speakers and listeners are likely to engage in a communicative endeavor with an implicit rule of thumb that what is said in word is what is meant. The speakers craft their messages and, in turn, the listeners comprehend them with this rule of thumb in mind. Thus, for example, when someone says "Yes," the listener ought to construe, first, the utterance to mean an affirmation of some kind. Only after this initial assignment of meaning may an adjustment be made on the basis of other contextual cues, including the attendant vocal tone. Once socialized in such a linguistic and cultural system, individuals develop a well-practiced attentional bias that favors verbal content.

In contrast, in high-context cultures and languages, both speakers and listeners are likely to engage in a communicative endeavor with an implicit cultural rule of thumb that what is said makes best sense only in a particular context. The speakers craft their messages and the listeners, in their turn, comprehend messages with this rule of thumb in mind. Thus, for example, when someone says "Yes" in a relatively reluctant tone of voice, the tone of the voice should figure more prominently, along with other available contextual cues, for the listener to infer the "real" meaning of the utterance. Once socialized in such a linguistic or cultural system, individuals develop a well-practiced attentional bias that favors vocal tone.

If the culturally divergent attentional biases predicted above are overlearned through recurrent engagement in one or the other mode of daily communications, they should be quite immune to intentional control to nullify them. Kitayama and Ishii tested this possibility with a Stroop-type interference task. Two specific predictions were advanced. First, suppose individuals are asked to ignore the verbal content of an emotional speech and, instead, to make a judgment about its vocal tone. Under these conditions, native users of English (the low-context language) should find it relatively difficult to ignore the verbal meaning. In comparison, native users of Japanese (the high-context language) would find it relatively easy to do so. Second, consider a reverse task, in which individuals have to ignore vocal tone of the speech and, instead, to make a judgment of its verbal content. Under these conditions, the native Japanese users should find it relatively difficult to ignore the vocal tone. In comparison, the native English users should find it relatively easy to do so. Native Japanese and English users made a speeded judgment of either vocal emotion or word evaluation of an emotionally spoken evaluative word. Word evaluations and vocal emotions were orthogonally manipulated and, furthermore, they were comparable in extremity in the two languages. In support of the hypothesis, an interference effect by competing word evaluation in the vocal emotion judgment was significantly stronger in English than in Japanese. In contrast, an interference effect by competing vocal emotion in the word evaluation judgment was stronger in Japanese than in English.

Social Explanation

Let me now move on to examine certain psychological consequences of naive theories about agency. Initial evidence was provided by Joan Miller (1984) in her study of social explanation in the United States and India. She found that whereas Americans explained another person's behavior that had either good or bad consequences predominantly in terms of either good or bad qualities or other corresponding trait terms, Hindu Indians explains similar behaviors in terms of social roles, obligations, and other contextual factors. Contextual attributions were twice as frequent for Indians as for Americans; dispositional explanations were twice as common for Americans as for Indians. Of particular importance, Miller provided evidence that the culturally divergent attributional tendencies develop gradually through socialization. Thus American and Indian adults were much more unlike each other in their mode of inference than were American and Indian children.

Morris and Peng (1994) also showed that causal inference differs across cultures. They took advantage of two parallel tragedies that had recently occurred in the United States. In one, a Chinese Ph.D. candidate at a Midwestern university, angry at what he regarded as ill treatment at the hands of his adviser, shot and killed the adviser and several bystanders. At about the same time, a postal worker in Detroit, angry at what he regarded as ill treatment by his superior, shot and killed the supervisor and several bystanders. Morris and Peng analyzed accounts of the two murders in English-language newspapers and in Chinese-language newspapers. Whereas the American accounts speculated almost wholly on the presumed mental instability and other negative dispositions of the two alleged murderers, the Chinese accounts speculated on situational, contextual, and even societal factors that might have been at work. Morris and Peng then showed that the same attributional patterns were obtained when Chinese and American university students were asked to explain the events. Chinese subjects were more likely to prefer contextual explanations, but Americans were more likely to prefer dispositional ones. These tendencies were demonstrated whether subjects were explaining the behavior of the American murderer or the Chinese murderer.

Correspondence Bias

The studies cited above suggest that there exists considerable cultural variation in the tendency to make dispositional attributions in person perception. Social psychologists have long known that this tendency is quite strong and pervasive in European American cultures. When people observe another person's behavior, they often immediately draw inferences about the person's internal attributes, such as attitudes, personality traits, or motives, that correspond to the observed behavior. Furthermore, this is the case even when there exists an obvious situational constraint or social inducement for the person to behave in that way. This bias in social information processing, which gives undue weight to personal factors in lieu of factors that surround him or her, has been called *the fundamental attribution error* (Ross, 1977) or *the correspondence bias* (Gilbert and Malone, 1995; Jones, 1979; see also Heider, 1958).

One experimental paradigm employed to demonstrate the correspondence bias involves an inference of a true attitude of someone who composed
an essay that states a pro or anti position on a social issue. In the original
demonstration of the correspondence bias, Jones and Harris (1967) had
American college students infer the true attitude of a hypothetical person who
allegedly wrote an essay that either supported or denounced Castro in Cuba.
In the free-choice condition, subjects had been informed that the target person wrote the essay by choosing for himself the stated position. Not surprisingly, in this condition the subjects ascribed to the target a strong attitude that
corresponded to the stated position. In the no-choice condition, the subjects
had been informed that the target person was assigned to one or the other
position by a coach of the debate team. Despite the fact that there was an
obvious social constraint on the target's behavior, the subjects still ascribed to
the target an attitude that corresponded to the stated position. Thus, the
subjects failed to take into full account the effect of social constraint.

Subsequent investigations in Eastern cultures have demonstrated similar
effects (see Choi et al., 1999; Fiske et al., 1998, for reviews). At first glance,
these initial findings are inconsistent with the notion that Asians are attuned
to situational or contextual information. However, some recent studies have
suggested one important caveat. Easterners, but not Westerners, are inclined
to refrain from dispositional attribution from a socially constrained behavior
as long as this latter information is made "salient enough."

Choi and Nisbett (1998) followed the procedure used by Snyder and
Jones (1974) in which subjects, before making judgments about the target's
attitude, were required to write an essay themselves and were allowed no
choice about which side to take. Furthermore, in one of the conditions they
were provided with a set of arguments to use in the essay. Subjects were
subsequently given an essay allegedly written by another person and told that
this target person also wrote the essay, just as they did. As in the Snyder and
Jones study, Choi and Nisbett found a robust correspondence bias in the
American sample. Korean subjects, in contrast, made much less extreme
inferences. In another attempt to increase the salience of the situational
constraint, Masuda and Kitayama (1999) used a modified version of the procedure devised by Gilbert and Jones (1986). Subjects chose one of two enve-
lopes that contained essays to be read by a target person. The target person
then read the essay in front of a video camera. Thus, it should have been very
obvious to the subjects that the target neither wrote nor chose the essay he
read. As in the Gilbert and Jones study, Masuda and Kitayama observed a
reliable correspondence bias even in these conditions for the American subjects. Yet for the Japanese, the correspondence bias entirely vanished. These
findings are consistent with the notion that Asian cultures cherish naive theories in which individuals are attuned to and sensitive to others or to situational constraints. These naive theories enable Asians to recognize the full

implications of information about social constraints so long as it is made cognitively accessible.

IMPLICATIONS FOR AGING RESEARCH

What effects will aging have on the performance of analytic versus holistic tasks? Will these effects differ across cultures? Given that many of the basic cognitive processes implicated in these tasks are almost always culturally saturated and, furthermore, that cultural knowledge and practices implicit in the pertinent cognitive skills and processes vary across cultures, the answers to these questions are most likely to be yes. Although the exact forms of such effects or cultural variation have yet to be empirically determined, some important predictions have been advanced by some leading aging researchers.

To begin with, Baltes and colleagues have distinguished between cognitive mechanics and cognitive pragmatics (Baltes, 1993). Cognitive mechanics are fluid cognitive capacities that reflect the biologically based "hardware" of the mind, whose function is strictly determined by biological potential. Baltes and colleagues assume that these capacities are indexed, for example, by psychometric intelligence tests designed to measure speed of information processing, working memory capacity, processing resources, and the like with materials that are relatively free of specific cultural content. Furthermore, the researchers reason that because the fluid mechanics of the mind depends mostly on the neurobiology of development, these capacities may be expected to increase up to a certain point, say, until early adulthood, and then gradually decline as a function of age. In contrast, cognitive pragmatics are relatively crystallized cognitive capacities that reflect the culturally learned "software" of the mind. They are based on "the bodies of knowledge and information that cultures provide in the form of factual and procedural knowledge about the world" (Baltes, 1997:373). The researchers assume that these crystallized capacities are indexed by a variety of culturally saturated skills and processes, including reading, writing, many forms of inference, decision making, behavioral regulation, planning, grasping the meaning of life, and so on. Evidence obtained by Baltes and colleagues has indicated that cognitive mechanics tend to decline steadily, but cognitive pragmatics are often well maintained in older age.

Although the distinction between the two forms of cognition is useful, there are some unresolved problems, and two issues should be pointed out. First, because the neurobiology of cognition is fairly invariant across cultural groups, performance in cognitive tasks designed to measure cognitive mechanics should be expected to be relatively invariant across cultures. In reality, however, pure measures of cognitive mechanics are hard to obtain. Even when a task seems culture-free at first glance, closer scrutiny may reveal otherwise. For example, a digit comparison task is quite simple, involving universal stimuli (i.e., pairs of digits), and thus may seem to be culture-free. However, arithmetic is emphasized more in some cultures than others in early socialization and, furthermore, digits are signified with varying ease in different languages. Hence, the task in fact may hardly be culture-free (see Hedden et al., 1999, cited in Park et al., 1999). If so, the same task may show a very different rate of cognitive decline in older age in different cultures. Second, Baltes and colleagues assume that performance of culturally saturated tasks is maintained fairly constantly throughout the life course. This, however, is not always the case. For example, consistent with the American processing bias that favors individual features rather than a whole scene, Park and colleagues found that performance in a feature-matching task is much better for American young adults than for their Chinese counterparts. Feature-matching is clearly culture-saturated. Yet performance declined considerably especially for Americans as a function of age. The processing advantage conferred on Americans by their cultural system dissipated as a function of age. It might then be suggested that the distinction between cognitive mechanics and pragmatics cannot be drawn too sharply. More often, any psychological function may emerge out of the actualization of innate potential through one's active participation in culture. If so, we may expect that in any basic cognitive functions, including inference, memory, and judgment, both the mechanics and the pragmatics of cognition are inseparably interwoven.

More recently, drawing on the large database amassed by Baltes and colleagues as well as U.S.-China comparison studies of their own, Park and colleagues have argued, consistent with the cultural psychology perspective presented earlier, that some tasks that have traditionally been viewed as culture-free in fact implicate culture in ways that are hitherto largely unexplored (Park et al., 1999). Furthermore, on the basis of the cross-cultural evidence that suggests a more analytic focus for Americans and a more holistic focus for Chinese, these researchers predicted superior performance in analytic tasks for Americans over Chinese and superior performance in holistic tasks for Chinese over Americans. Yet they also suggest that these cross-cultural differences can happen either because culture encourages a relatively *automatic* processing bias that is either analytic or holistic, or because culture encourages a relatively deliberate, *resource-demanding* strategy in processing that is either analytic or holistic. Furthermore, it may be supposed that, as one gets older, more cultural skills and operations are likely to be internalized and automatized, but fewer and fewer cognitive resources are left available. Accordingly, Park and colleagues hypothesize that cultural differences in relatively automatic cognitive operations (e.g., bias to spontaneously attend to figure versus context) should become more pronounced, but cultural differences in relatively deliberate cognitive operations (e.g., the relative ease of

Americans in feature-matching) should be attenuated as a function of age. Although evidence is still partial, a hypothesis like this will lead to a number of testable cross-cultural and developmental predictions.

CONCLUDING REMARKS

Biological aging occurs necessarily in a particular cultural context. Depending on the specific nature of the context, it can have quite divergent consequences. Imagine, for example, that aging is a series of failures to act, intelligence and rationality as an ability to quickly arrive at a solution to a well-defined problem, and well-being as an individual accomplishment. For many people in the contemporary West, these conceptions are natural in part because they fit so well with the implicit mode of thought. Alternatively, however, imagine that aging is a series of age-graded life tasks—preparations for death and therefore for rebirth; intelligence and rationality as holistic, encompassing, and wisdom-like; and well-being as a more collective product, shared and sustained by relation-ality rather than individuality. In Asian cultures, these conceptions are accompanied by a holistic mode of thought that confers considerable intuitive appeal on them. In both cases, cultural ideas about aging, rationality, and well-being are perceived to be real, which in turn may cause the reality of aging to change in accordance with the respective cultural world views.

Much more research is necessary in the future to examine issues surrounding aging from the wide-angle perspective engendered by cross-cultural considerations. The effects of aging on cognition must be examined in terms of more holistic, encompassing, relation-centered, and wisdom-like cognition as well as more analytic, object-focused, and individual-centered cognition. Furthermore, they must be studied as a function of cultural and social belief systems surrounding the notion of aging and related ones, such as rationality and well-being. Fortunately, theoretical frameworks that can produce testable predictions are beginning to emerge; the theories of Baltes, Park, and colleagues are notable examples.

Finally, further examinations of cognitive consequences of aging in a wide variety of cultures would entail much broader theoretical ramifications for the behavioral and social sciences in general. Indeed, this area offers a wonderful opportunity for investigating how cultural beliefs and practices and mental processes and structures make each other up, forming a particular psychocultural complex that has real consequences for the lives of all people in the culture. As noted earlier, it is the goal of cultural psychology to understand human psychology as part of such cultural complexes, and this perspective should be at the forefront of social and behavioral science research to attain a better and more comprehensive understanding of human psychology.

REFERENCES

Ambady, N., J. Koo, F. Lee, and R. Rosenthal
    1996   More than words: Linguistic and nonlinguistic politeness in two cultures. *Journal of Personality and Social Psychology* 70:996-1011.

Baddeley, A.
    1986   *Working Memory*. New York: Oxford University Press.

Baltes, P.B.
    1993   The aging mind: Potential and limits. *The Gerontologist* 33:580-594.
    1997   On the incomplete architecture of human ontology: Selection, optimization, and compensation as foundation of developmental theory. *American Psychologist* 52:366-380.

Baltes, P.B., and U.M. Staudinger
    1993   The search for a psychology of wisdom. *Current Directions in Psychological Science* 2:75-80.

Barnlund, D.C.
    1989   *Communicative Styles of Japanese and Americans: Images and Realities*. Belmont, CA: Wadsworth Publishing Company.

Borden, G.A.
    1991   *Cultural Orientation: An Approach to Understanding Intercultural Communication*. Englewood Cliffs, NJ: Prentice Hall.

Brown, D.E.
    1991   *Human Universals*. New York: McGraw Hill.

Brown, P., and S. Levinson
    1987   *Politeness: Some Universals in Language Usage*. Cambridge, England: Cambridge University Press.

Cantor, N.
    1994   Life task problem-solving: Situational affordances and personal needs. *Personality and Social Psychology Bulletin* 20:235-243.

Choi, I., and R.E. Nisbett
    1998   Situational salience and cultural differences in the correspondence bias and actor-observer bias. *Personality and Social Psychology Bulletin* 24:949-960.

Choi, I., R.E. Nisbett, and A. Norenzayan
    1999   Prediction and perception of causality across cultures. *Psychological Bulletin* 24:949-960.

Cole, M.
    1996   *Cultural Psychology*. Cambridge, MA: Harvard University Press.

Cutler, S., and A. Grams
    1988   Correlates of self-reported everyday memory problems. *Journal of Gerontology: Social Sciences* 43:582-590.

Durham, W.H.
    1991   *Coevolution: Genes, Cultures, and Human Diversity*. Stanford, CA: Stanford University Press.

Fiske, A.P., S. Kitayama, H.R. Markus, and R.E. Nisbett
    1998   The cultural matrix of social psychology. Pp. 915-981 in *Handbook of Social Psychology*, 4th ed., D.T. Gilbert, S. Fiske, and G. Lindzey, eds. New York: McGraw-Hill.

Geertz, C.
    1973   *The Interpretation of Culture: Selected Essays*. New York: Basic Books.

Gergen, K.J.
    1973   Social psychology as history. *Journal of Personality and Social Psychology* 26:309-320.

Gilbert, D.T., and E.E. Jones
    1986   Perceiver-induced constraint: Interactions of self-generated realities. *Journal of Personality and Social Psychology* 50:269-280.
Gilbert, D.T., and P.S. Malone
    1995   The correspondence bias. *Psychological Bulletin* 117:21-38.
Gould, S.J.
    1981   *The Mismeasure of Man.* New York: W.W. Norton and Company.
Greenfield, P.M.
    1997   Culture as process: Empirical methods for cultural psychology. Pp. 301-346 in *Handbook of Cross-Cultural Psychology*, 1st vol., J.W. Berry, Y.H. Poortinga, and J. Pandey, eds. Boston: Allyn and Bacon.
Hall, E.T.
    1976   *Beyond Culture.* New York: Doubleday.
Hedden, T., D.C. Park, R.E. Nisbett, L. Ji, Q. Jing, and S. Jaio
    1999   Cultural Invariant Tests of Neuropsychological Function across the Life Span. Unpublished manuscript. University of Michigan.
Heider, F.
    1958   *The Psychology of Interpersonal Relations.* New York: Wiley.
Heine, S.J., and D.R. Lehman
    1997   Culture, dissonance, and self-affirmation. *Personality and Social Psychology Bulletin* 23:389-400.
Ikegami, Y.
    1991   "DO-language" and "BECOME language": Two contrasting types of linguistic representation. Pp. 285-326 in *The Empire of Signs: Semiotic Essays on Japanese Culture*, Y. Ikegami, ed. Philadelphia, PA: John Benjamins Publishing Company.
Iyengar, S.S., and M.R. Lepper
    1999   Rethinking the value of choice: A cultural perspective on intrinsic motivation. *Journal of Personality and Social Psychology* 76:349-366.
Jones, E.E.
    1979   The rocky road from act to disposition. *American Psychologist* 34:107-117.
Jones, E.E., and V.A. Harris
    1967   The attribution of attitudes. *Journal of Experimental Social Psychology* 3:1-24.
Kashima, E.S., and Y. Kashima
    1998   Culture and language: The case of cultural dimensions and personal pronoun use. *Journal of Cross-Cultural Psychology* 29:461-486.
Kitayama, S., and K. Ishii
    1999   Word and Voice: Spontaneous Attention to Emotional Speech in Two Cultures. Unpublished manuscript. Kyoto University.
Kitayama, S., H.R. Markus, H. Matsumoto, and V. Norasakkunkit
    1997   Individual and collective processes of self-esteem management: Self-enhancement in the United States and self-depreciation in Japan. *Journal of Personality and Social Psychology* 72:1245-1267.
Lindenberger, U., and P.B. Baltes
    1994   Sensory functioning and intelligence in old age: A strong connection. *Psychology and Aging* 9:339-355.
Lutz, C.
    1988   *Unnatural Emotions: Everyday Sentiments on a Micronesian Atoll and Their Challenges to Western Theory.* Chicago: University of Chicago Press.
Markus, H.R., and S. Kitayama
    1991   Culture and the self: Implications for cognition, emotion, and motivation. *Psychological Review* 98:224-253.

Markus, H.R., S. Kitayama, and R.J. Heiman
    1996   Culture and "basic" psychological principles. Pp. 857-913 in *Social Psychology: Handbook of Basic Principles*, E.T. Higgins and A.W. Kruglanski, eds. New York: Guilford.
Masuda, T., and S. Kitayama
    1999   Culture and Correspondence Bias. Unpublished manuscript. University of Michigan.
Masuda, T., and R.E. Nisbett
    1999   Culture and Attention. Unpublished manuscript. University of Michigan.
Menon, T., M.W. Morris, C. Chiu, and Y. Hong
    1999   Culture and construal of agency: Attribution to individual versus dispositions. *Journal of Personality and Social Psychology* 76:701-717.
Menon, U., and R.A. Shweder
    1998   The return of the "white man's burden": The moral discourse of anthropology and the domestic life of Hindu women. Pp. 139-188 in *Welcome to Middle Age! (and Other Cultural Fictions)*, R.A. Shweder, ed. Chicago: University of Chicago Press.
Miller, J.G.
    1984   Culture and the development of everyday social explanation. *Journal of Personality and Social Psychology* 46:961-978.
    1994   Cultural psychology: Bridging disciplinary boundaries in understanding the cultural grounding of self. Pp. 139-170 in *Handbook of Psychological Anthropology*, P.K. Bock, ed. Westport, CT: Greenwood Publishing Group.
Morris, M.W., and K. Peng
    1994   Culture and cause: American and Chinese attributions for social and physical events. *Journal of Personality and Social Psychology* 67:949-971.
Park, D.C., R.E. Nisbett, and T. Hedden
    1999   Aging, culture, and cognition. *Journal of Gerontology: Psychological Sciences* 54B:75-84.
Peng, K., and R.E. Nisbett
    1999   Culture, dialectics, and reasoning about contradiction. *American Psychologist* 54:741-754.
Plath, D.W.
    1980   *Long Engagements, Maturity in Modern Japan*. Stanford, CA: Stanford University Press.
Ross, L.
    1977   The intuitive psychologist and his shortcomings: Distortions in the attribution process. Pp. 174-220 in *Advances in Experimental Social Psychology*, 10th vol., L. Berkowitz, ed. New York: Academic Press.
Ross, L., and R.E. Nisbett
    1991   *The Person and the Situation: Perspectives of Social Psychology*. New York: McGraw Hill.
Ryan, E.B.
    1992   Beliefs about memory across the life span. *Journal of Gerontology: Psychological Sciences* 47:41-47.
Sampson, E.E.
    1977   Psychology and the American ideal. *Journal of Personality and Social Psychology* 35:767-782.
    1988   The debate on individualism: Indigenous psychologies of the individual and their role in personal and societal functioning. *American Psychologist* 43:15-22.
Schaie, K.W.
    1994   The course of adult intellectual development. *American Psychologist* 49:304-319.

Seymour, S.C.
  1999 *Women, Family, and Child Care in India: A World in Transition*. Cambridge, England: Cambridge University Press.
Shweder, R.A.
  1991 *Cultural Psychology: Thinking Through Cultures*. Cambridge, MA: Harvard University Press.
Shweder, R.A., ed.
  1998 *Welcome to Middle Age! (and Other Cultural Fictions)*. Chicago: University of Chicago Press.
Shweder, R.A., and E.J. Bourne
  1984 Does the concept of person vary cross-culturally? Pp. 158-199 in *Culture Theory: Essays on Mind, Self, and Emotion*, R.A. Shweder and R.A. LeVine, eds. New York: Cambridge University Press.
Shweder, R.A., and M. Sullivan
  1993 Cultural psychology: Who needs it? *Annual Review of Psychology* 44:497-523.
Snyder, M., and E.E. Jones
  1974 Attitude attribution when behavior is constrained. *Journal of Experimental Social Psychology* 105:585-600.
Solomon, S., J. Greenberg, and T. Pyszczynski
  1991 A terror management theory of social behavior: The psychological functions of self-esteem and cultural worldviews. Pp. 93-159 in *Advances in Experimental Social Psychology*, 24th vol., L. Berkowitz, ed. San Diego, CA: Academic Press.
Sternberg, R.J.
  1985 *Beyond IQ: A Triarchic Theory of Human Intelligence*. Cambridge, MA: Cambridge University Press.
Tardif, T.
  1996 Nouns are not always learned before verbs: Evidence from Mandarin-speakers' early vocabularies. *Developmental Psychology* 32:492-504.
Taylor, S.E., and J.D. Brown
  1988 Illusion and well-being: A social psychological perspective on mental health. *Psychological Bulletin* 103:193-210.
Triandis, H.C.
  1989 The self and social behavior in differing cultural contexts. *Psychological Review* 96:506-520.
  1995 *Individualism and Collectivism*. Boulder, CO: Westview Press.

G
Functional Magnetic Resonance Imaging of the Brain in Nonhuman Primates: A Prospectus for Research on Aging

Thomas D. Albright

WHAT IS FUNCTIONAL MAGNETIC RESONANCE IMAGING?

In general terms, the goal of functional brain imaging is to obtain a spatially and temporally localized measure of neuronal activity through noninvasive means. By relating such activity patterns to behavioral measures of sensory, perceptual, cognitive, or motor events, it becomes possible to identify the neuronal structures and events that underlie these processes. Notwithstanding the fact that the brain lies within a closed cavity, the last 50 years have seen the development of a variety of noninvasive techniques for assessing brain activity (e.g., electroencephalography, magnetoencephalography, positron emission tomography). All have severe limitations, owing to the indirectness of the measurements.

An ingenious new technique, known as functional magnetic resonance imaging (fMRI), has emerged as the best and most promising tool for this purpose. This technique exploits variations in magnetic susceptibility that arise from molecular binding of oxygen to hemoglobin, which can be used to detect blood flow changes associated with neuronal activity. These neuronal activity-related signals can be isolated with a spatial resolution (1-2 mm) approaching columnar structure in the neocortex, and temporal resolution compatible with most perceptual and cognitive operations. In other words, fMRI is an extraordinary new window through which one can probe the neural machinery of cognition.

To date, the three principal research areas of fMRI application have been sensory (primarily visual) processing, memory, and language, all of which depend on brain systems that are at risk for varying rates of change with aging. In the field of sensory processing, a major development has been the identification of a hierarchy of functionally specific visual processing areas in the human brain (Sereno et al., 1995), which may be homologues of areas that have been studied extensively at the cellular level in nonhuman primates. Not only does this knowledge provide a solid foundation for the interpretation of a large body of existing neuropsychological data on human brain function (with concomitant clinical relevance), but it sets the stage for the first direct and in-depth comparisons between human and nonhuman primate data. In the field of memory, several recent studies have identified brain regions that are active while volunteers hold specific types of information in short-term memory (e.g., Smith and Jonides, 1998) Other studies have demonstrated changes in the nature of the fMRI response—expansion of the zone of activation, for example—associated with the learning of new sensorimotor tasks (e.g., Karni et al., 1998). These observations provide direct evidence for selective plasticity of neuronal structures as a substrate for learning. Finally, language has become a special focus of fMRI investigation, as it addresses issues that are difficult if not impossible to approach using animal models. Several studies have explored the functional modularity of language processing areas by these means (e.g., Posner and Pavese, 1998).

WHAT IS THE RELEVANCE OF fMRI TO UNDERSTANDING THE AGING BRAIN?

Inasmuch as an understanding of the relationship between the aging process and the brain must be built on a general understanding of brain organization and function, all of the functional imaging applications cited above are of relevance to aging research. In addition, there are specific areas of research in which functional imaging can make a unique contribution. Perhaps the most obvious of these is the use of imaging technology to compare brain organization and function across different age groups, as a complement to psychological and neurological characterization of normal and pathological states. Indeed, this is an area of tremendous potential owing to the unprecedented ability offered by fMRI to identify specific brain abnormalities associated with age-related sensory, motor, memory, and language dysfunction.

LIMITATIONS OF fMRI FOR STUDIES OF THE HUMAN BRAIN

The reasons for the rapid development of fMRI techniques and their application in studies of human brain function are obvious. In spite of the many realized and potential gains, however, and the fact that fMRI stands to significantly advance research on aging of the brain, there are some notable limitations to this approach when it is applied strictly to humans. These limitations exist because practical and ethical considerations preclude using fMRI in conjunction with other powerful techniques that have been developed for use in studies of nonhuman species. Two of the most salient examples illustrate the point.

First, manipulation of the genome (i.e., creation of transgenic animals) and subsequent controlled expression of specific genes are becoming extremely valuable tools for assessing the functional contributions of specific cells, subcellular components and signaling pathways (see Picciotto, 1999, for a review). Methods of this type are now applied routinely using germ-line transgenic manipulations in mice, and their enormous relevance to research on the aging brain is only hinted at by recent highly publicized demonstrations that gene-induced alterations of neurotransmitter receptor concentrations has a marked influence on learning and memory (e.g., Mayford et al., 1996; Tang et al., 1999). To completely understand the underlying mechanisms and implications of such findings, brains that have been functionally altered will be probed using many standard anatomical and physiological techniques. To that list of techniques we can now add fMRI, which can be applied to rodents with very high spatial resolution, and which offers a view of global changes in brain organization and function that result from genetic manipulations.

In the near future it will also be possible to extend this genetic approach to other species, including nonhuman primates, by exploiting the capacity of genetically engineered viruses to introduce novel genes into the brains of adult animals. Moreover, this pairing of techniques from molecular biology and functional imaging will provide a powerful means to investigate both the contributions of specific cells or cellular components to age-related changes in brain function and to evaluate genetic intervention as a means to influence the course of such changes. None of this research can be performed using humans as subjects.

A second realm in which great potential exists for using fMRI in conjunction with other methods is single- and multiunit electrophysiology in nonhuman primates. The technology for this type of physiology, which is often profitably coupled with behavioral analysis, has evolved over the past 40 years to become a preeminent experimental approach in the field of cognitive neuroscience (e.g., Hubel, 1988). Its applications in the field of aging research are few to date, but when combined with fMRI in nonhuman primates, this approach promises to tie functional imaging data on age-related changes in the brain to a firm foundation of cellular physiology. The next section focuses specifically on this potential, considering the likely gains from it and how it can be realized.

fMRI IN NONHUMAN PRIMATES: WHAT DO WE HAVE TO GAIN?

Ironically, it is the evident value of fMRI for human studies that occasionally prompts concerns about its utility in nonhuman primates. Monkeys, after all, have long been subject to fine-grained analyses of structure and function using other techniques that are unsuitable for work with humans. It would thus appear that monkey fMRI both fails to exploit the considerable advantages associated with the use of human subjects and lacks the power of existing techniques appropriate for monkeys. These concerns overlook, however, the enormous potential associated with *combined application* of fMRI and more traditional techniques *in the same animal*, which can be accomplished only with nonhuman primates. This next section begins by outlining the benefits to neuroscience generally of combining these approaches. It is followed by specific illustrations of what can be gained by studying the aging brain.

The focus of this discussion is on rhesus monkeys (*Macaca mulatta*) and other macaque species as animal models for aging studies, largely because (1) they have been the most well-studied nonhuman primates in the field of neuroscience, (2) there is extensively documented evidence of their similarity to humans with respect to a wide variety of sensory, perceptual, and cognitive functions, and (3) they are particularly amenable to the sorts of experimental manipulations commonly used for studies of the brain bases of cognitive decline with aging. Nonetheless, there may be specific advantages associated with the use of other nonhuman primates, including some great apes and prosimians. For example, the rhesus monkey life span (in captivity) is 25-30 years, which makes life-span studies prohibitive. The mouse lemur (*Microcebus murinus*), in contrast, is a potentially attractive subject for study because of its small size, rapid aging, and ease of breeding. Such benefits must, of course, be weighed against the fact that there are far fewer details known of brain anatomy and physiology in these species in comparison with macaques, but a case can sometimes be made for their use in studies of the aging brain and, hence, for fMRI studies of aging in nonhuman primates.

General Benefits for Neuroscience

As indicated above, fMRI has already begun to demonstrate its worth for understanding the neuronal substrates of sensory, motor, and cognitive function. Such an understanding is of obvious relevance to aging research, even if age-related changes are not the primary subject matter. Likewise, much of what we expect to learn from the merger of fMRI with other neurobiological techniques in nonhuman primates has general relevance to neuroscience, which is addressed here. Specific application of this general knowledge to aging research, and a consideration of new paradigms for aging research afforded by these research tools, follows in a later section.

Evaluation of Cellular Events That Underlie the Vascular Signals of fMRI

The fMRI technique enables quantification of local changes in cerebral blood flow. The use of these measures as an index of neuronal function is predicated on the assumption that there is a specific relationship between neuronal activity and the magnitude of the hemodynamic response. While that assumption is a reasonable first-order approximation, the broad nature and potential import of claims resulting from human fMRI studies demand that the relationship between fMRI signal change and neuronal response be investigated thoroughly. Studies using fMRI in nonhuman primates will make this possible.

A primary goal of such studies will be to characterize directly the relationship between the magnitude and temporal dynamics of the magnetic resonance (MR) response (e.g., to a sensory, perceptual, cognitive, or motor event) and the corresponding properties of a neuronal response (i.e., a change in the frequency of action potentials). In practice, this can be accomplished by recording both MR and neuronal responses under conditions that are identical and computing the correlation between the observed responses. If the correlation is significant and largely invariant over a range of conditions in nonhuman primates, it should be possible to draw quantitative conclusions about the nature of the neuronal response elicited in humans when only the MR signal is available.

The possibility also exists that the relationship between the vascular MR signal and neuronal activity varies in a context-specific manner—over time (in a circadian and/or age-related manner), cognitive demands, and/or attentional, motivational, or motor state. To the extent that this is true, correlational measures of the MR/neuronal relationship are valid predictors only if they have been assessed in the same context in which a prediction is to be made. In principle, knowledge of context-specific correlations will enable one to compute a normalized index of neuronal function across different contexts.

Linking Human Neuropsychology to Fine-Grained Measures of Neuronal Function

Historically, studies of brain function in humans have focused on the behavioral or cognitive effects of focal brain lesions in clinical populations, while animal studies using electrophysiological techniques have enabled fine-grained investigation of the cellular substrates of sensory, perceptual, cognitive, or motor events. fMRI will allow an unprecedented comparison of functional activity patterns in monkeys and humans engaged in identical tasks, which will, in turn, permit identification of functional homologies and the ability to directly relate the vast literature on cellular response properties in monkeys to the field of human neuropsychology.

Use of fMRI as an Adjunct to Traditional Methods Used in Nonhuman Primates

There remains much to be gained from the application in nonhuman primates of traditional experimental techniques, such as single-cell electrophysiology, anatomical tract tracing, and behavioral analyses of the effects of focal brain lesions. fMRI offers a valuable means to guide such experiments. For example, cortical regions that are active under specific perceptual conditions can be rapidly identified, and that information can then be used to guide the positioning of single-cell microelectrodes for more in-depth analyses. Similarly, fMRI can be used to identify functionally specific zones for injection of anatomical tracers or placement of focal lesions.

Specific Benefits for Research on the Aging Brain

General knowledge of brain organization and function is obviously needed to understand the aging brain, and fMRI is a valuable method to obtain that knowledge. Moreover, as we have seen, the joint application in nonhuman primates of fMRI and traditional research methods offers a means to accurately interpret human fMRI data on the aging brain, and to link a vast human neuropsychological literature on aging to cellular structures and events. In addition, there are questions specifically directed at aging phenomena that can be profitably addressed only by using fMRI in nonhuman primates. Generally speaking, the richness of this approach for aging research is found in the fact that it offers a means to *interpret* the cellular substrates of fMRI signals seen at different points in an animal's lifetime and, furthermore, to *manipulate* substrates identified by these means and evaluate the consequences of doing so for cognitive function.

Do fMRI Signals Change as a Function of Age?

fMRI signals reflect blood flow. Any attempt to assess neuronal function across different age groups using MR signals as a dependent measure is likely to be confounded by the fact that brain tissue undergoes significant age-related changes in vascularization (both vascular patterning and responsiveness), tissue volume, shifts in receptor subpopulations and signaling, among many other phenomena of tissue remodeling. In other words, because of such changes, the correlation between MR signal and neuronal activity may change as a function of age. A potential consequence of this confound is the possibility that an MR signal seen in a 20-year-old human may have an altogether different neuronal origin than the same signal in a 60-year-old, which—if unrecognized—could have profound implications for research and clinical diagnosis. fMRI in nonhuman primates offers a means to eliminate this confound. Specifically, by evaluating the correlation between the MR signal and neuronal response (outlined above) as a function of age, it should be possible to establish "normalization factors" that can be used to appropriately compare MR signals across different age groups.

In addition to their use for data normalization, any observed age-related changes in the MR-neuronal response correlation may be of interest in their own right. Such changes may be indicative of a decline in the metabolic requirements of specific cell groups and could perhaps be diagnostic of early age-related loss of function. Data informative of the correlation between MR signal and the activity of specific cell populations can be obtained only in nonhuman species.

Use of fMRI Signals to Guide and Evaluate Manipulation/Intervention Studies

Because fMRI reflects neuronal activity with good spatial and temporal precision, it promises to be a valuable tool for the identification and characterization of age-related loss of function and specific brain pathologies. Once age-related neuronal changes are detected, experiments can be designed to address hypotheses about their origins or to evaluate intervention intended to promote recovery—in each case using the characterized MR signal as a dependent measure. For example, one might use the MR signal as a means to evaluate the effects of estrogen administration on the activity of specific cell groups as a function of age. Perhaps the most exciting and promising prospect in this domain is the use of genetic manipulations (i.e., creation of transgenic animals and selective expression of novel genes in targeted cell populations) to alter cell signaling, metabolism, or firing rate in a precisely targeted manner, with the goal of promoting recovery from selective age-related loss of function. As indicated above, genetic manipulations of this type will soon be possible in nonhuman primates using genetically engineered viruses for introduction of novel genes. As a dependent measure, the MR signal can provide a repeated and highly localized assessment of the effects of such manipulations on brain function. Perhaps one day successful interventions can be employed in humans. At the present time, nonhuman primates provide an ideal model for studies of this type.

fMRI IN NONHUMAN PRIMATES: OVERCOMING METHODOLOGICAL CHALLENGES

What Are the Challenges and How Can They Be Approached?

There are a number of significant technical challenges involved in carrying out fMRI experiments in monkeys. While apparatus and procedures for behavioral control, and for immobilization of animals in a confined space, have been well developed for single-cell electrophysiological experiments and can be adapted for use in fMRI, there are some novel components that must be introduced to satisfy the constraints of the magnet environment. Solutions to many of these problems have been attained and are described thoroughly in published reports of initial studies (Stefanacci et al., 1998; Logothetis et al., 1999). These technical problems and solutions are summarized briefly here.

To begin with, most conventional fMRI facilities use a horizontal bore magnet. The methods that have been refined over the years for single-cell electrophysiology in alert monkeys involve restraining the animal in a natural "sitting" position, in which the vertebral column is vertically oriented. Monkeys are particularly receptive to behavioral conditioning under these conditions, and the vertical body orientation (compared to a horizontal, or "crouching" posture) frees the hands for use in making behavioral responses. A vertical bore magnet is thus preferred for use with nonhuman primates, particularly if the same animals are to be trained for use in single-cell electrophysiological experiments. Vertical bore magnets are now commercially available, but they are costly and highly specialized. A less satisfactory solution involves restraining (through a combination of behavioral conditioning and apparatus) the alert animal in a horizontal position to accommodate the bore of the magnet. Stefanacci et al. (1998) have demonstrated that this is a feasible, though suboptimal, alternative.

A second challenge arises from the fact that the magnet itself is a significant source of audible noise. Such noise poses two problems. First, to exploit the potential of fMRI in nonhuman primates, the experimenter must extract a measure of the subject's sensory, perceptual, or cognitive state, which can only be accomplished via some sort of behavioral response. Audible magnet noise is distracting and/or annoying to such a degree that it can interfere with expected cognitive events and the performance of animals on complex behavioral tasks. Second, unattenuated audible noise may preclude any clean investigation of auditory processing by the brain. These problems may be overcome using a combination of habituation to the magnet environment and noise attenuation devices. Recent studies have demonstrated the potential effectiveness of these solutions (Stefanacci et al., 1998; Logothetis et al., 1999).

Third, the magnet environment demands that the apparatus for restraining the subject must be made from nonferrous materials that do not interfere with fMRI signal acquisition. To meet this demand, Stefanacci et al. (1998) designed and constructed a specialized restraint device constructed entirely of plastic parts (e.g., nylon screws), which successfully avoided distortion of the magnetic field.

Finally, owing to both space limitations and magnetic interference, specialized devices must be designed for sensory stimulation and measurement of behavioral responses. Problems of this variety are similar to problems faced in human fMRI, but there are a number of unique constraints associated with the size and behavioral repertoire of monkeys. Initial studies have begun to offer workable solutions to these problems (Stefanacci et al., 1998; Logothetis et al., 1999).

Initial Evidence of Feasibility and Validation

fMRI research with nonhuman primates (rhesus monkeys) has thus far focused solely on development and validation of the technology. The initial target of investigation has been the visual cortex. Research progress is described thoroughly in published reports of initial studies (Stefanacci et al., 1998; Logothetis et al., 1999). Highlights of that progress are briefly summarized here.

Signal Acquisition and Identification of a Specific Locus of fMRI Response

This first step in validating the fMRI technique with nonhuman primates was recently accomplished independently by two groups (Stefanacci et al., 1998; Dubowitz et al., 1998). The MR signal was measured in the visual cortex in response to a stimulus known to elicit robust responses from individual cortical neurons. The MR measurements were low resolution and intentionally nonspecific, but cortical MR signals were robust and confined to regions known to exhibit significant neuronal responses to the stimuli presented. The observed correlation, though not precisely quantified, appeared quite high.

Spatial Precision of the fMRI Response

The second step in the validation process, which was recently undertaken by two additional research groups (Vanduffel et al., 1998; Logothetis et al., 1999), involved establishing the correlation between *specific spatial patterns* of MR and neuronal signal activation in the visual cortex. This step exploited the known topographic mapping of the visual field onto the cerebral cortex:

the spatial topographic pattern of neuronal activity known to be elicited by a given visual stimulus was directly correlated with the topographic pattern of MR activation elicited by the same stimulus. Initial results suggest that the degree of correlation is quite high.

WHERE DO WE GO FROM HERE?

The future of this approach to understanding brain function rests on: (1) continued validation of the methodology, (2) identification of the limits of the approach, and (3) application of the methodology to important and feasible scientific goals, including understanding the aging process.

Continued Validation of the Methodology

Having established that the correlation between the fMRI signal and neuronal activity is both modality and spatially selective, the third step in the validation process will involve measurements of the magnitude and time course of both MR and neuronal signals as a function of some stimulus dimension, such as contrast. (A similar approach has been used successfully to identify the relationship between neuronal and intrinsic optical signals recorded from visual cortex—Everson et al., 1998.) The observed correlation in nonhuman primates will provide a means to predict the magnitude and time course of the neuronal response in humans, given only the MR signal.

What Are the Limitations of fMRI for Use in Nonhuman Primates?

The maximal spatial resolution of fMRI obtainable with magnetic field strengths suitable for use with humans and nonhuman primates has improved by a factor of ~5 over the last decade, from around 1 cm in 1990 to around 2 mm today. Foreseeable changes in technology will improve this to approximately 0.5 mm over the next decade (Chen and Ugurbil, 1999), which is on the scale of functional columns in the sensory cortex. Despite these welcome advances, fMRI will never *replace* cellular electrophysiology as a means to investigate the neural foundations of cognitive function—there are physical upper bounds on the spatial and temporal resolution that can be achieved. However, as summarized above, fMRI is an extremely valuable complement to more conventional cellular studies of neuronal activation and patterns of connectivity. Indeed, it is primarily because fMRI in nonhuman primates lends itself (unlike human fMRI) to such combined use of techniques that it is an approach with enormous potential.

Scientific Applications

The preceding sections have reviewed specific types of scientific applications. The next section speculates briefly about what these applications are likely to reveal.

General Benefits for Neuroscience

The promise of monkey fMRI is considerable, but research efforts to date have achieved nothing more than validation of specific aspects of the technology. The next few years should see use of this technology—in conjunction with traditional electrophysiological, anatomical, and behavioral analyses—to topics ranging from the nature of sensory representations in the cerebral cortex and the neuronal mechanisms for plasticity of those representations, to mechanisms of memory storage and retrieval, to the cellular substrates of decision making, motor control, and even consciousness. Because this methodology provides a "global" view of brain events associated with cognition, it is likely to lead to many new discoveries regarding the interactions between major brain systems, such as those responsible for vision and memory, and the manner in which different sources of information (sensory, mnemonic, etc.) are integrated to yield coherent perceptual experience and behavior. This knowledge is a foundation on which a better understanding of age-related cognitive changes can be built.

Specific Benefits for Research on the Aging Brain

As indicated above, one can identify two general types of scientific applications of fMRI in nonhuman primates that are of relevance for an understanding of the aging brain and cognition: (1) collection of data that will serve as a basis for normalization of the MR signal across different age groups and (2) use of fMRI as a dependent measure for evaluation of the effects of specific manipulations of brain neurochemistry, organization, or function. The likely outcome of the first of these applications is straightforward (although the data may be complex in detail), and it will be invaluable for MR signal interpretation as an adjunct to cognitive studies of aging.

The concrete potential of the second type of scientific application is obviously dependent on specific hypotheses about the origins of age-related cognitive decline and the prospects for intervention. Nonetheless, the point can be illustrated briefly by a fantasy experiment that is not too far removed from reality. Consider, for example, the hypothesis that one aspect of age-related cognitive decline is linked to down-regulation of a specific subtype of postsynaptic neurotransmitter receptor in a specific brain region. fMRI data obtained from aged nonhuman primates confirms that the activity level in that brain region, in association with a specific cognitive task, is lower than what is observed in younger animals. An intervention study is planned, whereby a genetically engineered virus is packaged with recombinant DNA that codes for the expression of the down-regulated receptor, along with genes that will enable temporal control of expression and spatial restriction of expression to the specific cells in question. The virus is injected into the relevant brain region, whereupon it infects cells and results in the transgenes being inserted into the host DNA. Gene expression is subsequently activated to produce the receptor protein, which is thus up-regulated to levels present in younger animals. At this point, one needs an assay of neuronal activity to determine whether the manipulation has had the desired functional effect. fMRI provides such a dependent measure, which can be compared with the preintervention state. Moreover, when obtained in conjunction with a behavioral index of cognitive function, the MR signal can be used as a basis for identifying the neuronal substrates of any cognitive gain. An intervention approach of this sort will soon be possible using new molecular genetic tools, and will clearly have broad applicability in conjunction with fMRI.

In sum, the great richness of fMRI in nonhuman primates—for aging research and for neuroscience generally—lies in the fact that the method can be applied in conjunction with many other techniques that cannot be used for research on human subjects. The "whole" that we stand to gain from such conjunctions is surely far greater than what can be learned from each technique on its own.

REFERENCES

Chen, W., and K. Ugurbil
  1999 High spatial resolution functional magnetic resonance imaging at very-high magnetic field. *Topics in Magnetic Resonance Imaging* 10:63-78.
Dubowitz, D.J., D.Y. Chen, D.J. Atkinson, K.L. Grieve, B. Gillikin, W.G. Bradley, Jr., and R.A. Andersen
  1998 Functional magnetic resonance imaging in macaque cortex. *Neuroreport* 9:2213-2218.
Everson, R.M., A.K. Prashanth, M. Gabbay, B.W. Knight, L. Sirovich, and E. Kaplan
  1998 Representation of spatial frequency and orientation in the visual cortex. *Proceedings of the National Academy of Sciences of the United States of America* 95(14): 8334-8338.
Hubel, D.H.
  1988 *Eye, Brain and Vision.* New York: Scientific American Library, W.H. Freeman.
Karni, A., G. Meyer, C. Rey-Hipolito, P. Jezzard, P., M.M. Adams, R. Turner, and L.G. Ungerleider
  1998 The acquisition of skilled motor performance: fast and slow experience-driven changes in primary motor cortex. *Proceedings of the National Academy of Sciences of the United States of America* 95:861-868.
Logothetis, N.K., H. Guggenberger, S. Peled, and J. Pauls
  1999 Functional imaging of the monkey brain. *Nature Neuroscience* 2(6):555-562.

Mayford, M., M.E. Bach, Y.Y. Huang, L. Wang, R.D. Hawkins, and E.R. Kandel
    1996   Control of memory formation through regulated expression of a CaMKII transgene.
            Science 6:1678-1683.

Picciotto, M.R.
    1999   Knock-out mouse models used to study neurobiological systems. *Critical Reviews in
            Neurobiology* 13(2):103-149.

Posner, M.I., and A. Pavese
    1998   Anatomy of word and sentence meaning. *Proceedings of the National Academy of
            Sciences* 95:899-905.

Sereno, M.I., A.M. Dale, J.B. Reppas, K.K. Kwong, J.W. Belliveau, T.J. Brady, B.R. Rosen, and
R.B. Tootell
    1995   Borders of multiple visual areas in humans revealed by functional magnetic reso-
            nance imaging. *Science* 268:889-893.

Smith, E.E., and J. Jonides
    1998   Neuroimaging analyses of human working memory. *Proceedings of the National
            Academy of Sciences* 95:12061-12068.

Stefanacci, L., P. Reber, J. Costanza, E. Wong, R. Buxton, S. Zola, L. Squire, and T. Albright
    1998   fMRI of monkey visual cortex. *Neuron* 20:1051-1057.

Tang, Y.P., E. Shimizu, G.R. Dube, C. Rampon, G.A. Kerchner, M. Zhuo, G. Liu, and J.Z. Tsien
    1999   Genetic enhancement of learning and memory in mice. *Nature* 401:63-69.

Vanduffel, W., E. Beatse, S. Sunaert, P. Van Hecke, R.B.H. Tootell, and G.A. Orban
    1998   Functional magnetic resonance imaging in an awake rhesus monkey. *Society for
            Neuroscience Abstracts* 24:11.

H

Biographical Sketches

COMMITTEE AND STAFF MEMBERS

LAURA L. CARSTENSEN (*Chair*), is professor and vice chair of the Department of Psychology at Stanford University and also the Barbara D. Finberg director of its Institute for Research on Women and Gender. Her research focuses on life-span development, gender, and emotion. She is a fellow of the American Psychological Association, the Gerontological Society of America, and the American Psychological Society. In 1994, she was president of the Society for a Science of Clinical Psychology and, in 1996, served as chair of the behavioral sciences section of the Gerontological Society of America. She has received the Richard Kalish award for innovative research and the Stanford University Dean's award for distinguished teaching. She has a Ph.D. in clinical psychology from West Virginia University.

PAUL B. BALTES is a senior fellow (Mitglied) of the Max Planck Society for the Advancement of Sciences and director of the Center for Lifespan Psychology of the Max Planck Institute for Human Development in Berlin, Germany. His current research interests include theories and models of human development, interdisciplinary perspectives on gerontology, cognitive aging, and the psychology of wisdom. He is a member of numerous scholarly organizations, including Academia Europaea, the Berlin-Brandenburg Academy of Sciences, the Gerontological Society of America, the International Society for the Study of Behavioral Development, and the Society for Research in Child Development. His numerous awards include the International Psychology Award of the American Psychological Association, the Aristotle Prize of the European Federation of Psychological Associations, the Novartis Prize for Gerontological Research of the International Association of Gerontology, the Robert W. Kleemeier award in recognition of outstanding research in the field of gerontology of the Gerontological Society of America, and honorary doctorates from the University of Jyvasksla, Finland, and the University of Stockholm, Sweden. He has a Ph.D. in psychology from the University of Saarland, Germany.

DEBORAH M. BURKE is the W. M. Keck distinguished service professor and professor of psychology at Pomona College. Her research investigates aging and cognitive functioning, especially in memory and language, focusing on mechanisms responsible for maintained and impaired language performance in old age. She has written extensively on word retrieval, tip-of-the-tongue experiences, and aging. She received a MERIT award from the National Institute on Aging and several Wig distinguished teaching awards from Pomona College. She currently serves on the editorial board of *Psychology and Aging* and *Cognition and Consciousness*. She has served on the National Science Foundation Graduate Panel on Psychology of the National Research Council and is currently on the Integrative, Functional, and Cognitive Neuroscience study section at the National Institutes of Health. She has a Ph.D. in developmental psychology from Columbia University.

CALEB E. FINCH is director of the Alzheimer Disease Research Center (NIA) and the Kieschnick professor in the neurobiology of aging at the University of Southern California. His major research interest is inflammatory mechanisms in aging. He is the author of two major books on the biology of aging: *Longevity, Senescence, and the Genome* (1990) and *Chance, Development, and Aging* (1999). He chaired the National Research Council's Workshop on Bioindicators of Aging (1999). He received the Robert W. Kleemeier award in 1985 and the Sandoz premier prize in 1995. He participates on 10 editorial and national scientific advisory boards and is a fellow of the American Association for the Advancement of Science and the Gerontological Society of America. He has a Ph.D. in cell biology from Rockefeller University.

REID HASTIE is professor of psychology and director of the Center for Research on Judgment and Policy at the University of Colorado. He taught at Harvard and Northwestern Universities before moving to his present position. His primary research interests are in the areas of judgment and decision making (legal, managerial, medical, engineering, and personal), memory and cognition, and social psychology. He is best known for his research on legal decision making and on social memory and judgment processes. He is currently studying the role of explanations in category concept representations (including the effects on category classification, deductive, and inductive inferences), civil jury decision making, the role of frequency information in probability judgments, and the psychology of reading statistical graphs and maps. He has served on review panels for the National Science Foundation, the Office of Naval Research, and the National Institute of Mental Health, as well as 12 editorial boards for professional journals. He has a Ph.D. in psychology from Yale University.

RICHARD J. JAGACINSKI is professor in the Department of Psychology and the Department of Industrial, Welding, and Systems Engineering of Ohio State University. He is a fellow in the Division of Applied Experimental and Engineering Psychologists of the American Psychological Association and of the American Psychological Society. He is an associate editor of the journal *Human Factors* and serves on the editorial board of the *Journal of Motor Behavior*. He currently serves on the National Research Council's Committee on Human Factors. He has a Ph.D. in engineering psychology from the University of Michigan.

HAZEL ROSE MARKUS is the Davis-Brack professor in the behavioral sciences at Stanford University and has been a professor of psychology at that university since 1994. She is also co-director of the Research Institute for Comparative Studies in Race and Ethnicity. Prior to that, she was a faculty member in the Department of Psychology and a research scientist at the Institute for Social Research at the University of Michigan. Her research has focused on the role of the self in regulating behavior. She has written on self-schemas, possible selves, the influence of the self on the perception of others, and the constructive role of the self in adult development. Her most recent work in cultural psychology explores the mutual constitution between psychological structures and processes and sociocultural practices and institutions. She has served on the editorial boards of numerous journals and study sections at both the National Institute of Mental Health and the National Science Foundation. She is a fellow of the American Psychological Society and the American Psychological Association. She is also a member of the MacArthur Research Network on Successful Midlife Development. She was elected to the American Academy of the Arts and Sciences in 1994. She has a Ph.D. in psychology from the University of Michigan.

TIMOTHY A. SALTHOUSE is Regents professor of psychology in the School of Psychology at the Georgia Institute of Technology. His research concerns the effects of aging on various aspects of cognitive functioning, including what is responsible for the adult age-related declines reported in many measures of memory, reasoning, and spatial abilities, as well as the role of experience and knowledge in minimizing the impact of age-related cognitive declines in work and other real-world activities. He is a fellow of the American Association for the Advancement of Science, the American Psychological Association, the American Psychological Society, and the Gerontological Society and a member of the Psychonomic Society. He received the APA Division 20 Distinguished Contribution award in 1995, and was named an American Psychological Society William James fellow in 1998. He was editor of the journal *Psychology and Aging* from 1991 through 1996. He served on the National Research Council's Panel on Human Factors Research Needs for an Aging Population. He has a Ph.D. in experimental psychology from the University of Michigan.

LARRY R. SQUIRE is a professor of psychiatry, neuroscience, and psychology at the University of California, San Diego as well as a research career scientist at the Veterans Affairs Medical Center in San Diego. He is known for his research on cerebral memory systems, the development of theory related to cerebral memory, and the delineation of the brain-based dichotomy of procedural and declarative memory. He has made contributions toward defining the role of the hippocampus and associated structures in the memory of humans and other primates. He became a member of the National Academy of Sciences in 1993 and currently serves on the National Research Council's Board on Behavioral, Cognitive, and Sensory Sciences. His honors include a distinguished scientific award from the American Psychological Association, the McGovern award from the American Association for the Advancement of Science, and the Lashley award from the American Philosophical Society. In 1994, he served as president of the Society for Neuroscience. He has a Ph.D. in psychology from the Massachusetts Institute of Technology.

PAUL C. STERN is study director of the Committee on Future Directions for Cognitive Research on Aging at the National Research Council, a research professor of sociology at George Mason University, and president of the Social and Environmental Research Institute. In his major research area, the human dimensions of environmental problems, he has written numerous scholarly articles, coedited *Energy Use: The Human Dimension* and *Global Environmental Change: Understanding the Human Dimensions,* and coauthored the textbook *Environmental Problems and Human Behavior.* He has also authored a textbook on social science research methods and coedited several books on international conflict issues. He is a fellow of the American Psychological Association and the American Association for the Advancement of Science. He has a Ph.D. in psychology from Clark University.

RUDOLPH E. TANZI is director of the Genetics and Aging Unit in the Department of Neurology at Massachusetts General Hospital and professor of neurology at Harvard University. He has been investigating human neurodegenerative disease at the genetic, molecular biological, and biochemical levels since 1980, when he participated in a pioneering study that led to the discovery of the Huntington's disease gene in 1983. Subsequently, he has focused on studies of Down syndrome and Alzheimer's disease and went on to isolate the first familial Alzheimer's disease (FAD) gene, the amyloid beta protein precursor (APP) in 1986. He was also involved in the subsequent identification of three other Alzheimer genes, presenilins 1 and 2 and alpha2-macroglobulin, and the Wilson's disease gene. He has received numerous awards for his work, including the French Foundation fellowship award; the Pew scholar in biomedical sciences award; the Nathan Shock award; the Metropolitan Life Foundation award for medical research; the Potamkin prize for research in Pick's, Alzheimer's and related disorders; and the Alzheimer's Association T.L.L. Temple award. He has a Ph.D. in neurobiology from Harvard University.

KEITH E. WHITFIELD is assistant professor in the Department of Biobehavioral Health at Pennsylvania State University. His current research focuses on individual differences in aging in African Americans. Specifically, current projects include a study of the impact of health and personality on cognitive functioning and a study of health, cognitive, and psychosocial factors in the study of older African American twins. Some recent publications cover the topics of individual differences in aging among African-Americans (*International Journal of Aging and Human Development*), evaluating a measure of everyday problem solving for use with African-Americans (*Experimental Aging Research*), and the effect of race and health-related factors on naming and memory (*Journal of Aging and Health*). He has a Ph.D. in lifespan experimental psychology from Texas Tech University.

WILLIAM A. YOST is a professor of hearing science and an adjunct professor of psychology and otolaryngology at Loyola University Chicago. He is also director of the Parmly Hearing Institute at Loyola University. He specializes in psychoacoustics and auditory perception and has conducted research on sound source determination and segregation. He currently serves on the Board on Behavioral, Cognitive, and Sensory Sciences of the National Research Council, has served several terms on the Committee on Hearing, Bioacoustics, and Biomechanics, and was a member of the Panel on Classification of Complex Nonspeech Sounds. He has a Ph.D. in experimental psychology from Indiana University.

OTHER CONTRIBUTORS

THOMAS D. ALBRIGHT is professor and director of the Systems Neurobiology Laboratories at the Salk Institute for Biological Studies, as well as an investigator of the Howard Hughes Medical Institute. He is also adjunct professor of neurosciences and psychology at the University of California, San Diego, and director of the Sloan Center for Theoretical Neurobiology at the Salk Institute. His research is aimed at understanding the neuronal bases of visual perception and visually guided behavior in primates, using physiological, behavioral, and computational approaches. His work has focused on the influence of context on the neuronal representation of visual features and on the neuronal bases of visual perceptual experience.

CARL W. COTMAN is director of the Institute for Brain Aging and Dementia and professor in the Departments of Neurology and Neurobiology and Behavior at the University of California, Irvine. His research concerns synaptic plasticity and functional stabilization after injury in the mature and aged central nervous system. The goal of this work is to determine the nature of natural healing processes in the nervous system and to develop new therapeutic interventions.

DONALD L. FISHER is professor in the Department of Mechanical and Industrial Engineering and director of the Human Performance Laboratory at the University of Massachusetts, Amherst. His work involves improving the design of the human-computer interface for older adults. Recently, he has focused on the design of the interfaces that are just now appearing in automobiles and telecommunication systems. More generally, he is interested in the effects of aging on the microstructure of cognition and the implication of these effects for practice.

MELISSA L. FINUCANE is a research associate with Decision Research in Eugene, Oregon, and a visiting scholar at the Institute for Cognitive and Decision Sciences at the University of Oregon. Her research interests are in human judgment and decision making, affect, and risk perception. Currently she is studying the way affect helps people to make sense of complex financial and health information and is developing a multidimensional measure of decision-making competence.

SHINOBU KITAYAMA is associate professor on the faculty of Integrated Human Studies of Kyoto University in Japan, as well as a visiting associate professor on the Committee on Human Development at the University of Chicago. In his work, he approaches the issues surrounding culture, self, and emotion from a cultural psychological perspective. His research explores the ways in which psychological systems and cultural systems constitute each other. In particular, he is currently studying how divergent forms of agency are shaped and maintained by an assortment of cultural processes.

DONALD G. MacGREGOR is senior research associate at Decision Research in Eugene, Oregon. His research focuses on risk perception and communication, as well as human judgment and decision making. He is currently studying a number of applied issues in human judgment, particularly issues in behavioral finance and financial decision making.

JOHN H. MORRISON is a neurobiologist at the Mount Sinai School of Medicine, where he is professor and co-director of the Fishberg Research Center for Neurobiology, Willard T.C. Johnson professor and vice chairman of geriatrics and adult development, and director of the Kastor Neurobiology of Aging Laboratories. His work incorporates very basic neurobiological research on neuronal specialization and the biochemical coding of brain circuits with the application of such principles to human neuropathology, in order to illuminate the cellular events that lead to dementia. Recently, his research has dealt with the neurobiological events that accompany normal aging and the important differences between these events and those that accompany Alzheimer's disease.

ELLEN PETERS is a research associate at Decision Research and an adjunct professor at the University of Oregon in Eugene, Oregon. Her research examines the affective and analytical processes underlying the decisions that people make in an increasingly complex world. She studies decision making as an interaction of characteristics of the decision situation and characteristics of the individual. In one line of research, she investigates the conscious and less-than-conscious processes by which affect influences choice. In other work, she examines how aging influences the role of affect in choice.

PAUL SLOVIC is a founder and president of Decision Research in Eugene, Oregon. He is also professor of psychology at the University of Oregon. His work involves studies of judgment and decision processes with an emphasis on decision making under conditions of risk. In his research, he examines fundamental issues in the study of preference and choice, as well as the factors that underlie perceptions of risk and attempts to assess the importance of these perceptions for the management of risk in society.

SHARI R. WALDSTEIN is associate professor of psychology and director of the behavioral medicine program at the University of Maryland, Baltimore County. She is also research assistant professor of medicine at the University of Maryland School of Medicine. Her research applies the principles and methods of neuropsychology, behavioral medicine, and psychophysiology to the study of cardiovascular disease. In her work, she examines neuroanatomical, neurophysiological, biomedical, and psychological predictors of neurocognitive performance in older adults and conducts studies of individual differences in the magnitude and patterning of acute cardiovascular responses to psychological stressors.

Index

I

Imaging data, 5, 13, 17, 44-45, 56, 61-62, 204
  animal research, 5, 51, 57, 62, 63
    primates, nonhuman, 5, 51, 62, 238-250
  magnetic resonance imaging, 5, 19, 44-45, 51, 59, 61-62, 238-250
  memory, 46, 238-239, 248
Inference, 48, 224, 225-226, 229-230, 231, 232
Inflammation, 15-16, 17, 18, 19, 114, 116, 119, 122, 124-125
  anti-inflammatory agents, 117, 124
Infrastructure, research, 5, 56-62
Intelligence, 23-24, 38, 206-207, 218, 233
  artificial intelligence, 55, 56
  hypertension and, 195
  sensory-motor decline and, 40-41
Interactive interfaces, 175-177, 179
  automated teller machines, 29, 170, 174, 175, 180
Interdisciplinary research, 4, 11, 13, 34-35, 54-56, 62-63
  funding, 4, 36, 55-56, 62-63
  neural circuits, 89, 97-100
  nonneurological health status, 204, 205
  sensory-motor functions, 42
  technological aids, 35-36, 179-180, 181
Interfaces, 174-177, 179
Intervention strategies, 18, 19, 44, 85, 134-135, 192-193
  anti-inflammatory agents, 117, 124
  antioxidants, 7-8, 18, 40, 117, 128-129, 130, 134, 191
  behavioral, 6-8, 13, 17, 20, 121-122, 134
    environmental enrichment, 22-23, 104, 121-122, 134
    physical exercise, 4, 7, 8, 37, 50, 104, 121, 134, 191, 194
  biochemical, general, 17-18; *see also* Drugs
  cardiovascular disease, 44, 192, 198, 200, 202-203
  cultural, 8, 13
  environmental enrichment, 22-23, 104, 121-122
  estrogen replacement therapy (ERT), 32, 96-97, 100, 104, 244
  genetic engineering, 100-103, 249
  hippocampus, 103-105
  homeostatic processes, 114, 116, 121-122, 134; *see also* Antioxidants
  hypertension, 192, 198, 200, 203
  initiation of brain aging and, 121-122, 134
  magnetic resonance imaging in evaluation of, 244, 248-249
  medical and surgical treatments, 203, 205
  neural circuits, 17, 83, 85, 91, 100-105, 106
  physical exercise, 4, 7, 8, 37, 50, 104, 121, 134, 191, 194
  stem cells, 102-103
  transplantation strategies, 100-103
  see also Drugs; Technological factors

J

Judgment, 9, 29, 144-165
  heuristic processing, 146-151

L

Language abilities, 1, 8, 38, 45, 56
  cultural factors, contextual effects, 225-229, 232
  defined, 206
  hearing, 40-41, 42, 166
    aids, 29, 42, 170, 172, 173
  hypertension, 195
  magnetic resonance imaging, 238-239
  regional impacts on brain, 26
  speech, 46, 173, 206, 227-228
  see also Hearing
Learning processes, 31
  conceptual framework of study at hand, 9
  cultural learning, 218
  decision processes, 159